# STAY YOUNGER LONGER

Bronwen Meredith

# STAY YOUNGER LONGER

Michael Joseph·London

For my mother who seems to get younger and younger

Design by Craig Dodd

First published in this Mermaid Books edition
by Michael Joseph Limited
44 Bedford Square, London WC1
1985

This book was first published in Great Britain
by Elm Tree Books/Hamish Hamilton Ltd
Garden House, 57-59 Long Acre
London WC2E 9JZ

British Library Cataloguing in Publication Data
Meredith, Bronwen
   Stay younger longer.
   1. Women—Health and hygiene
   I. Title
   613′.04244    RA778

ISBN 0-7181-2574-6

Typeset by Servis Filmsetting Ltd, Manchester
Printed and bound in Great Britain by
R. J. Acford, Chichester, West Sussex

# Contents

# Acknowledgements

It is always very difficult to know where to begin and end the
thank yous in a book like this. I am particularly grateful to all
the busy professionals who spent time on interviews and
explained in details their various specialities, to the institutions
and librarians who sifted through learned papers to find just
what I wanted and to those who worked closely with me all the
time – my editors at Elm Tree, Connie Austen Smith, Kyle
Cathie and Caroline Taggart; Janine Wadlow who helped in the
fashion research; Chris Motley who typed the manuscript – and
a big pat on·the back for artist Edward Cairns who managed to
interpret all my rough sketches with amazing skill and style.

The author and publishers would like to thank the following people for
their contribution to the photography in this book:

Models: Annabel Schofield, Keith van Hoven, Scott Mackenzie, Erika Pek

Make-up: Teresa Fairminer, Cheryl Phelps-Gardiner

Hair: Steven Carey

Clothes: Browns (South Molton Street)

Special thanks to Teresa Fairminer for her contribution

Food photography is by Tessa Traeger and first appeared in Vogue

Thanks also to the following health spas for the use of photographs:

Champneys at Tring Health Resort (p. 220, 226, 233)
Forest Mere (p. 236/7)
Grayshott Hall (p. 223, 238)
Henlow Grange (p. 240)
Inglewood Health Hydro (p. 225, 241)
Shrubland Hall Health Clinic (p. 246)
Tyringham Clinic (p. 248)

# Foreword

First face the facts: despite the feminist movement, despite the many barriers that have been broken down, the truth is that our society continues to dismiss women when they are no longer young and attractive. Do you want it to happen to you? We all know it's not fair, but nor is it enough to fight back with words and indignation alone. A compromise has to be reached whereby there's an acknowledgement that looks do matter as much as minds, and that health and attitude affect both. Deploring the youth cult doesn't help: you have to meet it half way – for your own benefit. If you feel younger and have an air of energy and optimism about you, you are going to look younger. Bodies do age, and once we are in our thirties they start to let us know very quickly when we abuse them. However, it is possible for you to take control of your health and looks as never before. Caring for yourself is a wise investment; women in their thirties, forties, fifties and beyond still have a great many options in their lives, and decades in which to take them up. Age is no longer a limitation to change, but the later you leave it, the harder the work needed to get results, to undo years of bad habits. So much is possible. I am not talking about unreal goals of looking super glamourous, being super fit or super slim. Those are the magazine images and have little to do with everyday living. But you can become younger in all sorts of ways with knowledge and some effort. In the end there has to be a balance between the major preventive things such as eating right, doing a degree of exercise, keeping tabs on health risks, having enthusiasm for life – and the fun things of clothes, make-up, perfume, a little self indulgence. This is the story on the pages following: a balanced approach to the ways to stay younger longer – for your benefit, for the many years ahead.

# Resources, Referral Centres and Registers

The following list of societies and organizations is a guide as to where to find general information on health and also on specific therapies. Apart from literature of public interest, where applicable lists are available of practitioners who have undergone training up to a certain standard at recognized establishments. With a written enquiry, it is usual to send a stamped-addressed envelope. It is up to you to personally check out the premises and qualifications of any recommended practitioner. Bona fide therapists are happy about such individual integrity. Some of the following are charity organisations, some membership associations, while others are professional institutions.

Action on Smoking and Health
(ASH),
27/35 Mortimer Street,
London W.1.

Alcoholics Anonymous,
P.O. Box 514,
11 Redcliffe Gardens,
London S.W.10.

The Arthritis and Rheumatism
Council for Research,
41 Eagle Street,
London W.C. 1.

Association for New Approaches
to Cancer,
231 Kensal Road,
London W.10.

Dr Edward Bach Centre,
Mount Vernon,
Sotwell, Oxon.

Bates Association of Eyesight
Training,
49 Queen Anne Street,
London W.1.

British Acupuncture Association
and Register,
34 Alderney Street,
London S.W.1.

British Association of
Psychotherapists,
121 Hendon Lane,
London N.3.

British Chiropractors' Association,
5 First Avenue,
Chelmsford, Essex.

British College of Acupuncture,
44 New Market Square,
Basingstoke, Hants.

British College of Naturopathy
and Osteopathy,
Frazer House,
6 Netherhall Gardens,
London N.W.3.

British Holistic Medical
Association,
23 Harley House,
Harley Street,
London W.1.

British Homeopathic Association,
27a Devonshire Street,
London W.1.

British Hypnotherapy Association,
67 Upper Berkeley Street,
London W.1.

British Wheel of Yoga
80 Lechampton Road,
Cheltenham, Glos.

BUPA Women's Unit,
Battle Bridge House,
300 Gray's Inn Road,
London W.C.1.

Centre for Autogenic Training,
15 Fitzroy Square,
London W.1.

The Chest, Heart and Stroke
Association,
Tavistock House North,
Tavistock Square,
London W.C.1.

College of Health,
18 Victoria Park Square,
London E.C.2.

Forty-Plus Career Development
 Centre,
High Holborn House,
49–51 Bedford Row,
London W.C.1.

Health Education Council,
78 New Oxford Street,
London W.C.1.

International College of Oriental
 Medicine,
Green Hedges House,
Green Hedges Avenue,
East Grinstead, Sussex.

Institute of Complementary
 Medicine,
21 Portland Place,
London W.1.

Institute of Group Analysis,
1 Bickenhall Mansions,
Bickenhall Street,
London W.1.

International Institute of
 Reflexology,
P.O. Box 34,
Harlow, Essex.

The Keep-Fit Association,
16 Upper Woburn Place,
London W.C.1.

Mastectomy Association,
25 Brighton Road,
South Croydon, Surrey.

National Institute of Herbal
 Medicine,
148 Forest Road,
Tunbridge Wells, Kent.

Naturopathic Private Clinic for
 Women,
11 Alderton Crescent,
London N.W.4.

Register of Osteopaths,
1–4 Suffolk Street,
London S.W.1.

Research Council for
 Complementary Medicine,

37 Bedford Square,
London W.C.1.

Rolf Institute,
P.O. Box 1868,
Boulder,
Colorado 80302, U.S.A.

Society of Teachers of the
 Alexander Technique,
3b Albert Court,
Kensington Gore,
London S.W.7.

The Sports Council,
16 Upper Woburn Place,
London W.C.1.

Vegetarian Society,
53 Marloes Road,
London W.8.

Women's League of Health and
 Beauty,
Beaumont Cottage,
Ditton Close,
Thames Ditton, Surrey.

Women's National Cancer Control
 Campaign,
1 South Audley Street,
London W.1.

## Australia

Acupuncture Association of
 Australia,
159 Victoria Road,
Gladesville, N.S.W.

Acupuncture Specialist
 Practitioners Association,
76 William Street,
Sydney, N.S.W.

Alcoholics Anonymous,
127 Edwin Street,
Croydon, N.S.W.

Arthritis and Rheumatism
 Council,
Wynyard House,
291 George Street,
Sydney, N.S.W.

Association of Natural Health
 Practitioners
12/17 Knox Street,
Double Bay, N.S.W.

Australian Cancer Society,
Trust Building,
55 King Street,
Sydney, N.S.W.

Australian Chiropractors
 Association,
81 Strathallan Road,
Macleod,
Melbourne, Victoria.

Australian and International Yoga
 Association,
185 Pitt Town Road,
Kenthurst, N.S.W.

Australian Foundation of
 Alcoholism and Drug
 Dependence,
2nd Floor, T and G Building,
London Circuit,
Canberra City.

Australian Hypnotherapists
 Association,
562 St Kilda Road,
Melbourne, Victoria.

Australian Natural Therapies
 Association,
Roche Street,
Hawthorn, Victoria.

Australian Osteopathic
 Association,
551 Hampton Street,
Hampton, Victoria.

Australian Vegetarian Society,
45 Fourth Avenue,
Klemzig, S.A.

Co-ordinating Council for Health
 and Environment,
26 Russell Street,
Camberwell, Victoria.

Health Action,
P.O. Box 340,
Carlton South,
Victoria.

Herb Society of South Australia,
P.O. Box 140,
Parkside, S.A.

Homeopathic Association of
 Australia,
7 Hampden Road,
Artarmon, N.S.W.

Institute for Fitness and Training,
64 MacKinnon Parade,
North Adelaide, S.A.

National Fitness Council,
24th Floor,
570 Burke Street,
Melbourne, Victoria.

Natural Health Society of
Australia,
131 York Street,
Sydney, N.S.W.

South Australian Women's Keep
Fit Association,
121 Carvington Street,
Adelaide, S.A.

Whole Earth Healing,
13 Fairmont Road,
East Hawthorn, Victoria.

Women's Health Care Association,
92 Thomas Street,
West Perth, W.A.

## Canada

Acupuncture Foundation of
Canada,
10 St. Mary Street, Suite 503,
Toronto, Ontario.

The Arthritis Society,
Suite 420, 920 Yonge Street,
Toronto, Ontario.

Canadian Association for Health,
Physical Education and
Recreation,
333 River Road, Tower B,
Vanier, Ontario.

Canadian Cancer Society,
77 Bloor Street West, Suite 401,
Toronto, Ontario.

Canadian Chiropractic
Association,
1900 Bayview Avenue,
Toronto, Ontario.

Canadian Council on Health
Education,
71 Bank Street, Suite 605,
Ottawa, Ontario.

Canadian Council on Smoking
and Health,
725 Churchill Avenue,
Ottawa, Ontario.

Canadian Institute of Stress,
121 Hazleton Avenue,
Toronto, Ontario.

Canadian Osteopathic Aid
Society,
575 Waterloo Street,
London, Ontario.

Mental and Drug Dependency
Information and Counselling
Service,
818 Portage Avenue, Suite 205,
Winnipeg, Manitoba.

## New Zealand

Alcoholics Anonymous,
Box 6458,
Wellington.

Arthritis and Rheumatism
Foundation of New Zealand Inc.
Box 10–020,
Wellington.

Cancer Society of New
Zealand Inc.
Box 10–340,
Wellington.

International Yoga Teachers
Association,
25 Coverdale Street,
Napier.

Mental Health Foundation of New
Zealand,
Box 37–438,
Parnell, Auckland.

National Heart Foundation of
New Zealand,
Box 17–128,
Greenland, Auckland.

New Zealand Chiropractors
Association Inc.
Box 2858,
Wellington.

New Zealand Homeopathic
Society Inc.
Box 2939,
Auckland 1.

New Zealand Vegetarian
Society Inc.
Box 454,
Auckland.

## South Africa

Institute of Public Health,
Box 4623,
Johannesburg.

National Cancer Association,
Box 2000,
Johannesburg.

South African Medical and Dental
Council,
6115 Oranje-Nassau Building,
Schoeman Street,
Pretoria.

South African National Council
on Alcoholism and Drug
Dependence,
Box 10134,
Johannesburg.

South African Psychological
Association,
Box 4292,
Johannesburg.

South African Rheumatism and
Arthritis Association,
Namaqua House,
36 Burg Street,
Cape Town.

# HOW YOU CAN GIVE THE RIGHT IMPRESSION

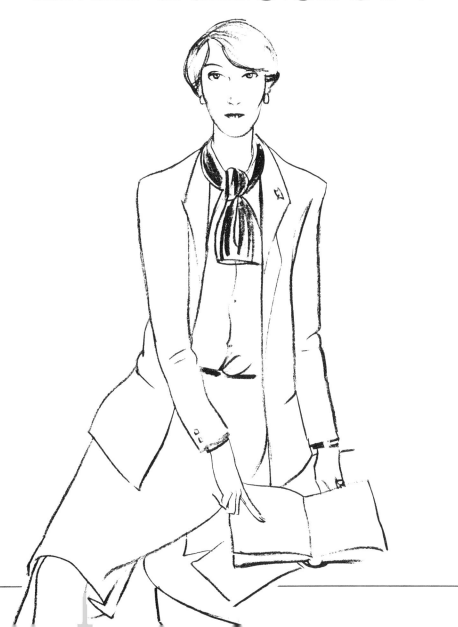

# ATTITUDE
## The best is yet to come

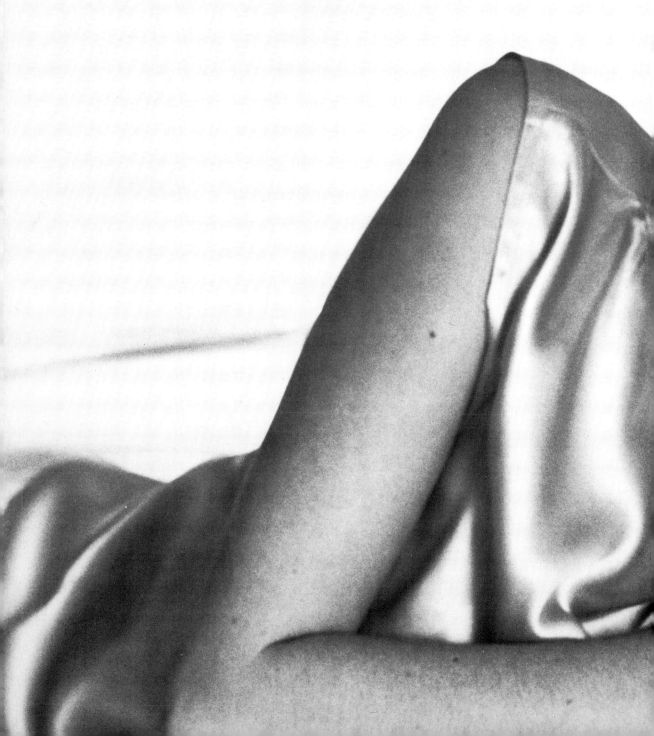

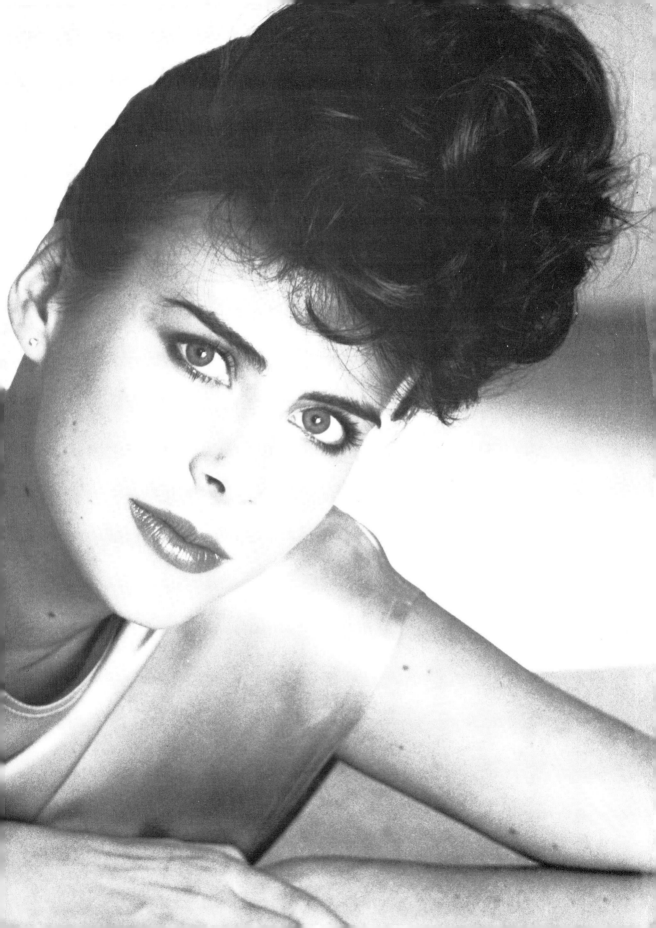

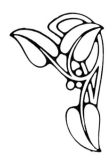

During the past fifteen years a revolution has taken place in our attitudes to age and aging. The stereotyped conceptions of age have gradually been dispelled and, today, your chronological age can be irrelevant to your looks, your attitude, your lifestyle. What you are supposed to look like in your twenties, thirties, forties, fifties etc. no longer means anything. Our whole concept of women and aging has changed dramatically – and attitudes have changed because of woman's new image and expanding role in society.

This new ageless point of view puts emphasis on health, vitality, optimism and achievement. It also has a lot to do with a woman's desire to balance the old traditions of marriage and family (where good looks and knowing how to keep them were considered important) and the new options of independence and a career (where good looks can't harm, but can't be relied upon either). Most of us want, if not the best of both worlds, at least something positive and rewarding from both.

Gone, thank goodness, are the rigid rules that assigned women to definite roles and definite images through the passages of life. The sequence is no longer career-girl to wife to mother to grandmother with its parallel images of sexy to smart to matronly to nothing. There is no accepted order any more which has as much to do with the mind as with the body. You can start off as a nothing and end up as a sexy grandmother running a business.

The Eighties is clearly the era of the indefinable woman. What age? What role? What slot? If you cannot be neatly categorized you can congratulate yourself on being on today's wavelength. What age you are is the age you project. If the vibes you send out are young and lively, that's what everyone will see. Women who've never thought about age in terms of passing years understand this perfectly – and they are invariably the women whose actual years come as a surprise. The trick is never to feel any age – never younger, never older, never in between.

How you feel, think and look at any particular moment is what's important. The roles that were once reserved for the young – career-girl, lover, mother – can now be undertaken almost throughout life. There are now first mothers in their forties, career starters in their fifties and lovers up to their last breath. What's more, these roles are performed with the poise and flair that can only come from experience in life, and with the polished looks that know no age.

There are millions of women who now stay young for what seems like an indefinite period. Who knows how old a woman is? Who really cares? Think of the women you know who look marvellous, not only the stars and celebrities, but a friend, the woman next door. Well, couldn't they be almost any age?

How do they do it? First of all they are interesting and alive. Their image, their projection has more to do with personality, presence, vital good looks and a breezy mind than actual beauty. Their appeal is that of pulled-together maturity, a word that now means self-confidence, knowing oneself and experience.

After a certain age, you get the body and face you deserve. Don't allow stress, discontent or self pity to get the better of you. It's very hard to look young and vital when these tensions are mirrored on your face.

Somewhere between thirty and forty your emotional life shows on your face – your character, your mind, your responses. There's a lot to be said for a sense of identity in a face; it's strong, it's individual and far superior to a stereotyped look that many women feel they should follow. Also by this time you know more or less what you look like, but do you accept it? Do you like it? The state of your body, the way you clothe it and the impact of your face all reveal your self esteem. Are you keeping track of your health, your fitness, your looks? This has nothing to do with being reed slim (though some weight control is desirable) or pressuring yourself into constant exercise and body treatments. It has everything to do with being sensible and observant and following daily routines that are realistic and realizing that it is your attitude to life that counts most of all.

It is your lifestyle that primarily dictates the length and health of your life. Studies around the world have revealed that these are the main contributing factors:

- a simple diet of natural foods, low in fat, high in vegetables, grains and fruits
- plenty of exercise or outdoor work
- a stress-free relaxed attitude with a philosophical view of events
- awareness of being useful, needed, loved
- a degree of genetic influence

## Looking on the positive side
## More years can mean more assets

If you think about it, older can be better. Many women like themselves better as they get older. It's really only logical, as the insecurities of youth invariably cause more anguish than the realities of later years. As the years add up, you learn to recognize and accept your minuses and pluses, and you learn how to deal with them. It is actually very reassuring.

How often do you hear today: she gets better-looking every year? The fact is that it is very often true. And it's not just because of the scientific and cosmetic aids; it's got a great deal to do with confidence and experience. It's also finally knowing who you are. You acquire a sense of self-respect which rounds off the sharp edges. There's a calmness that comes from security. There's the acceptance that you cannot be everything to everybody.

No one really likes looking older, but there's no point in wasting time worrying about the prospect of aging. Illusion is all, but it's an illusion that involves body and mind. Your younger image is not just a matter of retaining looks, it's discarding old attitudes, becoming flexible, involved, generous and outgoing. It's personality, it's spirit, it's being able to relax about age.

The great advantage of getting older yet staying young is to realize that specific physical faults are of little significance in the long run. It's the overall impression that counts, the interplay of looks and manner. A man – whether younger or older – is not going to worry about an extra pound here, a bit of cellulite there, if he finds an older woman fascinating. She, on the other hand, knows she can't compete physically with a girl of twenty, but in every other respect she's way ahead – she knows what life is all about and her attitude and image are young enough to withstand any challenge.

The future is wide open at any age. Confidence can pull you through many a situation, many a change. Confidence, though, is a strange thing. Once you have it, it's not necessarily there to stay, but must be resupplied daily – and you do that by keeping yourself up to scratch in every single way.

The basis of it all is coming to terms with your individual character. This is more than finding yourself, a path recommended by many feminists, and one that could lead to completely self-centred living. Knowing your character is recognizing good and bad points, realizing what can be controlled and what runs wild. It is learning to balance life's ups and downs and working out how to fit in with others close to you – how to love them, live with them, give and receive from them. Life is essentially a compromise and it's only as you grow older that you finally accept this as true. But from such a sound and realistic basis you can branch out in any direction.

Don't dwell on your imperfections. It is adolescent to be obsessed with what are invariably imagined major flaws. Take stock once and for all and decide what is realistic to change and set positive goals. In the frenzy to be thin, a lot of other values tend to get lost. Keep as slim and fit as possible, but don't let it ruin your pleasure or distort your mental attitude. Learn to like yourself and your body. How you feel about yourself is more important for your wellbeing than an extra inch or a pound of flesh.

### It may not be all in the mind but that's the control centre

Researchers are constantly hoping to find the key to perpetual youth in a chemical formula. However, all drugs have their drawbacks and the power of the mind in relation to their effectiveness is often underestimated. One man's elixir can be another man's poison depending on the messages sent from the control centre in the brain, and the individual interplay of body, mind and spirit. The role of human consciousness makes any search for a simple youth formula an ambiguous issue.

Many women now consider work vital for their wellbeing. If you do something rewarding, aging is more acceptable. Success shows – it's youthful.

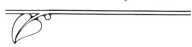

When one studies the habits of long-living people and looks into ancient philosophies, it becomes increasingly clear that the best ways of retaining youth are: natural good food, plenty of exercise, rest and relaxation, fresh air, pure water, light and sunshine, peace of mind, lack of stress and a positive attitude. All these are available to everyone and can all be achieved with the proper motivation and will.

The first step is a positive, health-orientated youthful state of mind. When the mind works negatively on the body, it can cause physical chaos. Emotional disturbances, stress and even just plain pessimism can bring about almost every ailment in the book, particularly manifested in circulatory and heart disorders, ulcers, skin conditions, rashes, asthma and breathing problems. On the other hand, the mind can also be the greatest healer of all. Your body is equipped with the most remarkable self-repairing system. All you need is to turn on the mental switch and take a good look at harmful daily habits. You can actually alter your life by altering your attitude.

Every woman should stop and take stock of herself. What have you done up to now? What's good and what's bad about your attitude, your mind, your health, your body, your looks? Don't brood over any mistakes, start new ways today and put your healthy future in your own hands. You don't need a professional, medical or otherwise, to tell you basically what's wrong. Look at yourself, listen to your body, and with the knowledge gained from this book, you'll know what to do. It does mean being convinced that it's never too late to start – and dismissing the conventional attitude to age. Only a few people actually pull themselves together to do something positive to delay the aging process. It can be done if you take a determined new direction – and there's no reason why you can't do it.

Certain mental attitudes are common in middle age. If you haven't achieved goals you aimed for in your twenties, you're bound to feel frustrated, disappointed and critical of yourself. On the other hand, if you have achieved all you wished for, you may very well feel life no longer has any purpose or meaning. If you've been a devoted wife and mother, who suddenly finds herself alone – children do leave the nest and husbands do often go off – it can be the most depressing time of your life. The problem is the actual entry into this transitional phase, coping with the initial upheavals when changes have to be made. Once past the starting post, you're usually all right.

Depression is centred in the mind and is triggered by your attitude to life. Once it takes hold, it is incredibly difficult to get rid of. It must be recognized for what it is – a symptom of your inability to face up to a problem with positive thought and action. It's not a disease in itself, but a manifestation of a negative attitude. A constructive remedy is to start taking positive steps and decisions about small things first, then working your way up to the more complicated issues. Work on your health and looks first. Are you eating right, exercising at all? Movement is a great antidote for depression. How are you dressing, could your face and hair do with a little more attention? This is not vanity, it's constructive care. You can gain confidence through feeling great and looking good, and then you are ready to take stock of yourself inwardly, to look at your life objectively and make decisions on the next move. Do you want to change a career, start working for the first time? Do you need to? You certainly don't want to sit around and mope for ever, do you? That is more aging than anything – and will only plunge you into greater depression.

The lack of confidence usually stems from decreasing energy. Suddenly we cannot cope, everything seems too much effort. And we all know that the less you do, the less you want to do and the less you are able to do. You can create energy by eating properly and starting to take exercise regularly. You also have to learn how to use energy most effectively. Don't throw it away on frustration and anger or self pity. Save it to push you forward in a positive way. To be confident you don't need to be aggressive – that in itself wastes precious energy; true confidence is a calm, sure attitude that commands respect.

Many of us waste energy on fear and anxiety – fear of the unknown, of poverty, of illness, of loneliness. Such fears are based on possibilities and not on fact. If you can learn to limit your concern for what is actually going on now, at this very moment, you are well on your way to having a young approach to life. In your teens did you worry about possible future disasters? No, you most likely looked on the bright side, thinking of things you could do and would do. That's one of the secrets of staying young.

---

If you think and act young, you will stay younger, longer. Be curious and creative, play games, enjoy yourself, dance, sing, see the world. Most of all keep on learning. Don't sit back and never think you've got more of a past than a future. You never know what might happen!

### How long you stay young depends more on lifestyle than on genes

In the 1980s the desire to stay young as long as possible is stronger than ever. Mankind has always searched for youth miracles, and today there are doctors, clinics, research teams and drug trials – all attempting to provide a realistic answer. But despite the advance and sophistication of genetic and biochemical studies, the single most important influence is your lifestyle. Mounting evidence indicates that it is your daily attitude to body and mental maintenance that will determine the quality and length of your life – and provide the outward signs of a younger person. It is how you cope with your environment that counts, your individual approach towards nutrition, exercise, stress, work and social roles, plus your attitude towards harmful habits such as smoking, alcohol and drugs. Like anything else, your body will show signs of aging according to the way it is treated. If you look after your body with care and keep your mind alert, they will serve you well. However good your inherited genes – and there's no doubt that some of us are better endowed than others – they won't help you that much if you treat your body thoughtlessly.

In the western world, a very large ratio of people die from heart disease, strokes, cancer or accidents. In all of these, lifestyle or behaviour patterns play an integral part. Bad eating habits, a sedentary existence, smoking and excess drinking all contribute to premature aging and possibly an early end.

Don't forget femininity. It gets lots of knocks these days, but it remains a woman's prime asset. We need to be tough and determined sometimes, but remember it's the natural gentleness of women that sets us apart, that offers something special and can be a source of strength.

Many of the world's great beauties are now over forty, yet they have all the outward signs of younger women

- sensuality
- health and vitality
- relaxed confidence
- thick shining hair
- smooth clear skin
- limber bodies
- casual clothes

They have learned to take care of themselves on a regular basis, to play up assets, play down faults.
The options are there for anyone to take up.
What's your attitude?

In modern societies women tend to live longer than men. This has been in part due to the role of the female hormones such as oestrogen, which, prior to the menopause, help protect the circulatory system and prevent heart disease. Now it is thought that longer life also had a lot to do with lifestyle and attitude. The combination of a woman being out of the mainstream of competitive working life, and at the same time being encouraged to be more passive than the male, resulted in a calmer everyday existence. Now that goals are changing, it is interesting to discover that when women are in stressful jobs, the protective effect of oestrogen is reduced. Women are fast moving into the same category as men, and when stress is combined with aggressive behaviour, alcohol and cigarette smoking, then they are subject to the same circulatory diseases as men. There has already been a marked increase in cancer of the lung since women started to smoke in greater

Maturity is not to be confused with old age. The main asset is that you can finally be yourself because you know exactly who and what you are. There is an ageless beauty in poise and there's a very special aura that shines from character. Your inner attitude comes to the surface and there it will glow.

numbers. It is ironic to think that woman's fight for equality in life and work is bringing equality in health risks and earlier death.

The sensible and practical way to stay young is to be vigilant about everyday living. Just saying this may very well cause apprehension because most of the dedicated health and fitness advocates recommend such strict regimens that many people are put off from the start. Moderation in all things can often take the joy out of life. We all have our excesses, our indulgences, our days of utter laziness. It is difficult to break old habits in one fell swoop; it is equally difficult to cut yourself off from the social stream by limiting your lifestyle. A health regimen that stipulates you give up all but the natural foods, push yourself when exercising, avoid the sun, never drink or smoke etc. is quite honestly too much for most of us to cope with. Including me. Granted, it may be ideal, but I believe it is not absolutely necessary, even in the interests of staying young.

The trick is balance. The body is amazingly recuperative and if you learn how to balance indulgences with immediate corrective tactics, you can afford to slip off the straight and narrow every so often. This particularly applies to food and drink, weight and shape. Keeping track of it on a daily basis is far superior to a frantic appraisal every six months or more. For example, if you indulge in a huge rich dinner one evening, try and eat just fruit the next day. If you've been drinking too much alcohol, help your liver by drinking lots of lemon juice diluted with mineral water (more details on page 94).

Fundamental to keeping young is to check on these points all the time – you need constant reminders to ensure you still have the right attitude:

**boredom** – this will age a person as quickly as a poor diet or lack of exercise. Try to lead a varied and complex life; seek out new experiences, start a career, learn something new, take up a creative hobby.

**weight** – if you keep your weight under control by watching it daily, you'll not only look agile and younger, but you'll keep at bay diseases that are related to overweight, such as high blood pressure, diabetes and hardening of the arteries.

**exercise** – lifelong exercise is essential if you want to keep your youthful figure. You don't have to push yourself to extremes, but it should be done on a regular basis which means ideally every day (even if it's only walking) but three times a week is adequate. It's important to find something you enjoy. Exercise is vital for health – it helps prevent circulatory and pulmonary diseases, it keeps bones in good condition which prevents early onset of arthritis and rheumatism, and is very good for morale.

**smoking** – just about the worst thing you can do for your health and aging process. Apart from the direct connection between smoking and lung cancer, it also contributes to coronary disease and chronic bronchitis. The skin of smokers also wrinkles much earlier.

**alcohol** – in our society it's difficult to avoid alcohol completely. In moderation it is all right, in fact is often recommended for low blood pressure and nervous disorders. It may be all right to drink spirits in your teens and twenties but as you grow older its important to cut down their consumption for health and weight reasons. Wine contains less alcohol and fewer calories.

**sex** – remaining sexually active is a known preserver of youth. Sexual desire is not just the prerogative of youth and it is no longer considered unseemly in middle age and beyond. You will also be more inclined to keep your body in good shape – and you'll be getting some exercise as well.

## Why are you interested in staying young?

- to simply look better than ever
- to retain current relationships
- to achieve career goals
- to feel healthy and active, full of spring and energy
- to remain sexually alluring – or to become more so
- to have the wisdom of years and the looks of someone younger
- to change your lifestyle, your ties, your work
- to get a new lease on life, using past experience for a positive future

Each and every one is a powerful and valid reason, and together they add up to a thoroughly optimistic view of life. Don't be shy about your ambitions. Being realistic about staying young is not self-centred vanity. It's reaching out for your full potential to please yourself and ultimately others.

'One should never trust a woman who tells you her real age. A woman who would tell one that would tell one anything.'
Oscar Wilde

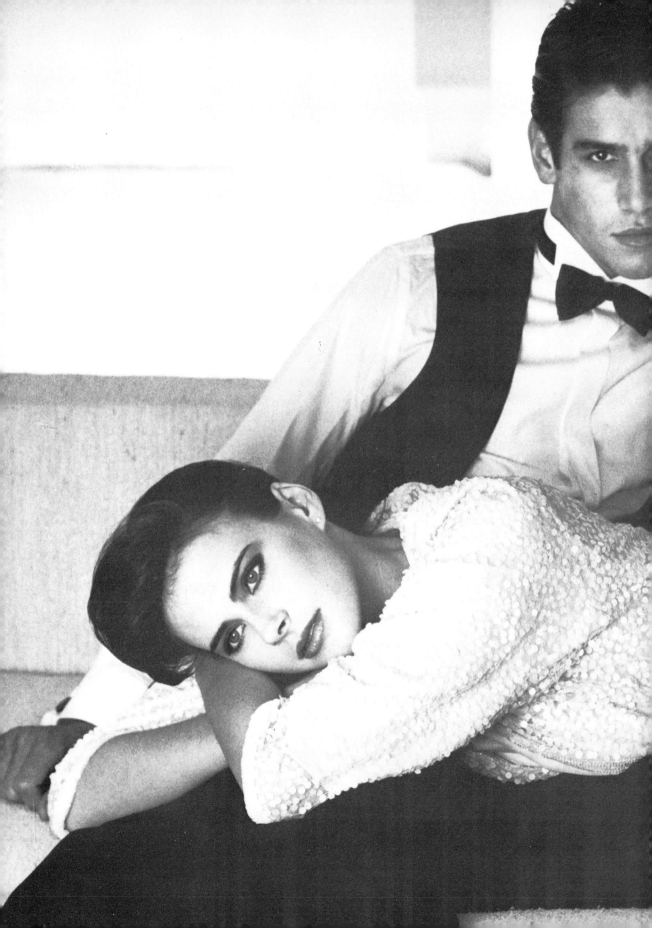

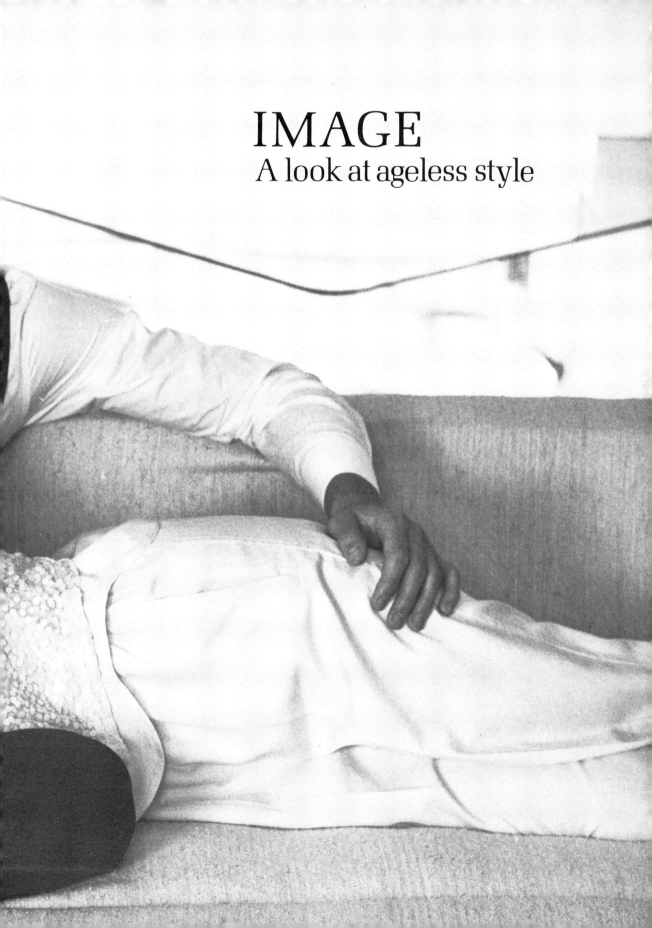

# IMAGE
## A look at ageless style

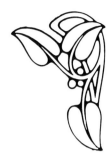

Any book about staying young cannot ignore the all-important issue of clothing. I am the first to stress the importance of health fundamentals, but if you are going to make effort with the basics, you need the fun of the icing on the cake. If you are feeling good, you want to express it in every way, and that means a bit of effort into pulling yourself together on the outside. Some women seem to make a point of being dowdy, as if being stylish might give the wrong impression and detract from so-called real values and character. Quite wrong. Never underestimate the power of personal style. It's not presumptuous to put your best image forward. You can actually take years off your looks in just one day by getting into the right clothes. Clothes are responsible for first impressions. Clothes communicate before words and minds.

Age used to enter into the choice of attire, but no more. The question used to be: is this correct for my age? Now it's: is this right for my figure, my idea of myself? Fashion today offers clothes for women who are fit and in good shape, not for women of this or that age.

The best thing is to create a definite style of your own. Style refers to much more than fashion. In fact it is often aging to be in fashion, to go for the currently trendy clothes. Many women make the mistake of sticking to a fashion that suited them years ago; this is extremely dating and bears no relation to knowing your own style and sticking to it.

This doesn't mean that all is possible – mini skirts and skimpy trousers should remain with the truly young – but in general, contemporary fashion can transcend the years. No woman need resort to matronly things. However, if you try to dress in a style that's too young, it can only be aging. Cute designs, little-girl prints, too many frills and gathers are out. Mutton dressed as lamb is a cruel joke and always will be.

A woman with style isn't usually a woman who slavishly follows fashion. She has found a look of her own, something that is comfortable, something that makes her look and feel good. It is invariably a certain way with the classics, a certain colour scheme, a length of skirt, a placement of waist, a height of heel. It's just right and as a central style should not be changed. But it can be adapted, varied, given colour and accessorized to make it move subtly with the times. It can be made more casual or more sophisticated, but that personal style, that individual stamp, remains. Once you find what suits you, you'll probably end up by continually buying a translation of the same outfit in different fabrics or textures – but they'll all appear different from the others, as well as definitely you.

How do you find your own style? First, you have to understand what you look like. That's the most difficult part. It starts by using your head and by being honest. Don't think in terms of age, but of figure. Look in the mirror in the nude and work out how best to handle your figure. Get to know your body type. Be objective, assess the good and don't skim over the bad. No one's perfect. Certain things can be changed by diet and exercise, but basic body structure cannot. Wide shoulders, a stocky torso, short legs, or thick neck are things you are stuck with. Face the fact they are there and keep them firmly in mind when selecting clothes.

Of course, there's more to style than coping with the physical. Your clothes should be a reflection of you, an expression of your feelings about yourself, a view into your personality, a clue for the others. Take another look at your image. Do you feel happy about it?

Style and flair are longer lasting than beauty. They can be acquired and never fade. Create your own aura and keep it for ever. Style doesn't age, it simply adjusts itself to time.

## Guidelines to youthful-looking clothes

**Comfort first** – you cannot move with youthful ease if clothes are constricting. What is young is anything that can make you forget you are wearing clothes. This doesn't mean sloppy attire – you'd be very conscious of that – but easy lines of the sort of fabric that moves with the body, such as the best wools, silks and cottons. Many synthetic fibres are rigid or irritatingly inclined to cling to the body; they can also be uncomfortably hot and sticky; they rarely move well.

**Simplicity is best** – the less contrived your attire, the more effective. Youthfulness in fashion has everything to do with simplicity – of line, of fabric, of colour, of accessories. Formal complicated designs are aging, so are stiff fabrics, elaborate weaves and busy prints. Solid-coloured clothes win all the time, and this includes muted tweeds and the tailoring cloths used for menswear. Stripes are fine and so are polka dots because there is something definite and crisp about them.

'Fashion works when it causes you to notice the woman. It fails when you notice what she's wearing.'
couturier Coco Chanel

**Stay with neutral colours** – clothes that work are those that are interrelated in colour. If you don't spread the colour around, you'll find you need far fewer things and you'll look more pulled together into the bargain. Begin with black and white, followed by grey and beige. Forget that old tale of black being aging; it can look superb. Decide on your neutrals and then take a man's approach to a wardrobe: build around classic shapes, suits, jackets, trousers, using accessories and splurges of colour to make them what you will.

**Sportswear looks younger** – this is because they are active clothes; they are casual, they are easy to wear and easy to put on – few encasing zippers, shaped bodices or definite waistlines. Sportswear provides the perfect balance of the tailored and the soft, and there's no better combination for a youthful look. The sharpness of skirts, trousers and jackets are offset by feminine shirts and sweaters.

**Accessories are major** – they can ruin an outfit or turn it into an absolute winner. They must be good; they must be kept to a minimum but with one item that stands out more than the others – a bright scarf, a stunning belt, special jewellery, a dazzling flower. Women of style know that to invest in one superb leather handbag, for instance, is a better investment than three lesser ones. Classic jewellery lasts for ever and always looks chic – pearl stud earrings, gold loops, gold chains, pearls, a really good watch.

**Aim for quality** – the young can get away with the cheap and cheerful, but it's a mistake to think that way later on. Look for quality of fabric and cut – this is how you will find the fluidity and movement that is an integral part of the younger look. It's worth it, because if you have properly worked out your basic personal style, items will stay in your wardrobe for years and years.

### Clothes can camouflage: here's how

Apart from the general principles that make fashion youthful, there are certain shapes that can play tricks on the eye, give the illusion of a better figure, put focus on the good points and allow the bad ones to fade away. Camouflage in itself, however, is tricky. It can't be overdone, otherwise it is blatantly obvious what you are up to. And there's always the chance of giving the impression that there could be something better underneath – which is hardly the point. A clever, discreet touch is needed. Here are some basic rules for the most common problems.

**waist** – an expanding waistline usually means bulges above and below it, so the whole midriff area has to be whittled away. Tunics and long easy sweaters are great, also dropped-waist dresses if your hips are in shape. Avoid anything that clearly divides you at the waist, such as contrasting colours top and bottom, or obvious belts. Stick to one shade throughout. Skirts can be straight or shaped, moderately flat-pleated; shirts should be bloused, whether tucked in or worn outside and narrowly belted. Skirts and trousers should have narrow waistbands or none. Select jackets like blazers. Leave those flowing-from-the-bosom dresses for ingenues or pregnant ladies. They just don't work except when floor length for evening.

**stomach** – again it's the tunic and the long sweater that helps. Blousing above the waist also lessens the thickness, particularly if it is low blousing that moves over the stomach area. A-shaped skirts are good, also those with stitched front pleats to around thigh level. Jackets and long loose cardigans are a boon, especially so when worn casually open. Out are straight skirts, fitted silhouettes, gathered skirts.

**thighs** – keep skirts to the A-line silhouette, but if your waist and stomach are small, gathered skirts and pleats work very well, and should be tightly belted. Draw attention upwards; wear blousey tops and sweaters, shorter jackets, scarves and interesting things around the neck.

*Christian Dior*
'A woman does not learn to dress well until she is over 35. One should remember that the most beautiful dresses in the world can be, literally, wasted on air if they are worn badly.'

**bosom** – watch this because no matter how effective an ample bosom can look when young, as you grow older even a medium one can start to look matronly. Loose-fitting shirts are the answer, easy sweaters, casual jackets. The rule is nothing clinging, but one can give a suggestion of decolletage in a casual discreet way. And if you wear a belt, be sure there's a visible area between it and your bosom. You are actually better off with a smaller bosom for a youthful line, as you can virtually wear anything. However, should your top area be much narrower than your bottom half, balance the silhouette with bloused and gathered tops, short jackets and waistcoats.

**upper arms** – flab around here is a sure sign of advancing years and not very attractive either. Sleeveless dresses should be avoided; short sleeves need to be much wider than the arm and as near to the elbow as you consider chic. Long sleeves are best, but they should be loose and banded at the wrist. And a rolled-up sleeve looks casual and very smart. Avoid strap sundresses, not only do they reveal all but because you are bare you'll be even hotter and your skin will suffer from the sun.

## What about underneath? How firm?

There are those who preach a firm foundation is everything, which is all very well for more control and a smoother silhouette pulling in the inches. But watch it, because too much upholstery is constricting. It can make you look too rigid, too held in place, thus losing that impression of body freedom essential for a youthful image. Fashion today doesn't require such a definite line.

Look for lightweight bras and firming panties. The idea is to remould and re-arrange, not squash flesh into the smallest area possible. One of the best things is the all-in-one body slimmer, which reshapes in the most natural way, and because it is based on swim, dance and exercise suits, it is supple and permits all movement with ease. The effect of any body shaper (bra, pantie or one-piece) depends on the fitting. You have to try and try before you buy. It's the most difficult piece of clothing to get right, and yet it is one of the most important. But if you get your under layer in order, it's so much easier to work out things on top.

Get your own image straight. It's not easy being just you, an individual you. Many women imitate looks, copy the models in the magazines. They are a great guideline, but set your own brand of style and stick to it.

Personal style begins by dressing to please yourself. No way can you ever work out your own individual look if you are wondering what others like, what would please *him*. Your own feelings, your intuition of what's right for you is more significant.

'Underwear is very important. The shape underneath makes all the difference to the shape in clothes. Although, I hate the armour-plated look with darts everywhere. There is no reason why a woman of any age cannot wear fashionable clothes, although a short skirt is a mistake. It is best to accentuate the best features – neck, legs, waist for example, and hide the rest.'
couturier David Sassoon

**Casual Looks** – the easiest way to keep a young image is to dress in a casual, off-hand way – roomy skirts, comfortable trousers, modest shorts, loose tops, roomy sweaters, sporty jackets and easy coats. Classic tailored shirts, jumpers and cardigans are basic and should be the mainstay of a casual wardrobe. Such separates as these can go on forever, with seasonal additions to update the look. Stick to neutral shades with the odd flash of colour for effect.

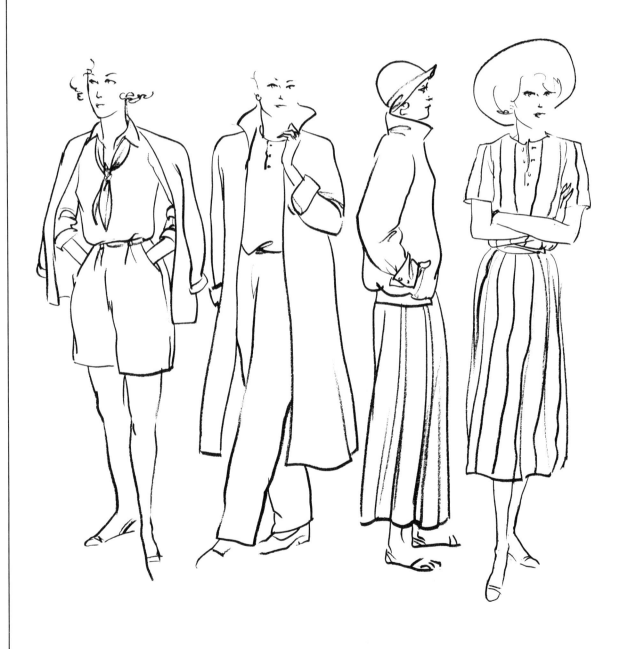

'It's a great mistake to try and look younger than you are by covering blemishes with too much make-up. Clothes that are showy are also a mistake. They must have an elegant line and then you fill in the gaps. One has to conform to fashion a bit but you must wear what suits you and you must never feel uncomfortable in what you are wearing.'

model and Vogue's ex Mrs Exeter, Margot Smylie

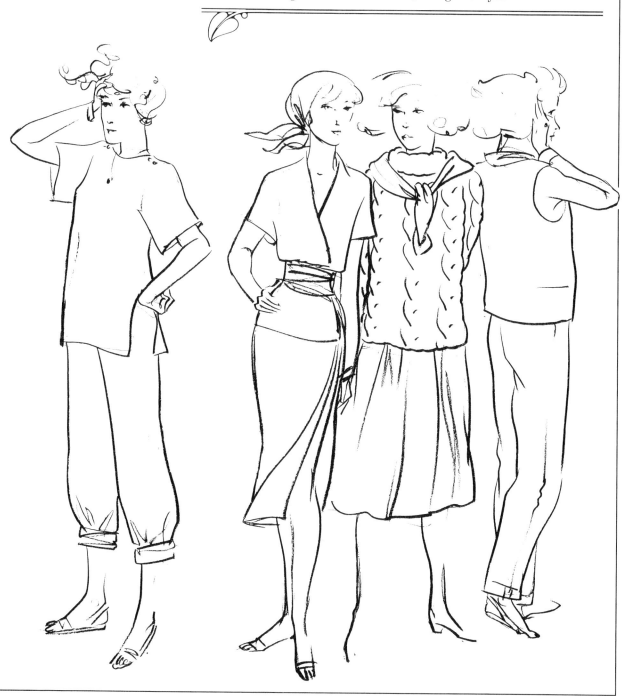

**Classic Clothes** – invest in the best – in cut, in fabric, in workmanship as these are going to be the clothes that last for years and years, no matter what fashion ideas come and go. They are also the styles that know no age – they are as effective when you are in your forties and fifties as in your twenties. Every woman needs a basic raincoat, a trenchcoat, a Chanel-type suit, a pleated skirt and blazer, a kilt and sweater, a simple shirtdress and a pair of flannel trousers to go with all shirts, sweaters and jackets. Build your classic wardrobe around one basic colour scheme and stick to wools, silks, linens and cottons.

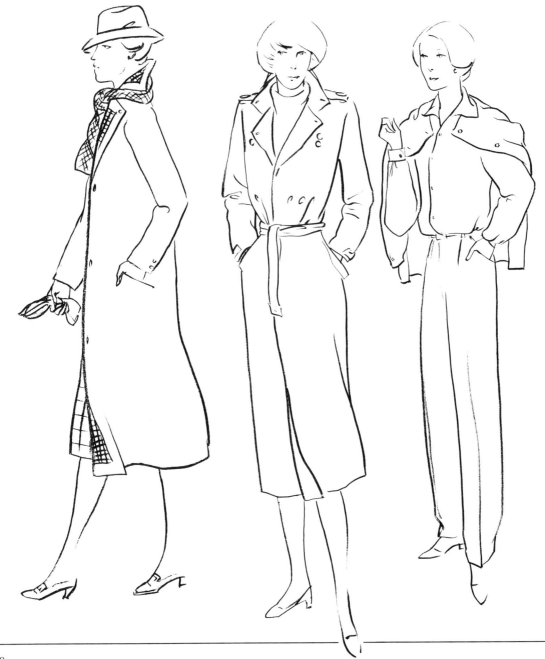

'If you want to preserve a harmonious total appearance, your dress should be as simple as possible and you should avoid the desire to protect yourself with scarves and a cluster of trinkets. Clothing should endeavour to show up favourably your good features and disguise your bad ones. The looser your clothing, the slimmer you will feel and the quicker your body will be able to move. There will be no strain on cloth which will hang gracefully and peacefully.'
couturier Hardy Amies

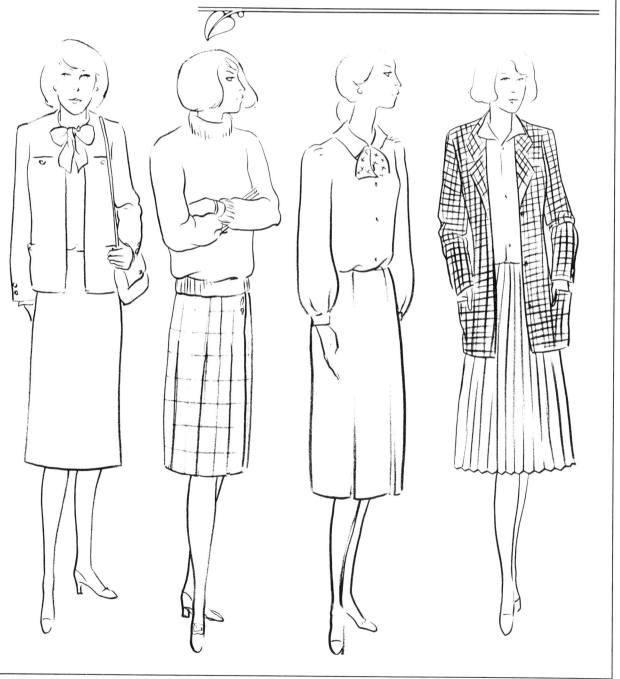

**City Dressing** – the most impressive looks are those that are essentially classic with a stamp of sophistication on them. This means sleek, tailored silhouettes that are crisp and curtailed, that provide a neat and finished body line. These are the sort of clothes that can be dressed up and down as you will – with accessories such as jewellery, scarves, hats, shoes, as their fundamental simplicity provides endless possibilities. Choose wools, silks and linens – choose from lines such as these which would look good in any city, any country.

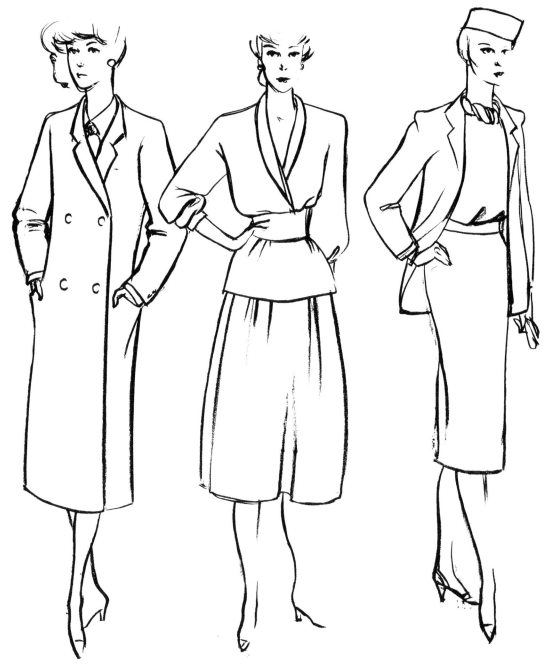

'I design for women with brains and careers – the sort of executive woman who wants to look smart in a suit, just as a man does. Chanel recognized the needs of career women in this direction back in the Twenties, and I am just carrying it on.'
designer Nino Cerruti

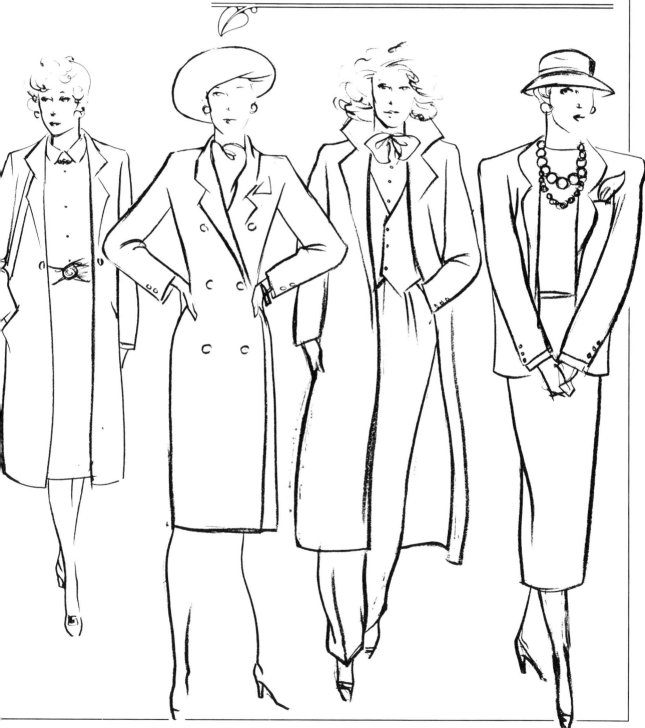

**Evening Glamour** – one great asset of maturity is that you can give way to glamour and look all the better for it – a thing that no young person could get away with. It is drama that counts, and that can really only come from stark, simple lines that put you into focus rather than the dress. Frills and fancies are best left to the very young – think in terms of cool, sophisticated lines that emphasize your assets, which are usually focused above the waist. It is often best to draw attention to the shoulder line with big sleeves, a décolleté, an alluring bareness. Waists can sometimes be a problem, a better solution is to go for long torso and blouson looks. And remember, plain fabrics – silks, chiffons, brocades, lace – are more impressive than most prints.

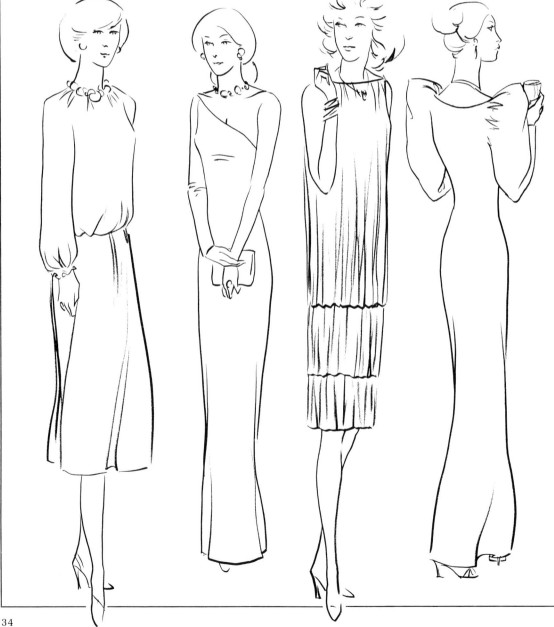

'It's egoistic to be careless of your appearance because you offend other people's eyes.'
designer and illustrator Erté

'The golden rule of fashion – that the essence of chic is elimination.'
couturier Balenciaga

'Fashion should always reflect a woman's mind, it can never dictate to her.'
couturier Jean Patou

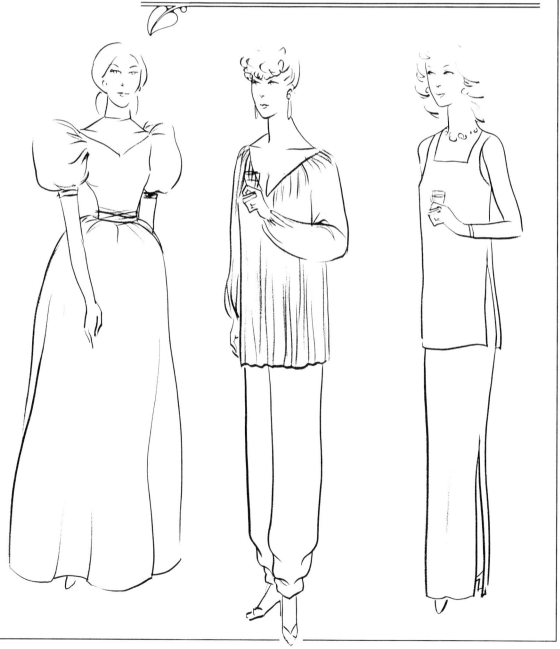

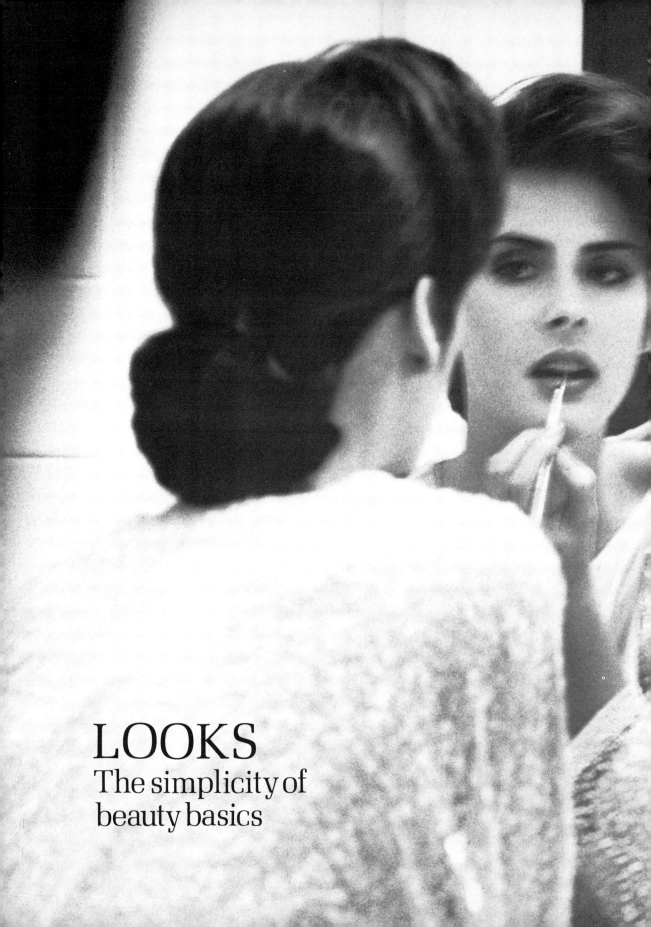

# LOOKS
## The simplicity of beauty basics

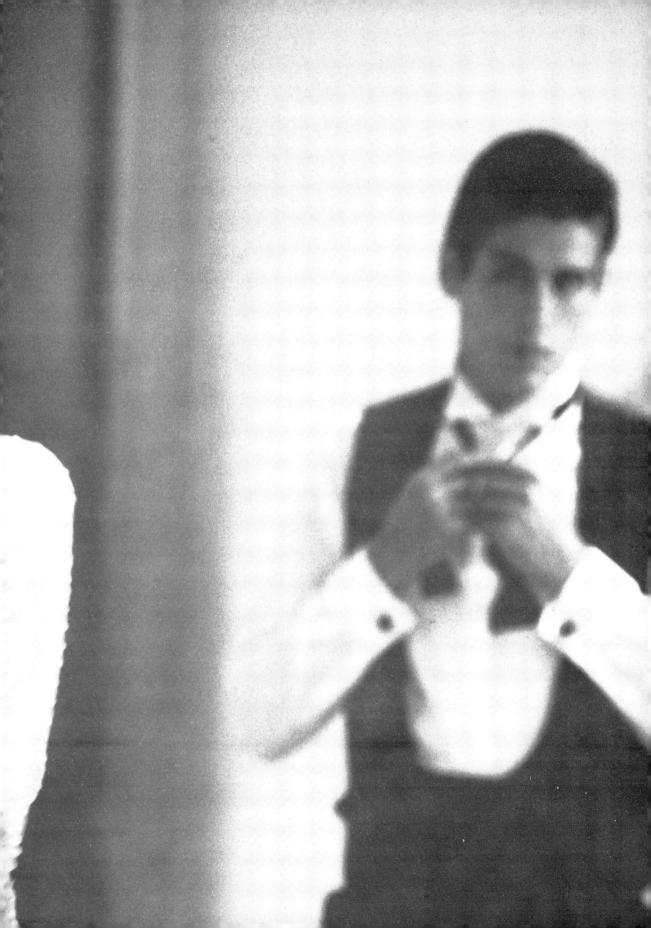

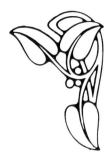

There is no doubt that looking good contributes enormously to confidence and the self-assurance of knowing that your appearance belies your years. Any woman who dismisses beautifying routines as unnecessary vanity in this age of equality is really only fooling herself. What is more, she is the one who is out of line, because she is using the old standards and values for her judgement. Attractiveness today is light years away from putting on a pretty face to please a man. It is still part of it, of course, and it's the honest women who admit it, but today's brand of good looks have to do with personal pride and self-respect, and are centred on the quality of your physical attributes, not the dressing-up of them. Is your skin in the best of condition? Is your hair shining and healthy? Is your body skin smooth and soft? Are your hands and feet immaculate? That is what beauty is about now – and these values embrace all age groups.

Pretending beauty doesn't matter is a delusion. Most women would like to be as beautiful as possible, but too many think in terms of standardized beauty which is completely wrong. There are so many dimensions to beauty, not the least being the special appeal of individuality, that it is nonsense to strive for a certain look. Being comfortable with who you are and what you look like is vital, but this doesn't mean that you should ignore the ways and means to make the very best of your external image. Staying younger, longer has a lot to do with how you present your package to others – all right, it may only be the outside wrapping, but it can say a great deal about your inner feelings and attitude. And it's fundamental to first impressions.

But back to the keyword: quality. The only way to achieve it is through care. Do I hear a groan at this point? Care to most women is synonymous with time, and time is something today's woman has precious little of. Who has time to spend on all those beauty routines? Few of us do, but this brings me to one of the most important facts about a beauty programme: it need not take up much time at all providing it is organized and continuous.

Women think a lot of time is necessary mainly because so much is written about beauty procedures and since cosmetic technology has become so highly scientific, explanations as to how and why products work are inclined to get involved to the point of a product's use appearing more complicated than it really is. In the Eighties we have the good fortune to have at hand incredibly sophisticated preparations, some of which go beyond being preventive and are actually restorative. The research laboratories of cosmetic companies are doing a remarkable job and it is due to them that we now have super-efficient soaps, cleansers, tonics, moisturizers, creams, treatments, oils, shampoos, conditioners, non-toxic make-up and longer lasting perfumes. The cosmetic industry gets lots of unfair knocks from independent dermatologists, yet in the battle against the visual aspects of aging, it is the commercial laboratories who are our allies, and they are responsible for bringing the new efficient simplicity in beauty basics.

Perfume is the most elusive of beauty resources, yet it is one of the most impressive because one is aware of a woman's perfume before one sees her, before one knows her, and it can uncannily provide an aura, create an image and a mood – and stir up emotions to a remarkable degree. You can argue that perfume is not necessary, that it is expensive, that it is frivolous, that it no longer plays an important role in a modern woman's attitude towards looks. And you'd be wrong on all counts, except the expense. The old thinking was to consider perfume as a means of sexual attraction, a tool of seduction and so on. You can still use it for that, of course, but all depends on the type of perfume. The heavy florals, the spicy, the sweet and the oriental aromatics should be left for the couch, or perhaps sprayed on it. Modern perfumes provide just the opposite effect; they are fresh and lively, giving off an air of dash and efficiency, of joyful activity and a youthful image. Now this all may sound like rather flowery language but such is the vernacular of perfume even when one is approaching it from a sensible and liberated point of view.

So what are the basics, the things that require continual beauty checks through minimum daily attention? Here is the essential list: the five factors of beauty care, details on the following pages as to the simplest and quickest ways to take care of them.

- body – its shape, posture and condition, bathing basics and perfume extras
- face – help structure and skin resilience through exercise
- skincare – easy daily routines for skin preservation
- make-up – the most from the minimum, done with speed
- hair – health and condition first, then style

## Body

The two fundamental check points for the body are posture and shape. In a way they are interdependent, because very often the way you hold your body can greatly influence its shape. But first of all, a word on body type, as it is important to accept the fact – even if you haven't up to now – that there are many things You can do to change the shape of your body by diminishing fatty deposits and building up muscles, but there is nothing you can do about your basic structure. Bodies have medically been put into three main categories: small frame with narrow shoulders, narrow hips with a slender side view; medium frame that can be rounded or athletic but with a certain degree of narrowness through the ribcage, waist and hips, though shoulders may be quite broad; a heavy build that is chunky with shoulders often narrower than the hips. It is being honest about this basic type that will enable you to check realistically on how your outward body is faring. Many women in their middle thirties haven't come to terms with such realism. You must.

Next step: check on posture. Good posture gives a better figure immediately. The way you carry and move your body affects its shape and the habit of good posture can mean you have a young-looking figure for life – it can reflect youth and vitality at any age. How do you stand and walk? When standing, think of a thread running through the vertebrae of your spine, then imagine it being pulled tautly from above your head; lift and stretch the whole body – it makes you feel much lighter, springier and younger. When walking be aware of an easy gait, of supple swinging limbs, of giving the impression of a jaunty air. Relax arms and allow them to follow the body naturally and with ease. You should walk using the full leg, not just the area from the knee down, and try not to swing from the hips. Keep the back straight, up and down hill, up and down steps – when you lean forward it's an old-looking movement.

The shape of your body depends, of course, on the amount of daily attention you give to your diet and your exercise. You know when you are carrying around too much fat without having to go on the scales, and it is true that it is more difficult to get rid of fat as you get older. Prevention and reshaping is possible, but what about that

## Perfume Choice

Perfumes can be grouped into categories according to content and impression. You usually find you prefer one type to another. The *florals* are by far the biggest group and can either by sharp single aromas (such as rose, lily of the valley, jasmine) or harmonious blends that would include such aromatics as gardenia, jonquil, narcissus, honeysuckle, lilac, carnation, orange blossom, violet, geranium. They can be fresh or sweet, but after your thirties it is best to stick to the fresh notes, as the sweet ones can often give the aura of lavender and old lace. The *greens* are fresh and woodsy, crisp and clean – perfect for the country and outdoor woman. The *modern* blends are bright and sharp and are usually favoured by career and stylish women because they are pleasant and effective without being overpowering, without making a too obvious statement of feminity. The *citrus* scents are blends of lemon, orange and bergamot essences. They are particularly sharp and fresh, perfect for warm climates as they are cooling and refreshing. (But a word of warning, be careful not to wear a bergamot blend when sunbathing, as this can often cause an allergic reaction; in fact it's wise never to wear perfume on the beach.) The *oriental* scents are sweet, heavy and quite exotic. They can imply glamour and sophistication, but they can also be rather overpowering, and are apt to underline any sultry image.

fearsome ogre – cellulite? Does it or doesn't it exist? Doctors continue to argue about this, but as far as the individual woman is concerned, it is a very real problem. Cellulite is fat that stubbornly stays even when other areas respond well to diet and exercise. It can often plague women who are basically thin. Hips, buttocks, thighs, knees, stomach and upper arms can all have it – lumpy fat which puckers like the skin of an orange when you squeeze it. It can develop at any age, but the highest percentage of women who get it do so around the start of the menopause. There is a definite hormonal link – on that all doctors agree; the controversy is whether it is a special kind of fat and what are the other contributory factors, such as a diet too high in refined carbohydrates, trapped toxic wastes, poor circulation and inefficient elimination due to constipation or weak functioning of the kidney and liver.

However, while the professionals carry on the debate, there are many preventive and recuperative steps you can take which have proved successful even though they are dismissed in medical terms. Try not to be obsessive about lean and lithesome looks; many women are naturally big without carrying excess fat; the widely promoted 'ideal body shape' is in reality difficult to achieve and for some quite impossible. Be honest about your body type and work within those boundaries. Daily vigilance is the best – and these are the things to watch:

- *diet* – if you follow the stay younger longer diet regimen (see page 92) you are cutting down on the starches, sugars and packaged foods that encourage cellulite. A good way to get rid of the trapped toxics faster is to go on a raw food diet (see page 109) and have daily drinks of celery and cucumber juice which are splendid eliminators and aid kidney function. If you haven't got a juice extractor (though this is a vital investment in the interests of general good health), eat a large cucumber salad every day. Cut out alcohol for a while, and instead of tea and coffee, drink herbal teas, plus a pint of mineral water every day.

- *exercise* – the significance of movement in relation to cellulite is in the way it increases circulation which helps clear the tissues of their toxic sludge. You can't firm up cellulite as such, but the slow build-up of muscle power will help prevent skin sag once the fatty areas have been reduced.

- *local stimulation* – the aim of this is again to step up circulation. Daily rubbing with a loofah or friction glove is good, so is massage, but don't do it too hard. A jet of water from the shower is a stimulating force, while the shock of alternate splashes of cold and hot water wakes up sluggish circulation. All of these can be done during daily bathing.

- *creams* – there are a few 'cellulite creams' on the market and research has produced proof of the efficacy of their use. If you massage them daily into affected areas you can often get good results.

# Bathing

Keeping clean, of course, is basic to good looks, yet most women so rush the whole bathing procedure (which naturally should be a daily one) that they don't get the extra benefits which contribute to the feeling of beauty as much as to the personification of it.

When you bathe you can help preserve and restore the condition of your skin – a treatment that takes no extra time out of your day because it is done at the same time as your essential bathing. As you get older your skin gets dryer, so it is imperative to counteract this, First of all don't lie around too long in the bath and don't have it too hot, as your skin will become dehydrated and shrivel up – crinkling of the tips of your fingers is the first indication. You need to lubricate or nourish your skin while you soak and to this end you are better off selecting the oily and powdered bath essences rather than the crystal fixed ones. Some of these are stimulating as well because of the herbal extracts or volatile essences they contain. Not everyone can afford – or wishes to spend money on – these commercial preparations, but there are equally good substitutes that can be worked out from kitchen items together with herbs and aromatic oils:

- *to lubricate*: a few drops of any oil in the bath helps dryness, but for a fragrant one mix together $\frac{3}{4}$ cup of almond oil or castor oil with $\frac{1}{4}$ cup of any aromatic oil (available at some health food shops and chemists) – best are rose, jasmine, lavender, lemon flowers. Shake well before each use, and a teaspoonful is ample for each bath.
- *to nourish*: the easiest method is a cup of powdered milk in the bath, but you can also fill a muslin bag with oatmeal, almond meal or bran, and let it soak in the bath by hanging it from the tap. It usually lasts for two or three baths.
- *to restore and tone*: once a week, before any type of bath, rub the entire body with salt, just ordinary kitchen salt – the coarser, the better – and rinse off; this clears the surface of dead surface cells and rubs away flaky top layers of skin. Herbal baths are restorative – either put herbs in a cheesecloth bag and soak in the bath, or make an infusion using 2 tablespoons of leaves or flowers and pouring over a pint (6dl) of water; let this steep for 15 minutes and pour all in the bath. Dried lavender is very effective, so is a mixture of rosemary, fennel, sage and yarrow; camomile is soothing to the skin; elder tones the skin and also helps to calm the nerves; if you have any scars and cuts that are healing slowly (a thing that happens as you get older), use an infusion of comfrey.
- *to condition*: always, always smooth in a body lotion after bathing, it's the best counter-measure for dryness; bath oil spray softens and scents the skin and is less drying than perfume; go easy on the talcum powder.

# Arms and Hands

As you get older, the upper arm tends to become flabby which is usually due to poor muscle tone, and it can sometimes have a mottled look because of bad circulation and a diet too high in refined foods. Check your diet to see if you are getting enough raw fresh food and unrefined grains. Aid circulation by rubbing vigorously with a loofah when bathing. Improve muscle tone by doing the following two exercises.

**Arm stretch:** sitting or standing, raise arms sideways to shoulder level, palms down, fingers stretched; push arms outwards as far as possible, then bounce up and down ten times; raise arms a little into a Y position, bounce ten times.

**Weight lift:** sitting or standing, take a dumbbell or heavy book and hold firmly in one hand; raise arm above head, keeping it close to your head, then bend the elbow and lower weight behind the head to touch the opposite shoulder; raise arm up again. Repeat ten times with each arm.

The skin on the arm is often sadly neglected; it needs plenty of moisturizing with a rich cream to prevent dryness and that crepy look. Pay special attention to the elbows to prevent a rough and ridged surface – if very rough and ingrained, first soften and cleanse with an oatmeal-and-water paste. Check on hair – if it is very dark, then bleach it; even a lot of hair can be minimized in this way. Removing hair from the arms is not generally advisable, but if you consider it necessary use wax or a chemical depilatory – never shave.

Hands reveal age more than any other area of the body, and once you have let them go, they are extremely difficult to resurrect. So don't let your hands tell your age when the rest of your body doesn't. The answer is prevention: daily caution and care from the very beginning. Hands respond quickly and well to exercise, creams and massage. And equally quickly they deteriorate when exposed to too much water, detergents, household chemicals, cold weather and burning sun. Check on these points to keep your hands in the best condition:

- exercise – clench fist tightly, hold to the count of three, then throw open the hand, widely spacing the fingers and stretching them, hold to the count of three. Repeat ten times. Another good exercise for graceful hands and supple wrists – rotate hands from the wrists, ten times in each direction.
- protection – wear gloves for all work, rubber ones for wet work, cotton ones for housework and gardening, warm ones when it's cold. And protect hands from the sun by using a sunscreen or wearing gloves if you are constantly out of doors working – this helps prevent the development of those small brown spots, called 'liver spots' but actually caused by the skin's reaction to excess ultraviolet rays. It is virtually impossible to get rid of these marks – only a cover-up make-up will camouflage them.

## Step by step Manicure

**1** Using an oily remover (never neat acetone) remove polish with a cotton pad, pressing it first against the nail to soften polish, then wiping off.

**2** File nails into an oval shape using long strokes from side to centre, being careful not to file too low at the sides. Use an emery board, not a metal file – it's too harsh.

**3** Rub a little cuticle cream into the base of each nail.

**4** Soak nails in warm soapy water for a few minutes; brush away any dirt and soften any hard spots with a pumice stone.

**5** Wrap cotton wool around an orange stick, dip into cuticle oil and smear around the rim of the cuticle.

**6** With another cotton-wrapped stick moistened in the soapy water, gently work at the base of the cuticle, lifting skin from the nail – never force it; smooth with finger into a curve.

- cleansing – wash hands thoroughly many times a day, rinse with clear water before patting dry; scrub fingers and nails with a brush. A pumice stone used with soap and water will remove rough skin and most stains, otherwise try rubbing with a slice of lemon.
- treatment – massage rich handcream well into the skin after each washing; if hands are very dry give them an extra creaming at night and wear cotton gloves to bed. A soak in warm olive oil is good for dryness, good for brittle nails too.
- beautifying – keep your nails in good order and condition and give yourself a weekly manicure. Remember hands are on show all the time. If nails are brittle, it may be because you are lacking sufficient B-6 vitamin and zinc – take brewer's yeast daily. Brushing with white iodine also helps. Treat nails gently, don't push too vigorously around the cuticle area, as once this is damaged it continued right up the nail during growth. Nails grow slowly and improvements take time. A good manicure is also a treatment for nails and helps prevent problems. Here's how:

**7** Clean under nails with cotton-wrapped stick (or cotton bud), dip hands in water, pat dry, and liberally apply hand lotion.

**8** Dip fingernails only into the water to get rid of any film of cream, then brush gently to ensure a really smooth surface.

**9** If you don't wear polish, an idea is to accentuate the tip of the nail, by running a white nail pencil under the surface.

**10** Not very often used now, but excellent for circulation – a nail buffer. Buff in one direction only – it brings colour to the nail because of increased circulation; it's a nail-health benefactor too.

**11** Apply varnish: first a base coat, then two layers of colour and finally a sealer. Apply in long straight strokes from the base to the tip, one down the middle, one either side.

**12** Clean up any smudging by dipping a cotton-wrapped stick into the oily remover and running it around the nail and under the tip. Give nails ample time to dry before using hands.

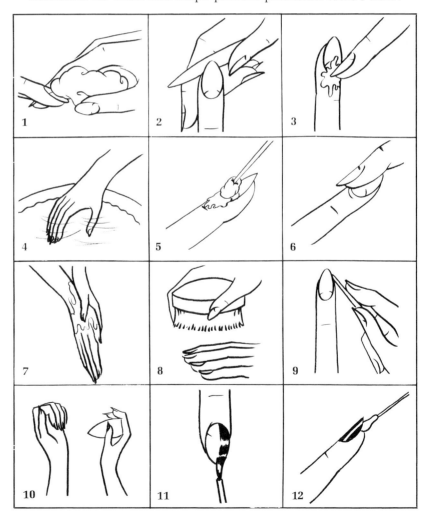

# Legs and Feet

If your legs and feet are looking the worse for wear as you age, it is most likely because you are neglecting elementary basic care and not because it is an inevitable aspect of aging. Apart from fretting about fat on the thighs, few women pay much attention to this area, and yet it is so important in maintaining a youthful image. However, if legs are exercised regularly (many routines on pages 128 to 143) and checked for cellulite (page 40) they can be kept trim and firm well into later years. Activity is particularly important, not only for shape and condition, but for suppleness and mobility – if you start to drag your legs, you immediately take on the air of someone getting on in years. Lack of exercise and a bad diet (plus overweight and badly fitting shoes) are invariably responsible for the onset of varicose veins; all these causes are self-corrective. Swollen ankles, too, are often due to an incorrect diet where fluid is retained, a condition aggravated through lack of exercise. Legs require some conditioning as by nature they are rather dry and become more so (sometimes to the point of scaliness) as we age. The best way to help is to exfoliate the skin (remove the dead surface cells) once a week by rubbing them with coarse salt and rinsing well. Afterwards apply a rich body lotion or cream. Legs should be moisturized this way every day. If legs are particularly dry and scaly, rub in honey, olive or baby oil, leave on for a few minutes, rinse away and cream. Hair on the legs can look unsightly. If there are not too many, bleach them, otherwise waxing is best – only shave in an emergency.

Feet contribute more to aging than you would think. If your feet hurt or ache, you not only move slowly and stiffly, but the pain they are causing shows on your face. It would seem that once tucked away in shoes or slippers, it is out of sight out of mind. Nothing could be worse. Feet need tender loving care, they need air and exercise and they need to be checked for problems such as corns, bunions, callouses, verrucas, ingrowing toenails and foot infections. And all of these need immediate professional help. A regular visit to a chiropodist is a basic essential, and sadly one that is usually completely overlooked. It's one speciality that is not very expensive and it's so worth while, because all foot problems get worse and are difficult to correct if left too long. Feet need these attentions:

- **exercise** – stand and take weight on one foot, raise heel of the other and bend the toe joints at right angles to the floor, hold to the count of three, lower. Repeat five times with each foot. Exercise the ankle by doing foot circles, ten times in each direction. Help toes by trying to separate and spread them, holding for the count of three, relax, repeat ten times.

- **protection** – by selecting carefully the most comfortable of shoes; the best heel height is between one and a half and two and a half inches; avoid pointed toes, stiletto heels (just occasionally for glamour) and low-cut sides. Best prevention of problems is to walk barefoot whenever possible and don't keep nylon stockings on all the time – they trap moisture as well as restricting feet.

- **cleansing** – wash daily, massage with a loofah, use a nail brush to get rid of stubborn dirt, check between toes, use a pumice stone on hard skin.

- **treatment** – massage a lotion into the feet, particularly around the heel area; dust lightly with powder if they are inclined to be sweaty, dab with surgical spirit if sweat is excessive. Give tired feet an Epsom salts bath – two tablespoons to a quart of lukewarm water; soak for ten minutes, then plunge into cold water, rub with alcohol or witch hazel, moisturize and prop up for ten minutes.

- **beautifying** – giving yourself a pedicure every ten days, which makes you even more conscious of the condition of your feet. Toenails are particularly prone to ridges and discolouration, so painted nails can only be an asset. It is not easy to master the skill of taking care of your own feet – even getting down there can be a problem – but with practice it can be done very well at home.

## Step by step Pedicure

**1** Remove polish with a cotton wad soaked in an oily remover: first press wad on the surface to soften, then wipe off.

**2** Trim nails with either scissors or clippers. Cut straight across because if you go down at the sides, nails are inclined to cut into the flesh, particularly when you wear shoes most of the time.

**3** With an emery board, smooth the edges of the nail.

**4** Soak feet in sudsy warm water for a few minutes, then with a brush scrub all over.

**5** Hard spots need special attention – the back of the heel, the sole and the ball of the foot – use a pumice stone or friction pad to soften and ease away the hard skin.

**6** Dip a cotton-wrapped orange stick in water and clean under and around the nails.

**7** Apply cuticle oil or cream at the base of the nail and massage in gently with fingers or a cotton-wrapped stick.

**8** Rinse foot in water, towel dry and check the skin area around the nail to see it is smooth; be sure to dry between toes very well.

**9** Massage in a hand or body cream, be liberal and remember the underfoot area and back of the heel; while massaging rotate ankle and pull toes individually with a jerk; also massage lower leg with firm upward strokes.

**10** Buff toes to help circulation.

**11** Separate toes with a strip of cotton wool or a folded tissue, weaving under and over the toes – this prevents smudging of polish.

**12** Apply polish, first a base coat, two coloured layers and a final sealer if you like. It looks best if you cover the entire nail. Tidy up any smudges with a cotton-wrapped stick dipped in remover.

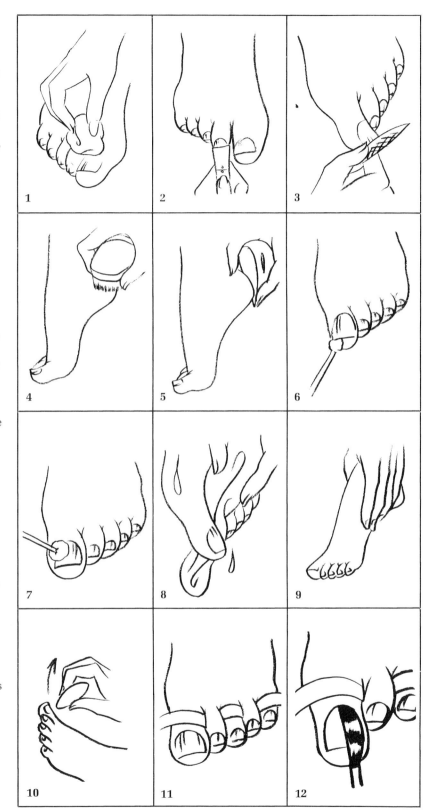

45

# Face

There is no avoiding it: everything you do, and sometimes what you don't do, shows on your face. The eyes may be the mirror of your soul, but your face is the reflection of your life and a telling indication of your health and general attitude towards yourself. All too often the face is treated as a superficial structure, as a blank canvas that can be changed through the various camouflage skills of make-up and hairstyle. Or it is thought of as an area of such important skin exposure that it requires special rituals and care. Both are part and parcel of projecting a youthful image, but what is sadly overlooked and frequently forgotten completely, is that the truly fundamental and vital things to do with a face are more than skin deep. And I'm not talking about inner feelings and glow etc., but about those very basic issues such as bones and muscles.

The shape of your face is, of course, determined by your bone structure, and you are stuck with that except to the extent of changing the shape of your nose through surgery, and helping the line of your chin the same way. The next contributory element to the look of your face is muscle – that essential underlying layer that literally holds the skin in place. It may come as a surprise to many women to learn that faces actually do have muscles – exercise routines rarely include facial movements – yet when a face begins to sag because of age it is as much due to loss of muscle support as to loss of skin elasticity.

Muscles actually help shape the face. It's a two way exchange: muscles regulate facial expressions, while facial expressions determine our features. All expressions are put into action through muscles – frowning, smiling, laughing, chewing, sulking, everything. All expressions stretch the skin to a degree and over the years lines and wrinkles are formed; these can denote joy or stress, can be downward or upward indentations, but they are there and they do increase as the years go by.

You can do something to counteract this gradual decline. And again, I stress, it doesn't take much time. The most important muscles from a stay-younger point of view are those which extend across the cheeks from the temples to the corners of the mouth. Learn the facial expressions routine on the opposite page and do it daily. Make it as automatic as cleaning your teeth.

Another simple, quick way to aid your face is to stroke away to ease the lines whilst you are cleansing or creaming. Both these treatments are daily skin-care essentials (see following page) and if you just take the extra trouble and a very little extra time to do the following specific strokes, you will be coaxing your face into a smoother surface. Results come slowly, but on a continual basis, stroking has been proved to work. It is rather like a delicate massage – the face must never be subject to rubbing or firm pressings – which gently increases the circulation and stimulates the underlying muscular structure. Just take an extra five minutes for both your two daily skin routines and use these strokes either to distribute the cleanser or to blend in the moisturizer.

## Facial stroking

- *cheek and mouth area* – purse the lips into an O-shape; with the first three fingers of each hand, gently stroke upwards from the outer corners of the mouth, going diagonally up across the cheeks to the outer corner of the eye. Stroke slowly, six times.
- *chin and mouth area* – purse lips and with the same three fingers, stroke upward from the centre of the chin diagonally to under the cheek bone; do six times.

## Skin essentials

Skin varies all the time, depending on health, nutrition, environmental factors and care. It is important that attention varies according to the condition, and the idea of a rigid routine is now considered out of date. It is what your skin is at any time that determines what you do to it. Skin care as you get older has to be flexible, but

Now we come to a real problem area when it comes to looking older: the neck. It, too, is often forgotten in the rush to get skin and make-up right, yet of all areas, the neck is one of the main tell-tale signs of age (together with the hands, as mentioned earlier). What can be done? Crepiness is caused through slackness of muscle and dryness of skin. Remember to moisturize and cream-treat your neck as much as your face. Remember that the elements of good posture help enormously to keep neck contours under control: stretch the neck, hold the head high, drop the shoulders. Then snatch a few extra minutes a day to do the following exercises – no need to make a special time, do them at the times indicated:

- *before rising –* stretch your body to get it into action for the day, one big stretch, then concentrate of your neck for just a minute; arms at sides, legs together, head flat on bed (toss pillow away); slowly raise the head by pulling on the neck muscles, hold to the count of five, slowly lower; repeat five times.

- *in front of the mirror –* before or after washing, face the glass head on, then without moving shoulders turn the chin slowly over each shoulder, first to the right, then to the left, keeping neck stretched; repeat ten times each side.

- *at your desk or at the sink –* relax and hold arms in front of the body, hands together at the lowest level; bend head forward so chin touches upper chest; then slowly raise head and at the same time bring up the arms and stretch to make a Y above the head, pulling the shoulders down and really making the neck stretch to give the widest gap between shoulders and chin; hold to the count of five; repeat five times.

## Skincare

Little affects the way you look, the way age shows, more than your skin. Skin aging lies in the genes, but you have certain controls that revolve around lifestyle habits, regular care and selective use of the new scientifically formulated preparations. Caring for your skin conscientiously in your twenties and thirties pays off. However, it is in your early forties that you really have to take a new look at the condition of your skin, re-evaluate its needs and organize a different type of programme because cell turnover rate slows down and the skin becomes noticeably drier. Fine lines appear around the eyes, on the forehead and radiate from the mouth. Skincare at this stage does not mean more time, it simply involves a change of regimen and a commitment to daily observation.

On a day-to-day basis, well balanced eating, regular exercise, adequate sleep and the know-how about counteracting stress are all factors that help maintain skin's condition and glow. Smoking is a skin-killer, so if you still haven't managed to break or control the habit, its negative aspects will start to become even more obvious.

## Daily Basics

The cleanse/tone/moisturize routine for facial skin should be second nature by the time you are in your thirties, and it has to continue to be the core of sensible protective care. This simple three-step system should be executed twice a day; it takes only a few minutes.

- **cleansing** – even though skin does become drier as you get older, there is still no need to shun soap and turn to oils and lotions. The majority of dermatologists consider soap and water the most effective way to get skin clean. It is a misconception that it's drying – but it must be done the right way with the right soap. There are so many soaps to choose from and frankly it is purely personal selection that can establish which is the best for you. Try the special facial soap bars, because these are the mildest of all, and although expensive can last for ages if just used on the face. Soap should be very gently massaged into the facial skin. Smooth circular movements – then rinsed away many times in clear water. It is the residue of soap that is drying, not the use of it.

- **toning** – because a toner is essentially a drying agent, a light freshener rather than the stronger astringent is advised for mature skin. Toning is actually not necessary if you rinse your face thoroughly, but many women like the fresh feeling it gives. A fifty-fifty mixture of rose water and witch hazel is a very good economical toner. What a toner does is: remove any last trace of cleanser, speed up the return of the protective acid mantle of the skin and temporarily tighten the pores to refine skin texture.

- **moisturizing** – regular moisturizing is essential for mature skin. It should be liberally applied and several times during the day if you are not wearing make-up, while a tinted moisturizer is a worthy alternative to a foundation. Creams and lotions do not add moisture to the skin, nor do they retard aging, but they do help keep the drying process in check and thus prevent premature aging signs such as lines and a leathery appearance. Moisturizers work best when applied to a dampened skin – pure water sprays are the most effective.

## Flexible Treatments

Apart from cleansing – everyone's basic need – you have to work out your own individual skin-care regimen with a product acting when and how the skin requires it to retain a youthful appearance. Available now are products that perform specific tasks, and the previous ideas of just having a daytime moisturizer and a rich nourishing cream for night are being replaced by the more sophisticated approach of using them together with biologically active energizers which stimulate cell metabolism and give you a second chance to look younger.

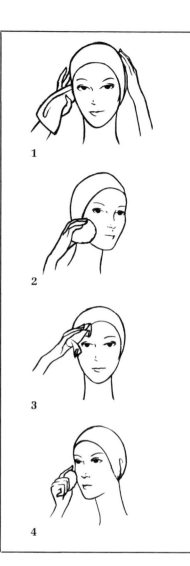

## The At-Home Facial

1. Smooth hair away from face and tie a band around the hairline for protection.
2. Remove make-up with soap or a cream cleanser, using small circular movements to massage the skin gently at the same time; this aids both circulation and muscular substructure.
3. Tissue or rinse off depending on the cleanser.
4. With cotton wool pad, apply a light freshener to remove last traces of the cleanser.
5. Dot a moisturizer all over the face and gently blend in.

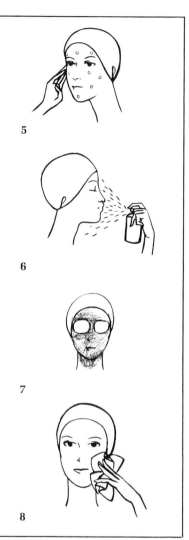

5

6

7

8

- **exfoliators** – recent research has revealed that in the battle against aging skin, it is very important to clear the surface of all dead cells and debris regularly, this not only gives the skin a brighter and clearer look, but also encourages new cell growth and activity. This is called exfoliation. It should be done every few days. There are several commercial 'scrubs' that are creams containing abrasive silicone grains, but it is also possible to get the same results by using ordinary fine salt. Dampen a face cloth, sprinkle with salt and very gently rub into the face. Rinse away with lukewarm water. Your skin will feel incredibly smooth. Afterwards always apply a moisturizer.
- **emollients**: these continue to have valid use as a way to lubricate dry skin. These are the classic night creams, newly modernized with such additions as collagen, hormones and proteins. Mature skin does require regular enrichments from such creams.
- **energizers**: this is the new word in skincare, a new concept too. Energizers are the result of today's scientific approach to beauty – and the technological advances in skincare products increase every year. There are now effective modern formulas geared for specific functions, but all to do with controlling signs of aging through encouraging increased cellular reproduction. Energizers usually come as fluids or oils and offer a kind of skin repair service. They are easy to use, quick to apply and supply very specific instructions as to quantities and regimen. It is up to you to go out and explore what is available for your particular needs. Meticulous care has gone into research and product development; energizers have been tested for performance and safety – and the implication by some sceptics that there can be no real results is quite wrong. Energizers carry on corrective work in the deeper cell structure of the epidermis and aid the earliest form of cell damage.

6. Spray on a film of pure spring water – or pat with clear water – though the finer layer achieved through spraying is preferable.

7. Apply masque all over the face and throat, leaving a free circle around the delicate eye area. Cover eyes with cottonwool pads soaked in milk or a non-alcoholic freshener. Relax, lying down for 10 to 20 minutes.

8. Remove masque with cottonwool pads soaked in lukewarm water. Splash on more water to remove all traces of the masque; finish by applying a thin film of moisturizer.

## Weekly Pick-up Facial

Giving yourself a facial is really very simple. It not only stimulates your face, but also forces you to relax for about twenty minutes. The point of a facial is to increase circulation and cleanse the skin thoroughly. Follow the step-by-step guide for your at-home facial. There are many commercial masques on the market, but here are some you can make yourself:

- **Brewer's yeast** – mix 1 teaspoon of powdered yeast in 2 teaspoons of warm water; adjust consistency so it spreads like paste.
- **The beaten white of an egg** – add $\frac{1}{4}$ teaspoon of lemon juice or cider vinegar.
- **An egg yolk** – mixed with a few drops of cider vinegar.
- **Honey** – 2 tablespoons with $\frac{1}{2}$ teaspoon of lemon juice or cider vinegar.

## Sun Awareness: The Most Vital Factor

When it comes to the relationship between skin and sun, doctors agree that if you don't want your skin to wrinkle, line and, to some degree, sag, then stay out of the sun – or protect your skin.

Sun damage is permanent because exposure to ultra violet rays starts a series of biochemical changes that doesn't stop even if you suddenly start to protect yourself. A tan is not a sign of health – it is nature's way of limiting the damage, and your body's defence mechanism. Rays penetrate the skin and cells to produce melanin, a brownish pigment which acts as a screen. But the ultra violet waves also release a chemical that affects the cell's normal metabolism. Apart from drying out the skin and all the subsequent aging effects, it is now certain that the sun can cause benign growths, premalignant tumours and two out of three skin cancers. It can also initiate herpes outbreaks. Most skin malignancies are curable, but they must be caught early. Look for loss of skin colouring, for a small pearly nodule or patch, for a change in colour or shape or a mole, for any small area that doesn't heal well.

Most women like to have some degree of a tan and it is impractical to think that everyone can be persuaded to stay out of the sun all the time. Also, it is ironic, that a touch of 'healthy' colour actually makes you look younger, more vital. One has to be sensible about it and get the balance just right. A very significant factor is skin colour. The darker your skin is naturally, the more easily and readily you can tan, and the less damage is caused. The key to protection is choosing the right sun screen and using it properly. Over recent years, the sun protection factor (SPF) has become a big issue. Previously suntan lotions were usually formulated to promote a tan, now it's the reverse. The SPF indicates the length of time required before the sun starts to harmfully burn you. For example, SPF 5 means that the result – tan or damage wise – would be the same after five hours under the sun with the screen as one hour without it. The SPF is a time indicator, a safety precaution but not an absolute protector.

A light tan is flattering, no doubt about it, and there's no need to panic over possible dangers. Like everything on the health and beauty level, obsessive concern is taking things too far. Remember sun exposure also has its benefits: it can clear up skin problems due to oiliness, it is relaxing and soporific, it is necessary for the assimilation of vitamin D and it does make you look and feel particularly good. A life without sun would be a sorry one, but there's no advantage to frying in it. The SPF numbers should be taken as a guide. They are worked out under static laboratory conditions and don't take into account the lessening of effect due to perspiration and water contact. The protective film can be broken in these ways, so it is best to re-apply lotion every few hours. Another point: don't think of sunscreens as isolated to sunbathing per se. Everyday outdoor jobs can cause cumulative damage even in temperate climates. If you garden a lot, for example, put a screen on your hands as well as your face; wear gloves, wear a hat. The same applies when participating in outdoor sports. And watch that winter sun – the reflection from snow can be as lethal as that from sand or water.

When selecting a sunscreen check the ingredients: the best are the para-aminobenzoic acids (PABA) and benzophenone derivatives. These should be clearly indicated on the labels. Unfortunately, the most effective sunscreens are often drying, so be sure to massage in a good amount of skin lotion afterwards.

*Linda Gray*
'I'm not one for half an hour in the bathroom with 900 splashes of Evian water, but I do take care of my skin. I have lots of laugh lines because I have a fabulous life. It's the frown lines people should worry about.'

## Daily Exercises to Save Your Face

Just like any other part of the body, the face can benefit from exercise and although it's bone structure that shapes your face, it is the network of tiny muscles that gives it expression. These can work for or against you – they can form frown and laughter lines, but they also can form a firm structure for the skin. If you run through this series of facial exercises each day, you'll help smooth out lines, stimulate circulation and tone up the essential muscles.

**1** Hold a book firmly under the chin, and against this pressure open the mouth wide, hold to the count of five, close. Repeat five times.

**2** Purse lips and at the same time fill cheeks with air, blowing them out as far as possible; then gently press the three middle fingers of each hand against the puffed-out surface, tap repeatedly to the count of ten, but don't let the air out. Repeat five times.

**3** Open mouth wide as if screaming, open eyes wide and staring at the same time; hold to the count of three. Repeat five times.

**4** Open mouth wide and fling head back, really stretching the neck and chin area; open and close mouth ten times.

**5** Stick your tongue out as far as possible, hold to the count of five; repeat five times.

**6** and **7** With lips together twist the mouth first to one side and then the other, swish it back and forth fifteen times.

**8** Finally allow yourself a big hearty grin, mouth a little open, relax; repeat five times.

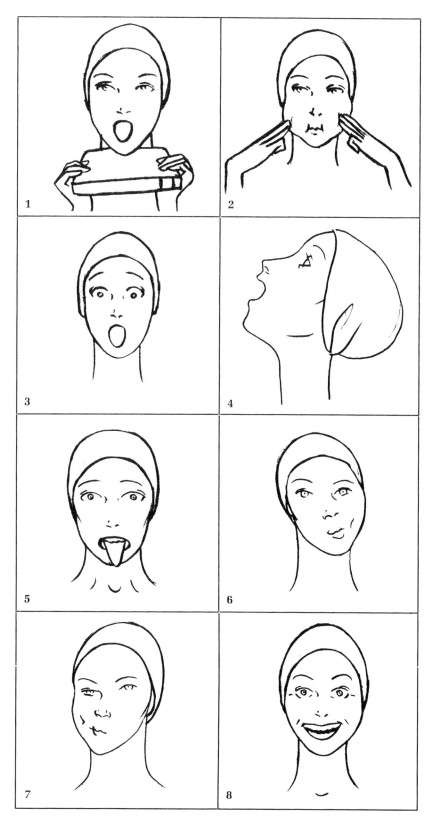

# Make-up

In your thirties you have to come to terms with your face. You know what looks good, what doesn't, the best colours, the way to shade and highlight. It is at this age that you can handle the most drama and exude glamour without looking or feeling overdone. However, as you ease into your forties, the cardinal rule is: less implies more. Make-up has to be toned down, but certainly not phased out. A mature face needs make-up, not necessarily to make it younger, but simply to liven it up.

There are two major mistakes that a mature woman frequently makes. Firstly, thinking that a lot of make-up will cover up give-away lines and impart an overall impression of a younger face. In fact, the opposite is true. Heavy make-up only exaggerates lines as it lodges in the crevices, and if you use too colourful a make-up you can end up looking rather clownish. This will only indicate a last attempt to look young – which in itself adds years. The second most common error is the tendency to stick with the same look and not move along with the times.

The use of colour is especially significant. Keep it all very neutral, stay away from too pinky foundations, from too definite eye colour, from rosy cheeks and brilliant lips. Any force of colour draws attention to defects. The art is in the blending – textures, tones, shadings, colours. Blending is mostly done with your fingertips, but for specifics it is more effective to apply make-up with brushes – it gives a softer look to eyes and lips in particular. By now you should be able to make up your face effectively in less than ten minutes even when you want to look quite special, and in even less time for a casual daytime look. Are you doing it right? Now is the time to check on your step-by-step make-up and to make note of the changes that will help an aging face.

- **Foundation** – use the sheerest coverage, a few dots all over the face blended in with damp fingers or a damp sponge. For a daytime make-up it is a good idea to substitute a foundation with a tinted moisturizer. Blend well into the hairline and over the neck and under chin area.
- **Erasing** – next step is to lighten up dark areas such as those under the eyes, and help ease away lines by blending in a light cover-up cream. This is heavier than a foundation but can easily be blended in with fingertips.
- **Fading** – correcting errors such as a wide nose or a heavy jaw by blending in a darker tint of your foundation. This has to be done terribly well so as not to be noticeable, and it is something you can get away with when you are young, but unless you are very skilful at it, camouflage attempts such as these are all too visible later on. Actually as you get older, physical faults are less important, simply because you are not so conscious of them. When one is young one wants to look perfect, but when one is older one wants to look younger, faults and all.

**Close-set** – concentrate shading at the outer corner, but work it in a crescent shape starting to fill out around the centre of the eye. Another check is to be sure of the widest possible division between eyebrows.

**Small** – work colour around the outer rims, beginning at the centre and swelling out in the corner. A great help is to add lashes to the outer corner – much more natural looking than doing obvious eye-liner extensions.

**Droopy** – a common problem as you get older, and if you use a subtle neutral colour an effective camouflage can be achieved by covering most of the lid, but with emphasis on the outer corner, where shadow should be winged upward to touch the brow line. It can also be helped by drawing a fake socket line with a crayon – a complete arc smudged.

**Puffy** – the best way to cope with this is to cover the lid entirely with a neutral colour and accentuate eyelashes as much as possible, either with several layers of mascara or an added false line on the top rim. Whatever you do, don't draw attention to the problem with strong shading.

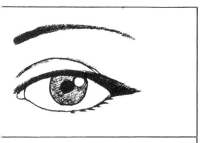

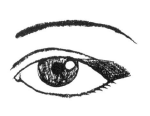

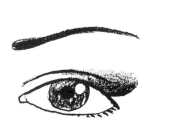

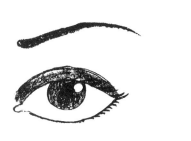

- **Cheek Colour** – don't overdo this, and stick with peach and tawny tones rather than the rosy and red ones. It often looks more natural if cheek colour is blended in as a cream, rather than applying later as a powder.
- **Powder** – use this only to stabilize make-up because too much powder can be very aging; do without it completely if you can as a shine on your face gives it a more youthful glow. If you powder, gently pat it on in many tiny circular motions using a fresh wad of cottonwool. Then take a big brush and flick downward over the face to remove excess.
- **Eye Colour** – forget obvious colour, stick to neutrals such as grey, taupe, brown and experiment with peach, gold and lilac as all these can be very effective. Colour has to be blended so well that it gradually fades away into the foundation and the standard rules of where to shade for eye emphasis and enhancement still apply (see illustrations), but you need to go softer on the colour and be more meticulous about blending than ever before. The best effects are achieved with a combination of thick crayons and powders. As for eyeliner, unless done with a crayon and smudged a little, the result is invariably too harsh; also use brown or grey pencils.
- **Eyelashes** – emphasized lashes really are effective and give a great boost to the mature face. If your lashes are still fairly full, use a lot of mascara on both top and bottom rims; if they are getting a bit sparse – which can happen – there's everything to be gained from adding false ones. Of course, don't have them too long or too thick. Apply mascara by starting with tips of lashes and working to the base for a natural feathery line. Brush upper lashes downwards from the top first, then brush up from below. Lower lashes up first, then down.
- **Eyebrows** – avoid harsh pencil lines and too dark a colour. Eyebrows ideally should be just a little darker than your hair. Define brows by brushing up, then across; check there are no straggly hairs; if you use a crayon be sure it is sharp and use in light tiny diagonal strokes. A natural looking alternative is to use a slanted eyebrow brush and apply powder colour.
- **Blusher** – peach and tawny shades are the best. Apply with discretion. Hollow-looking cheeks may have their appeal, but after a certain age the quality and shine of your skin is more important than the perfect undulations of your face. But if you want a touch of glamour, suck in cheeks and flick brush across the top of indent in upward strokes and blend into hairline.
- **Lips** – a possible danger area, because as those aging lines that radiate from the mouth begin to develop, it is necessary to keep track of 'bleeding' lipstick, because if anything is a sign of age, this is. It helps to powder the upper lip and the whole area around the mouth; another aid is first to outline the lips in crayon – a shade darker than lipstick colour. Lips also sometimes shrink with age, so to add fullness first use a white underbase. More accurate lines and a better look is achieved when lipstick is applied with a brush.

# Facial Checks

## Eyebrows
With age brows can get straggly and may require more definition and grooming. The brow should start at a point above the inside corner of the eye. Brush eyebrows into shape, up first then across. Pluck out stray hairs from underneath the brow lines, never from above. Apply a little lotion first, tweeze with a quick firm tug.

## Crepy Eyelids
Loose skin over the lids is aging and although it can be camouflaged to a degree with shadow, the only real solution is eyelid surgery (see page 201), a simple and very effective medical procedure.

## Superfluous Hair
Due to hormone changes, mature faces are inclined to become hairier, particularly on the upper lip and there's invariably the odd hair sprouting from the chin. It is not attractive at any age, so get rid of it all, preferably with electrolysis – the only permanent method of removal. Alternately, the single hairs can be plucked out as soon as they show, while the area above the lip can be regularly waxed. Caution: never pluck a hair from a mole; get professional attention or cut it off as close as possible to the surface.

## Firm Jawline
Exercise, massage and an ability to consciously remember to hold your head high are the three factors that help prevent a sagging jaw. Use long upward strokes to blend in a moisturizer or a richer emollient. Check out the particular neck exercises on page 47.

## Forehead Lines
These are almost inevitable and are caused as much by expression as by aging skin. Try to be aware of when you raise your eyebrows or crinkle up your forehead – and immediately correct it. Fingertip stroking in circular movements can help erase lines if done on a continual basis.

## Under-Eye Area
The skin is particularly delicate here and should be handled with care. There are special creams for around the eyes and they should always be gently patted on, never rubbed in. To help smooth lines temporarily, dab on a little white of an egg before applying foundation.

## Skin Condition
Its appearance has more to do with the amount of care you give it than your genes. Skin becomes drier and thinner as it ages, so the most important thing is liberal use of a moisturizer. The new fluid energizers offer a promising chance of skin repair and are more exciting in their function than regular night creams.

# Make-up Points

### Eyebrows

Beware of them looking too dark, too static, too painted on. A natural effect is achieved with a light brown or grey pencil and making lots of short and feathery strokes with a finely sharpened point. Sometimes just brushing with mascara or smearing with vaseline for gloss is more effective. As you get older it is often better to draw attention to the eyes and lashes, letting the brow be just a subtle frame.

### Eyes

What few women know or understand is that it is more youthful to emphasize the lashes rather than the lids. Bright shadows should be discarded for ever, as the very intensity of colour draws attention to lid imperfections such as crepiness. Soft natural tones plus peach, gold and lilac are effective. And remember that matching shadow to eye colour went out years ago. Use lots of dark mascara and extra eyelashes for futher fullness; in this way you can help detract from any lid heaviness or droop.

### Lips

Watch bleeding. As fine lines develop around the mouth, lipstick tends to travel along these little canals. It is only something that happens in your thirties and later and can give you a big black mark for looks immediately.

### Foundation and Powder

As light and sheer as possible, say the experts. Choose a liquid foundation that is quite oily and smooth it on with a damp sponge – or moist fingers. If your foundation is too heavy or too dry it only emphasizes lines and can give the face such a plastic look that it ages at once. As for powder, always use a translucent one, not a colour, and use sparingly – think of powder only as a means to keeping make-up under control, to prevent running of colour. A face with a certain amount of glow and shine is a young face.

### Blusher

Again as with all make-up – keep the colour low key. After your thirties ask yourself: do you really need that extra touch? Usually you don't, so go easy on cheek colouring and experiment with the creams that can be applied after the foundation as these blend in more easily, and frankly, you are not likely to get so carried away as you might be with a brush and powder.

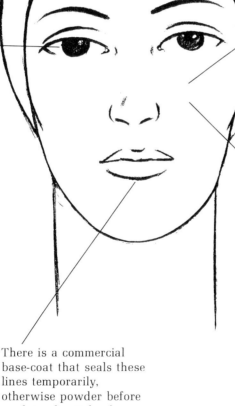

There is a commercial base-coat that seals these lines temporarily, otherwise powder before applying lipstick, also use a crayon for outlining and keep control of the lipstick itself by applying with a brush. Powder afterwards.

### Shading

Caution with contouring is the rule. In your youth you can get away with the shaded-in illusion of interesting hollows, but as you get older it looks too contrived, too desperate. What you can do is put on a darker foundation to soften the jawline, a lighter foundation to lift mouth and eye lines. The truth is you have to be very skilful to get away with it. An over made-up face usually looks an older face. A uniform skin colour often works best.

# Hair

At any age, one thing that is vital to your appearance and morale is the state of your hair. As you get older it becomes even more significant, because if your hair is working well it immediately attracts attention and can compensate for other shortcomings. Healthy hair is the first priority, before style, before colour. Two things you have to watch out for – dryness and hair loss. Dryness can be easily counteracted through sensible basic care, the use of conditioning treatments and controlled use of heat when styling. Hair loss goes on all the time and you can lose between forty and seventy hairs a day, but this is often accelerated during and after the menopause when the change in hormone balance affects the hair and scalp. The faster the menopause, the more obvious hair fall will be. With a longer menopause, the thinning will be more gradual and you probably won't notice it. There's no need to worry, because there is usually some reversal of hair loss, and with good care it can be kept in check.

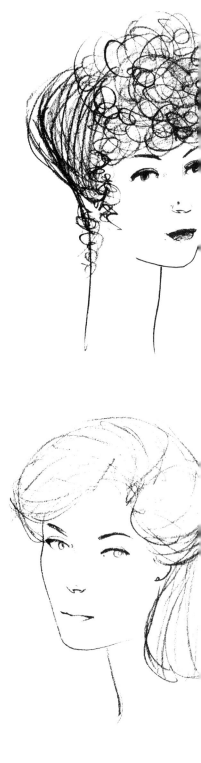

## Style

The big change in hair is that the old restrictions and traditions on age-related style are no more. Advice used to favour short hair after a certain age, but this was mostly because thinner hair was thought to look better this way. The point today is, that due to new awareness of basic care and conditioning, plus the superior products at hand, hair is much healthier and can look thick and lustrous almost indefinitely. Almost any style is possible at any age, providing it suits your personality and type of hair. I am not suggesting flowing tresses forever but it does mean that there are now many more options. Look over these sketches for some ideas; look in the latest magazines for others. Long hair can look very good and it is often easier to manage than that ubiquitous short frizz. There is no doubt that short, non-descript hair is aging. So are stiff coiffures. Long hair, however, when softly rolled up or simply braided can look effective without appearing overdone. Hair can be very glamorous. The rule is to make it look as natural as possible. Keep it easy and work out a style you can manage yourself. Simplicity is everything.

All the heated appliances are a boon for styling hair, but go easy on them. Dry hair becomes more of a problem, and overuse of electrical gadgets means more brittle strands and broken ends – and you will need a weekly deep conditioning treatment. Watch those blow dryers and electrical tongs; limit use of heated rollers. Other check areas: use combs with widely spaced teeth, brushes with widely spaced bristles; don't brush or comb too much. Treat hair very gently to preserve its health, its looks, its continued success. Moving hair is youthful hair, so give it the chance to swing, to fly around a bit but never in an unruly manner. Neatness is aging; unkemptness is aging. Find a way to strike the balance.

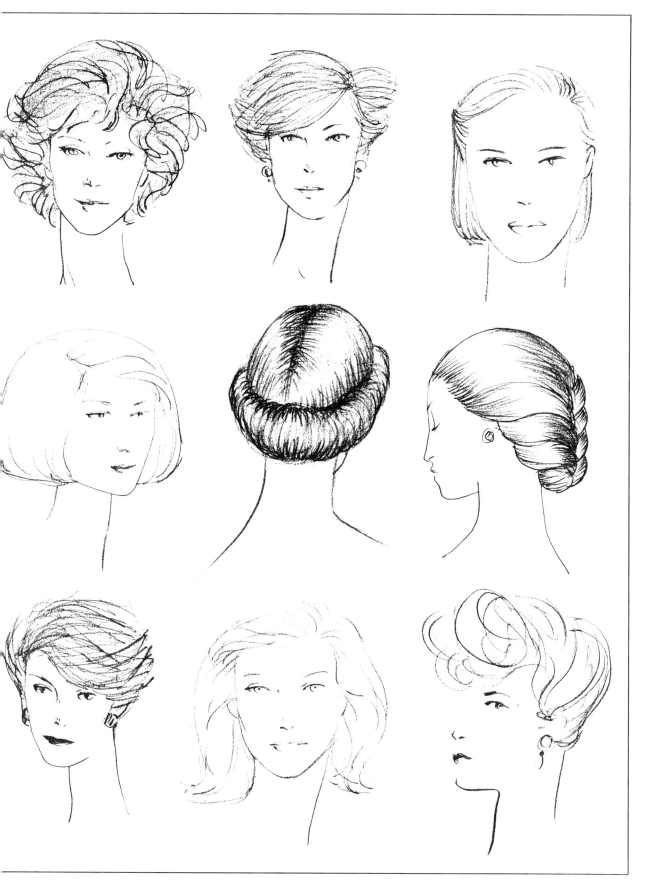

## Care

Hair must be kept clean, and because shampoos and conditioners are formulated for all types of hair, there is no harm in frequent washings, even if your hair is dry.

Brush hair gently before washing – this helps remove loose hairs; then massage scalp with smooth kneading motions – this encourages circulation and hair growth. Wet hair thoroughly with warm water making sure it is really drenched. Take a little shampoo and gently work into the hair – try not to rub hairs hard against each other. Most women use too much shampoo and get too assertive with the rubbing. Gently does it when it comes to hair. Rinse many times as any residue of soap will leave hair dull. Most older hair needs conditioning because of dryness and the use of chemical procedures. Commercial conditioners are massaged into the scalp, left on for a few minutes, then rinsed away. Sometimes the conditioner is incorporated in the shampoo.

## Colour

There is no average age when hair starts to lose its colour – there are grey heads in their twenties – but it is the first thing that changes with age; dryness comes later. There are only two ways to deal with it: wear it grey with great panache, or colour it. More and more women are opting for colour and the sophisticated formulas of today produce extremely natural results. The first thought is usually to recreate your natural colour, but the fact is that this is not always the best solution. Skin colour changes as one ages, and it is more flattering and more youthful looking to think about going lighter and softening the colour density. Bright reds, brassy blondes and jet blacks can age your face. The latest professional way of dealing with grey is to lighten the entire head so the grey blends in; highlighting, streaking and frosting are good camouflage tactics, so is adding streaks to the dark colour. On your own you have the choice of three colourings – temporary, semi-permanent and permanent.

Temporary rinses simply add colour to the hair shaft and are washed away at the next shampoo. They really don't work very well on grey hair, except to add a little colour; they cannot lighten.

Semi-permanent tints cannot lighten either, so again they are no good for softening dark hair, but they will give more cover to the grey; these tints will last through four to five shampoos. Finally the permanent colourings which do contain bleaches. Any colour change is possible as the colouring agent strips the hair shaft of colour and then adds the new one. Grey hairs can be completely changed. I think it is worth the investment to have this done professionally – after thirty-five you should be able to treat yourself to something. But if you want to try to do it yourself, check the label indications thoroughly for the colour effect on your particular shade of hair. You should also always do a trial patch test – the best area is behind the ear – twenty-four hours before complete use. Allergic reactions are rare, but it's a precaution that should be taken.

# HOW TO HELP YOURSELF TO HEALTH

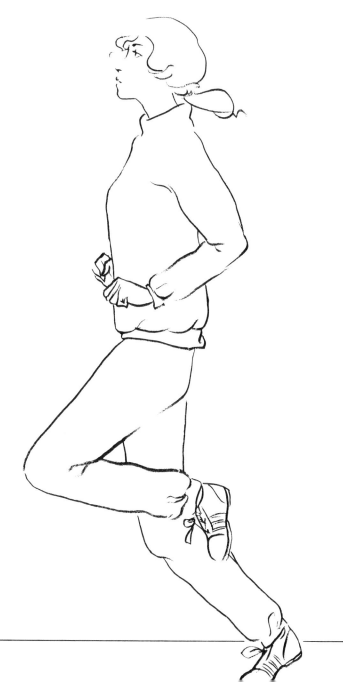

# BODY
## Know the risks of early aging

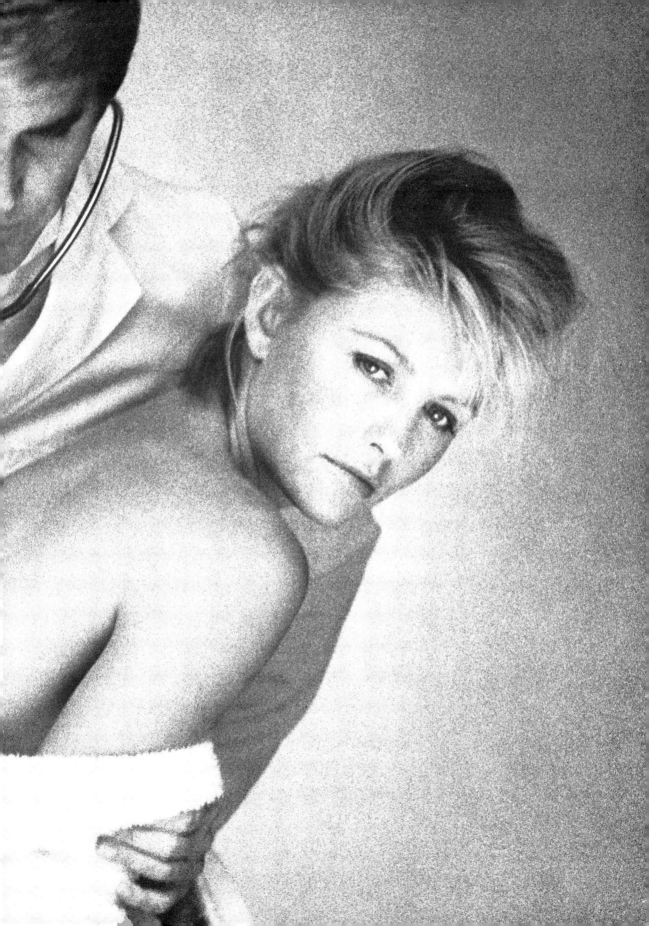

How long can you realistically live and to what degree of 'wellness'? There isn't any precise answer. Scientists are undertaking extensive studies to shed new light on the matter of life and death, but haven't come up with any startling discoveries. One thing is certain: our knowledge about the human body is expanding incredibly, but although researchers can now offer information on what chemical and metabolic reactions are performed in the body, they are rarely clear as to how and why – or more important, why not. It's the 'why-nots' that affect the aging process. We are finding out that the human mechanism is far more complicated than ever imagined, and related to this is the realization that the body has an amazing capacity to protect and heal itself. Outside interference is proving to be not necessarily the best thing.

Traditionally we are given a life span of three score and ten years, which is seventy. We are already going well over that and, after all, this ancient biblical estimate was at a time when hygiene was not so good and when virus infections could not be put under immediate control. Today, gerontologists are bold enough to say that we are programmed to live to around 110 or 120 years. There are several theories, but they fall into two main categories. The first is that the human body is genetically and biologically timed to die at a certain age, either due to the cessation of cell division or to the secretion of a 'final hormone' that puts the brakes on the endocrine system, thus diminishing all metabolic function to an ultimate end. The other belief is that we are designed to function indefinitely providing the style of life and environmental conditions are favourable. The reason why we don't go on 'ad infinitum' is because of biological and biochemical interferences that are brought into the body from the outside. There is a lot of reference to 'free radicals' – a name given to what can only be described as elements that are not bound into fixed chemical compounds but are at liberty to attach themselves to any available cellular matter in a destructive way. How to harness these 'free radicals' and keep them under control is not definitely established, though there are indications that a finely attuned vitamin and mineral balance is the answer. However, yet again science comes up against a problem: what is the ideal balance? We still don't know, but most likely nature does.

All these matters are being specifically explored in relation to aging, not only in the interests of prolonging life but also with the hope of getting a new perspective on the seemingly inevitable disorders of later life. What is emerging is fascinating, because although no magic formula has been found, evidence is building up to show that we are literally killing ourselves off by violating the basic rules of health and natural living. The degeneratory diseases are really diseases of our modern lifestyle and not of advanced years. When we are young we take good health for granted. But it is becoming increasingly evident that, even in our twenties, we may, by our lifestyle, be laying the foundations for the health problems that afflict us as we grow older. There is no pill to cure them, though there are aids to help them temporarily. The great hope of staying young actually lies within our own bodies and minds. If you develop a positive, health-orientated pattern of life and listen to your body when it sends out warning signals, you will get to the point of not only knowing what you have done wrong to give you symptoms of illness, but you'll instinctively know how to counterbalance it. For instance, once you start eating a healthy diet, the minute you have a heavy fried meal you can actually feel your body objecting and you will crave some fresh salad, raw vegetables or fruit. And once you get used to daily exercise, if you stop for only a few days you will feel sluggish and know that to bring back vitality you need fresh air in your lungs.

The real secret of living at a young level for as long as possible is simply to adjust your lifestyle so as to avoid the diseases that age you prematurely. In other words you have to: check you are eating right (see page 88), get enough exercise, avoid emotional stress, stop smoking, only consider chemical drugs in an emergency, don't allow yourself to be X-rayed unless absolutely necessary. (Many scientists are concerned about the possible damaging effects of radiation from X-rays.)

Assessing fitness: you may think you are fit enough to take on any kind of exercise, but as you grow older you have to be realistic about your capacity and not overdo it. If you gradually work up to a sensible level of fitness through the programme outlined on page 128 to page 135 then your body can cope, but if you are inspired to put your body through stiffer routines, then it is a good idea to take a fitness assessment test. Clinics in the private health sector have units that will measure heartbeat at rest, during exercise and at recovery; lung function is tested which reveals oxygen consumption, carbon dioxide production, cardiac and respiratory rates. All these things are measured during stationary running on a moving belt. Analysis indicates present fitness level and future potential. You are then given a programme to follow, which will get your body into better condition without the risk of over-taxing it. It is interesting to have a professional assessment of your fitness level, but if you consciously listen to your body and become aware of its capabilities, you will quickly be able to measure and plan activity to suit your metabolic rate.

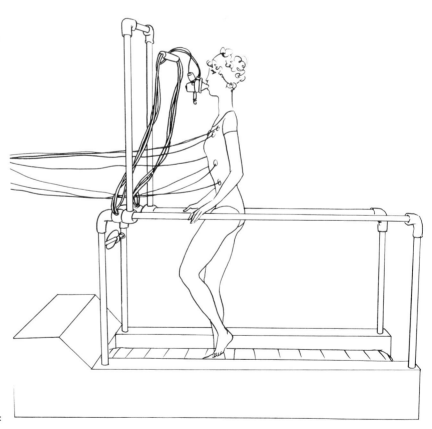

The fitness-assessment unit at BUPA.

Your health is your responsibility. No one cares about it as much as you and it is simply impractical to put it entirely in the hands of a doctor. There is no way a physician can wipe away years of misuse with a prescription. It is up to you to change your ways, and if you check on the common disorders of the thirties and upwards, you'll soon realize how you can go a long way to preventing them. If you want to keep young and active you need to know how to counteract the threats and to reduce the risks. It means believing in yourself and in body power; it means getting into contact with your body in an intelligent and knowledgeable way. Here are the most common ailments that can start as early as in your thirties.

## CIRCULATORY DISORDERS

Various diseases of the cardio-vascular system can become serious problems. In fact, heart disease is the killer epidemic of this modern age. It is the most common cause of death among men and although women are protected to a degree until after the menopause (due to the presence of female hormones) the mortality rate for women is now increasing, while related disorders are also becoming more prevalent. As the gap between the sexes narrows and there is more of an equal share of ambition, responsibility, habits and stress, the more equal is the chance of falling victim to heart disease. Why?

Over the years research has come up with definite risk patterns that have everything to do with lifestyle and personality – rather than sex or genes. The risk issues are: heavy smoking, high blood pressure, overweight and lack of exercise. On the dietary side, contributory factors are too much salt, too much saturated (animal) fat and too little dietary fibre. But what is emerging as the most significant aspect is the part played by emotional stress and general attitude to life. People who push themselves and are ambitious react adversely to any stressful situation with damaging, and sometimes fatal, effects on the circulatory system. More placid personalities cope with stress in a calmer, philosophical manner and therefore don't put undue strain on the body. However, there is no single factor that can be named responsible for heart disease – it could be any one, two or more or all. What is known though, is that those people who cut down on the risks, live longer.

**high blood pressure** – blood pressure is the force of the blood in the arteries together with a measure of the tension against the arterial wall. Two pressures are recorded – the output of the heart (systolic) and the resistance to flow by smaller arteries (diastolic); the former is written first, and is always greater. The latter, however, is the more important as this indicates the strain on the heart. Around 80 is normal, and anything over 100 needs immediate attention. An average healthy woman in her twenties or thirties would probably have a reading of 120:80.

A certain level is necessary for normal circulation and a higher one is required at times of physical or emotional demand. After exertion, however, the pressure should fall to normal. If blood

The heart is your body's main pumping station. It's about the size of a fist and weighs less than a pound ($\frac{1}{2}$kg). It is situated just to the left of the chest. It has four chambers, two for collecting blood and two for pumping – one of the pumping chambers sends blood through the pulmonary system (the lungs), the other supplies blood to the rest of the body. It is essential for the heart to get a constant and abundant supply of blood which comes through the arteries. The heart beats a two-fold sound, on the average seventy times a minute. With increased physical or emotional demand, the heart has to beat faster in order to supply more oxygen-rich blood to the necessary organs.

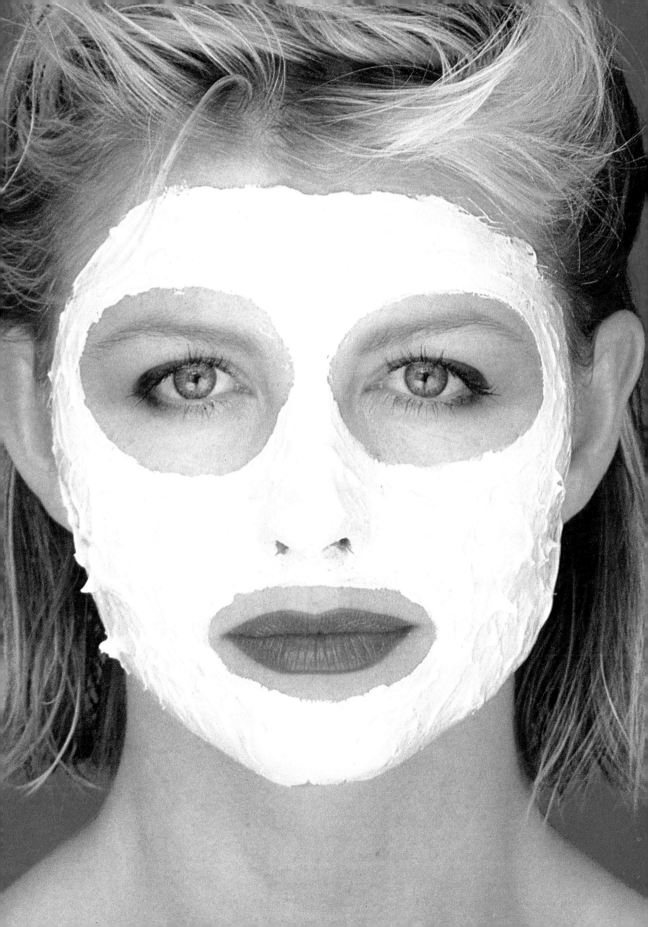

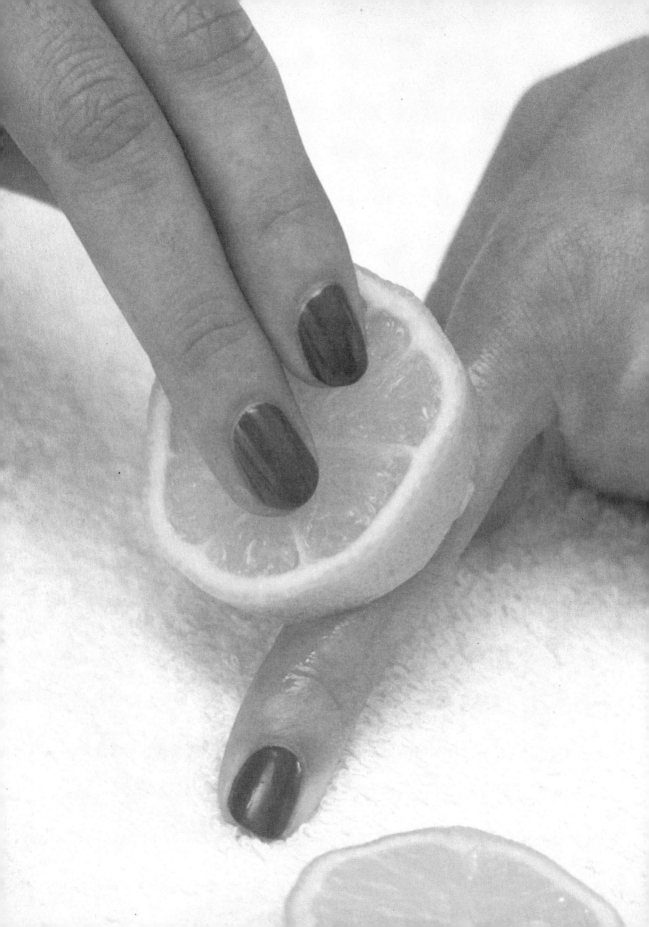

pressure is constantly high it overtaxes the heart, can lead to kidney damage and increases the risk of a heart attack or a stroke.

High blood pressure, also known as hypertension, is widespread but only a few women realize they are suffering from it, as in the early stages it produces no obvious symptoms. It also tends to affect women more than men, particularly during pregnancy and at the onset of menopause, when the physical and emotional stresses may be the reason as well as the reduction in oestrogen level. Blood pressure frequently increases with age, so it is important to have it regularly checked. Warning signs could be unnatural tiredness and shortness of breath.

Causes – apart from genetic factors – are now considered to be those bad lifetime habits of too much of the wrong food, smoking, overweight and stress. All are self-corrective. Natural therapists also treat high blood pressure by trying to find ways to remove tension. It can be reduced safely by any of the relaxation techniques (see page 168) used in psychological therapies. Biofeedback (see page 170) is particularly valuable as it has been shown that people can be trained to lower their own blood pressure and keep it down. Important also is to eat little salt and possibly take potassium supplements. Control of blood pressure levels on the orthodox level is not easy and the drugs that help often have unpleasant side effects, while the correct balance of drugs is only attained through many adjustments.

**coronary artery disease** – this is where cholesterol, a fatty substance in the blood precipitated by a diet too high in animal fats, is deposited on the walls of the arteries. The result is that the arteries become narrower and the flow of blood to the organs is greatly reduced, and could at one point be finally and fatally cut off. Again, the way to prevent this is to follow a low-fat diet (as outlined in the chapter on food), stop smoking and do some exercise.

**angina pectoris** – one of the unpleasant results of narrowed arteries, is that when the heart needs more blood for either physical or emotional needs, it cannot get an adequate supply quickly enough. When this happens a severe pain spreads across the chest like a tight band; it can also go up to the shoulders, sometimes down the left arm. If you rest or calm down for a few minutes it will stop, simply because the demand for extra blood has ceased. It often occurs after a meal, so many people mistake it for indigestion. It is actually an early warning sign that all is not well with the blood flow. The most practical way to help angina pectoris is to stick to a low-fat diet, calm down physically and emotionally – and if you're still smoking, stop it. Angina pectoris can cause heart failure.

**intermittent claudication** – cramp and pain in the calf muscles are also a sign of inadequate circulation due to blocking of the arteries. It can be very painful and only standing still or sitting will bring relief. It is much more prevalent in heavy smokers.

**coronary thrombosis** – this is when a blood clot forms inside the blood vessels. When the artery walls are smooth, this will not happen, but when they are uneven due to fatty deposits there's always a chance that a clot will form, cause an obstruction or be carried along to disrupt the blood supply at a vital point in a coronary artery. An agonizing pain is felt in the centre of the chest, sometimes spreading to the neck and left arm. It can happen in a flash, is not relieved by rest (as is angina pectoris) and is the true heart attack. A life can be saved with prompt action and extensive rehabilitation, but self care could have prevented a life reaching this point.

**varicose veins** – these develop because the veins of the legs are unable to return blood back efficiently to the heart against the force of gravity. Veins become dilated and prominent, the legs ache and feel heavy, they also tire very easily. The reason why the veins have trouble is either that the valves are not working properly and allow a back-flow of blood, or that the veins themselves have weak walls and little support from the surrounding tissue. What causes them? It has a lot to do with heredity, but also you are more likely to get them if you are overweight or standing a lot. Exercise is the great preventive, particularly walking, and the movement required from going up and down steps gives a push to the circulation. One good exercise is to lie on your back, lift the legs and do cycling in the air for five minutes. Varicose veins can be successfully treated; minor problems are eliminated by injection followed by the continuous wearing of bandages for about six weeks; more serious cases require an operation for the removal of the vein, but this involves only a brief hospital stay and within a few days you can walk fairly well – though bruising and swelling will take some time to go away.

## RESPIRATORY DISORDERS

The most prevalent are bronchitis, pneumonia and cancer of the lung. All of them are more common in smokers and city dwellers. Pneumonia develops when the body is not strong enough to counteract a cold-related virus, and if you have let your body power fall below par you are naturally more susceptible. Bronchitis is considered to be due to the combination of hereditary factors and environment. It flourishes in damp, cold climates; if you have had repeated colds as a child you are more vulnerable; smoking is lethal; air pollution in cities contributes greatly and so does any pollution contact at work. Avoiding the risk factors of climate, dwelling and work conditions is not always that easy, and you are hardly responsible for what happened in childhood. But there is no doubt that if you smoke the likelihood of either catching bronchitis or it becoming chronic is greatly increased. Also it is clear that lung cancer is a direct result of smoking. The good news – and this endorses the remarkable way in which the body can adjust and cure itself once left without outside irritants – is that even after years of heavy smoking, once you stop the risk of cancer is immediately diminished. Smokers may feel no benefit – if bronchitis is the problem – for months, but even chronic cases will improve with time. If you are lucky enough to have smoked without a trace of cancer, after several years of abstinence there is only a slight difference between you and a non-smoker as far as risk of cancer is concerned.

Orthodox medicine doesn't have a cure for bronchitis. Initially it was thought that antibiotics would do the trick, but finally it was realized that they only help a more serious infection. Natural therapists say that just as in a fever, the toxins should be allowed to come out of the body and the only path to take is to change the environment that causes the disease. A final point: watch your weight, because it has been shown that overweight people have problems expanding the lungs and thus trap irritants and infections.

## DIGESTIVE DISORDERS

It is not only the type of food that you eat but also your state of mind that influences the digestive system. Nerves affect all the digestive processes, so when you are agitated or upset, it is very likely that your stomach will suffer. The lining of the stomach can also be adversely affected by smoking, strong alcoholic drinks and some drugs. Digestive disorders range from constipation to cancer and include heartburn, ulcers, haemorrhoids, gallbladder problems and liver diseases. A lot are due to incorrect diet, particularly lack of fibre. Prevention starts right at the table, and bear in mind that many of the disorders get worse with constant use of pills and purges.

**constipation** – although doctors are not completely clear about the intricate workings of the bowel, it is generally agreed that constipation invariably stems from lack of fibre in the diet or dehydration caused by diarrhoea. All over-refined foods are absorbed in the first part of the intestines and yet it is very important that the bacteria in the lower end of the digestive tract get food to function, while the whole gut needs to be forced into action by pushing food through the entire intestinal channel. It is only the high fibre foods that do the complete journey. So check you are eating wholewheat bread, lots of vegetables and fruits. Muesli made from raw oats is still the best and far superior to the packaged bran cereals which usually contain phytic acid which is a mineral robber.

The answer to constipation is not a laxative, despite the fact that they are the most widely taken of all medicines. Laxatives work by stimulating the nerve endings in the bowel and this induces muscle contraction. If they are taken frequently, the nerve endings become less receptive and so even greater doses are required. It is a vicious cycle which can result in chronic diarrhoea – and that means dehydration and an upset in the delicate sodium-and-potassium balance vital to the proper functioning of major organs. Women use many more laxatives than men, and often this is related to dieting – a quick purge after eating too much. Continued laxative taking is potentially dangerous, as it can deprive any useful bacteria of nourishment to the extent that they may attack the bile acids and could produce carcinogenic substances.

What is perhaps the most basic point about constipation is that in itself it is not a high risk disorder. It is possible to continue for a week or more without emptying the bowels without dire consequences; it is just that most of us have been trained since childhood to think of it as a daily essential. Forcing the bowels to work through pills is potentially more hazardous than the constipation itself. The answer is simple: change your diet, possibly first cleansing out the intestines with a regimen of raw fruit and vegetables only.

**haemorrhoids** – these are often the result of constipation and the way in which it is treated with laxatives. They are often associated with other digestion disorders and obesity.

**gallstones** – middle-aged women are more prone to these than men of the same age group. If you are overweight the risk is higher and again it's most likely to be because of a diet high in refined carbohydrates – white flour, sugar and all its end products from cakes and pastries to sweets.

**ulcers** – it used to be men that suffered mostly from ulcers, but now that women are often under equal stress on account of work and emotional pressures, the gap is closing. They generally start between thirty and forty and it is the tense, nervous personality that is more prone. To avoid ulcers, the suggestion is try to take life more calmly, don't rush meals, cut down on spirits and smoking. Wholesome fresh food is recommended and herbalists say that helpful preventives are garlic, sage and nettle.

**diabetes** – this disorder can develop as you grow older and it is more prevalent in the overweight. It is the metabolic failure of the pancreas to utilize carbohydrates properly – the sugar is deposited in the urine and is thus lost. At risk are those with a diet high in refined carbohydrates and there is thought to be a psychosomatic element – blood sugar levels go up and down as emotions rise and fall. Correction of diet will help prevent and adjust diabetes that appears after forty-five – it is only when you are younger that there's the necessity for insulin.

Have you ever heard of air ions? You should know about them because they are now considered contributory to our general wellbeing. Most of the air we breathe is in the form of electrically neutral gas molecules, but a small number of molecules carry an electrical charge which is produced naturally by forces such as cosmic rays or ionizing radiation – only one molecule in every ten thousand million million carries a charge. Although this would seem insignificant – indeed that is the very reason why up to now any talk of the benefits of ionized air has been considered fringe medicine – it has now been shown that where negative ions are present, people tend to feel better in general and experience improved mental clarity. However, where they are absent – in the city air, heated buildings and cars – people are more listless, lack concentration, suffer breathing problems and get headaches more easily. Negative ions are more concentrated in mountain air and by the sea, both places long considered health recuperation areas. They are virtually non existent in polluted air. Ionized air, however, can now be reproduced artificially in a simple generator small enough to be placed in any room or on a desk. Research in office buildings has shown that there's all round improvement in physical and mental capacity when an ionizer is present. Why negative ions have such a positive effect is not clear, but they seem to stabilize cell metabolism and the central nervous system. If you can't get the natural ionized air, try the synthesized method.

# GYNAECOLOGICAL DISORDERS

As you grow older, periods often become heavier and more prolonged. It is important to keep a check on this and know that frequent floodings can lead to the risk of iron deficiency, anaemia and general tiredness. By the time you are in your late twenties or thirties, a regular menstrual pattern is established, so any change in it – heavy bleeding, intermittent spotting, different timing – should be reported to your doctor. After the menopause any bleeding from the vagina should be checked immediately.

A gynaecologist can find out a considerable amount from a physical examination of the abdomen, breasts, vagina and uterus. The uterus and ovaries can be felt when the doctor places one hand on the lower part of the abdomen and inserts one or two fingers of the other hand in the vagina. The neck of the womb and the walls of the vagina are examined by inserting a speculum and literally looking inside.

Unusual bleeding may be due to a simple polyp, which can be corrected with a 'D and C' operation (dilation and curettage) which is a scraping of the lining of the womb. Most causes of abnormal bleeding around the menopause or after can be corrected with this procedure. It is often used to take out cells for diagnosis, but in itself can be curative.

A 'D and C' operation is done under general anaesthetic and usually requires a night's hospital stay, but the actual procedure is very quick and can be done in a matter of minutes. The cervix is dilated and the lining of the womb removed in small strips. If any polyps are found, they are removed. Cells of the extracted matter are always sent to pathology for examination. After a 'D and C' there is a slight ache in the lower abdomen, which quickly passes and can hardly be called pain. There is usually slight bleeding for a few days and the first period afterwards may be heavy.

**fibroids** – these are swellings in the wall of the womb and are rather like muscles because they are firm. Most women have some, and if they are small it makes little or no difference to genital health. However, if they get bigger and thus provide a larger area to the womb, they can cause heavy periods. Other symptoms are a heavy feeling in the lower abdomen or pelvis area, or a sensation of pressure on the bladder or rectum. The only treatment for fibroids is surgery, usually a 'D and C', but if they are really enlarged, an hysterectomy is necessary. Fibroids, however, do usually reduce in size after the menopause.

**prolapse** – occurs when the pelvis muscular structure is weakened and because of lack of support, the uterus literally drops; it descends into the vaginal cavity and if serious can protrude from the vaginal entrance. Any degree of prolapse can only become worse over the years, especially if the level of oestrogen drops. It has to be checked as soon as possible. Early symptoms are a dragging feeling in the lower abdomen, an impression that there's some sort of lump in the vagina and lower back pain. A prolapse can also cause urinary problems – difficulty in emptying the bladder, signs of incontinence such as slight leaking of urine while laughing or sneezing, for example. If caught in its very early stages, a prolapse can be corrected by a regimen of exercises to strengthen the pelvic muscles. This only works if exercises are done efficiently and regularly. There is also a non-surgical method that has proven to be successful in many cases. It doesn't cure the prolapse but it does relieve the symptoms and to a certain degree helps prevent a worsening of the situation. A supporting ring pessary is fitted at the top of the vagina; this holds the uterus in a normal, or near normal, position. No anaesthetic is required. The ring has to be changed after a few months because it can become hard and dirty and cause infection.

It may be necessary to have an operation, which is actually only a repair job, because the only ultimate solution is an hysterectomy. The operation removes excess lining from the vagina and tightens up ligaments and muscles. It is done through the vagina, therefore there is no external scar. It does alter the size and shape of the vagina and it is important to discuss with the surgeon to what extent. It is easier to reconstruct a short vagina, but this can make sexual intercourse very tricky afterwards. If you have an active sex life, let the surgeon know, so that he can tighten the vagina and keep shortening to a minimum. The operation usually helps incontinence.

**hysterectomy** – this is a major operation and should never be undertaken lightly. It is the surgical removal of the uterus and sometimes the ovaries and fallopian tubes. Some years ago, particularly in the States, it was performed for no good reason; it was a sort of medical fad, and considered a preventive method against cancer. Today, surgeons are more conservative, having realized that the removal of any part of the body connected with sexuality can have a profound effect on a woman's life. Nevertheless, many gynaecologists are thoughtless and are more concerned with the mechanics of the operation rather than the emotional aspect. Women are timid about enquiring about the sexual implications, and even if they do ask questions, most doctors are reluctant to discuss it. Women are now demanding answers, so the situation is improving. An hysterectomy is an irrevocable step. After it you are sterile. If the ovaries are removed as well, you immediately go into the menopause and will need hormone replacement therapy (see page 160) to help you gradually to rebalance your endocrine system. Studies reveal that women are more prone to depression after an hysterectomy and there are psychological problems due to loss of fertility. Sex life and libido can be the same, and in some cases can be improved if constant bleeding was hampering sexual intimacy, but many women have reported that orgasm is not so intense even though the vagina remains fully functional. The reasons for having an hysterectomy have to be medically valid; these are: to remove cancer in the vagina, cervix, uterus, fallopian tubes and ovaries, to treat chronic pelvic infection, to stop uncontrollable haemorrhage and sometimes for severe disorders of the intestines or the bladder; it is also the only way to cope with large or multiple fibroid tumours, although these are not malignant. Doctors try to avoid removing the ovaries because of their vital hormonal role. If only the uterus is removed, although periods cease, the ovaries continue to function producing hormones in cycles so that symptoms of the menopause do not occur until they would naturally. An hysterectomy is done through the vagina, which leaves no scar, but if the uterus is enlarged it is removed through an abdominal incision. It takes several weeks to heal and intercourse should be avoided for about four weeks.

## ARTHRITIC DISORDERS

This is considered a wear and tear malady and not much progress has been made by medical authorities either for prevention or cure. It affects millions of people young and old alike. The side effects of drugs given for arthritis are sometimes worse than the disorder itself. Naturopaths, however, take the view that it can be prevented to a great degree by sticking to a simple fresh diet low in fats and avoiding meats. They also think that toxic drinks such as tea and coffee should be replaced by herbal beverages. Then there are the hydro and mud treatments available at many European clinics, which act on both the preventive and curative level. If you take regular exercise, you'll stand less risk of stiffening up in later years. Yoga (see page 138) is particularly valuable and can be done at any age. And have you heard of the copper protection? This is the wearing of an item of copper next to the skin – a bracelet, a strap lining, a necklace. Thousands of people swear by them, and it has definitely been shown to help counteract arthritic problems, but whether it works on a protective basis is hard to determine. Its use originated in South Africa, where it was discovered that the tribesmen who wore copper (at times in considerable amounts) were free from aches and pains. How did it work? Research revealed that arthritic sufferers had a copper deficiency and that indeed this essential trace element can penetrate the skin. It's an easy enough insurance anyway.

Arthritis affects more people than any other chronic ailment. The causes remain unknown and orthodox treatment is never completely successful. Drugs deal with symptoms, not the cause of the trouble, and many drugs have serious side effects. New hope comes in the form of vitamin C – daily megadoses from half a gramme to ten grammes taken in two sessions. Such an amount may not meet with the approval of the average doctor, though excess is not harmful as it is eliminated through the kidneys. Check with your doctor or consult a nutritional therapist before embarking on megavitamin C treatment.

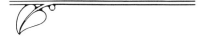

## CANCER

The most common cancers in women are those of the breast, the cervix and uterus, but it is the breast cancer that is not only the big fear but the big killer. Fear is so strong that most women take, on the average, six months to pluck up courage to go and consult a doctor about a lump. The attitude is that if you do nothing about it, it will miraculously go away. Unfortunately it won't, but not every lump is cancerous, in fact few are. Nevertheless, the bad news remains that it affects one in every seventeen women at some time in their lives, and one in thirty will eventually die of it. It is the leading cause of death for women between thirty-five and forty-five. There is proof that cancers detected early have a far better chance of being successfully treated. In the fight against cancer every woman should check the following:

- know your risk factors
- self examine your breasts every month
- have regular screening and cervical smears
- find out about the various types of treatment


### Risk Factors

The causes of cancer remain undiscovered, but evidence is mounting to reveal certain risk factors – race heredity, diet, environment and stress, plus the belief that there are certain cancer-prone personalities. The following are now considered the ones for breast cancer:

**age** – if you are over thirty-five, but the highest risk is over fifty.

**past history** – if you've already had cancer in one breast or in a hormone-related area such as the cervix, uterus or ovaries; also a previous benign condition of the breast.

**cancer in the family** – highest risk is if your sister has had breast cancer, slightly lower if your mother did. Other female relatives can be an influence, but the most significant factor is the age at which they contracted it. If late in life, then there's minimum risk, if prior to the menopause the risk increases, while if before thirty it is even higher.

**race** – if you are white the risk is highest, Latins have a lower incidence of cancer, while black women have even less.

**fertility** – highest risk is if you have no children, have never been pregnant or had your first child over the age of thirty-five. It is agreed that the more children you have, the less likelihood of cancer, but this is thought to be related to breast feeding. Another factor is menstruation – if you started early, or at the other end of the scale, if you had a late menopause then the risk factor is greater.

**diet** – naturopaths cite diet as the main culprit and even orthodoxy says there is a connection with breast cancer and a diet high in animal protein and dairy produce. There's also more of a risk if you are overweight.

**environment** – women in industrial cities run a higher risk, medium sized cleaner cities are next, but of course country living is best.

**personality** – women who hold in their emotions are now thought to be more cancer prone; tense personalities who bottle up anger and yet blame others for their frustrations are cited along with those who are overdependent on others and find little outlet for self expression.

## Self Examination of the breasts

Early detection starts with you and your discipline to give yourself a monthly check. It is very simple and once you get used to the feel of your own breasts you'll soon be able to spot any changes. At first, they may appear to be all lumps as it's the very nature of breast tissue to have many inundations. Follow the guide here and as soon as you feel or even sense a slight change, don't wait, but go to have it medically checked out.

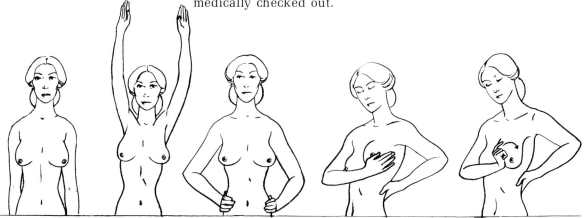

First do a visual check, get to know your breast shape and individual characteristics – the more thoroughly you do this, the easier it is to spot deviations early on. Stretch arms above the head, and observe how breasts fall in this position. Place hands on hips, check contours. Lie down and feel each breast in turn, starting at the nipple and working outwards in finger-traced circles. Still lying down, with flattened fingers feel the area at the sides of the breast and well into the armpit. It is only after many self-examinations and exploration that you actually be in touch with your breast structure and able to detect changes. Check for lumps – even the tiniest one should be looked at medically – check for any new prominence of veins, for puckering of the skin, for discharge from the nipples, for enlarged lymph glands at the side of the breast and under the armpit, for any moles or blemishes that seem to be changing shape or colour. Breasts should be examined once a month, and the best time is just after your period has finished.

### Breast Screening

It is prudent to have a manual breast check-up every year, but if you fall into the high risk groups it is recommended that at thirty-five you have a special technical screening; these are only done in certain hospitals or at women's clinics in the private sector. There are three methods: mammography, thermography and ultra sound. Mammography is the most efficient; it produces an X-ray of internal breast structures which reveals increased densities and calcification of tissue; these are signs of possible cancer. However, because of radiation exposure – though it is a minimum – the frequency of mammography should be limited unless the doctor particularly indicates otherwise. Thermography is a way to pick up any 'hot' spots through infra-red scanning; it is not as reliable as mammography. Ultra-sound provides pictures similar to X-rays through measuring the echoes of sound waves which vary according to the density of the tissue.

### Cervical Smears

Cancer of the cervix, or neck of the uterus, is responsible for five per cent of all cancer deaths in women and a quarter are in women under fifty. Yet if it is detected in time, the methods of treatment are swift and successful. This is because it has a feature that differentiates it from other cancers – a pre-period when it grows but doesn't spread widely or invade other tissues. This is called being 'in situ' and if caught at this point, it can be cured completely by surgery, heat or laser treatment. Detection method is through the cervical smear (the Pap test) which involves scraping cells with a spatula during an examination. It is quite painless. Cancer of the cervix is more prevalent in younger women, so if you haven't had a test by thirty-five start now and continue at two or three yearly intervals until you are sixty. However, if you have had genital herpes, you need annual check-ups.

### Treatments

There is considerable controversy at the moment about the effectiveness of the traditional orthodox treatments for cancer and some of the optional methods. No-one dares use the word 'cure'. However, it is worthwhile to explore the many avenues and not just accept the usual route of surgery, radiotherapy and chemotherapy which are the established methods. Opinion is mounting that neither surgery nor radiation influence the final effect of the disease, in fact there are some people who think they might actually accelerate it. Then in breast cancer, many surgeons are now skeptical over the advantages of a mastectomy (complete removal of the breast) to simply removing the tumour. Cutting out cancer doesn't necessarily mean cutting out the disease. The new idea is that something in the body's central homeostatic mechanism is out of control and it becomes incapable of stopping the invasion of unwanted tissues. Chemotherapy is another choice, based on the idea that drugs could attack cells throughout the body. Unfortunately the side effects of these

A recent development in help for cancer is Visualization therapy developed in America by Carl Simonton, a doctor practising radiotherapy. The idea is that the patient develops a mental picture of how the disease looks in the body and then visualizes how the malignant cells can be destroyed. In regular sessions, a patient first practises relaxation and deep breathing, then moves on to visualization. This mind over matter therapy is used in conjunction with standard cancer treatment, and there have been some amazing results.

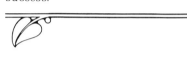

drugs can be so terrible, that many patients prefer to die.

The public is desperately trying other avenues, all of which are outside the realm of orthodoxy and therefore medically dismissed, it would seem, on principle. Yet one constantly reads of individual successes. All optional therapies take the attitude that it is a failure of the vital force that causes cancer, and this can be stimulated by physical, psychological or psychic means to check the spread of cancer and possibly reverse it. How else can one account for 'miracle' cures?

Check the sources for optional therapies (see pages 7–9 for helpful references) and talk to a practitioner. The naturopath says that anyone who follows a healthy diet and lifestyle will rarely get cancer. Others offer special curative diets, megavitamin therapy or enzyme injections. What is building up to a remarkable degree is evidence that cancer is a disorder of the psychosomatic-stress syndrome and should be treated accordingly. Mind over cancer does get results, particularly when Visualization therapy is employed. All offer a message of hope.

## EYES

Most people with normal eyesight will find increasing difficulty in reading small print at the normal distance of ten to twelve inches with age. This is called presbyopia and is considered normal, though naturopaths say a proper healthy diet and special eye-training (see below) can improve eyesight so long as it is failing from age only.

The reason why the eyesight weakens is that the lens within the eye becomes less flexible as the ciliary muscle loses its power to shape the lens to focus on the retina such small shapes as print. The usual practice is to wear glasses with a weak magnifying lens for close work and reading only. The eyes continue to change so a check-up every few years is recommended. If you are slightly short-sighted, you will find your eyesight gets better. Unfortunately, two pairs of glasses are finally required, or bifocals. Is this inevitable?

The theory that vision defects are irreversible because of the deterioration of the eye's lens was challenged more than sixty years ago. An American eye physician, Dr William H. Bates brought a whole new dimension to eye treatment and cured thousands of cases. His system had remarkable results, but it was never taken up by the profession as a whole, although individuals who have followed his methods strongly vouch for it. Any woman who finds her eyesight going should look into it (association reference on page 8) because most of us who wish to feel and appear younger would agree that glasses for reading are a clear sign of aging. Bates argued that eye muscles like any other muscles can be trained. You first learn how to relax them, then you find the way back to automatic responses naturally and gradually. It is preferable to be taught by a qualified Bates practitioner so the first few sessions are long and intensive, then less frequent. You also need time to benefit

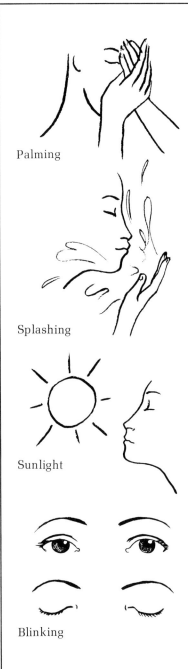

Palming

Splashing

Sunlight

Blinking

from this eye-training technique, but it has an impressive record in short-sightedness due to age, and vision that becomes blurred either near or far. It's a great preventive measure, so here are some steps you can take on your own.

**Palming:** Eyes can be helped by simply relaxing them. Close eyes, but because light can penetrate the lids, it is important to cover the eyes with the palm of the hand, fingers overlapping on the forehead and putting pressure there instead of on the eyeball. Relax for five to ten minutes, two or three times a day.

**Splashing:** Each morning splash your closed eyes with warm water twenty times, then cold water for twenty times. Do the same before going to bed, but first with cold, then with warm.

**Sunlight:** Sunlight is necessary, but this does not mean looking into the sun nor staying in it for a long time. Close eyes and allow the sun to warm the lids for a few minutes, moving the head from side to side. Afterwards, palm the hands over the eyes to shut out the light for a moment. Repeat two or three times a day.

**Blinking:** The normal eye blinks gently and frequently, yet one with defective vision not so much. Force the eyes to blink, particularly when reading, every ten seconds. It trains them to do it automatically and the exercise itself can often clear vision, if only for a moment.

**Swinging:** The eye usually remains fixed on a point for a fraction of a second, if it stays longer the eye is strained and vision impaired. To make the eye dart from one point to another, Bates devised a body swing that forces the eye to continually look at something different. The rhythm of the movement is gradually transmitted to the nerves that control the eye muscles. If done for long enough the eye automatically takes up the pattern. To swing, stand with feet a little apart, turning on the left foot to move the body to the right, then swing to the left side using the right foot as a pivot. The head and shoulders should be aligned, only the torso moves. Be careful not to watch anything in particular. The stationary objects around you will appear to move. Swing for five minutes.

## Eye Disease

When eye diseases begin to develop it is often so inconspicuously that you are not conscious of symptoms until it is almost too late for a possible cure. It is sensible to have eyes tested every two years after the age of forty. The disease that needs to be specially screened for is glaucoma as this affects about one person in a hundred over that age and must be caught early for the most effective treatment. Glaucoma can be hereditary, so if you have any relative with it, you are at particular risk and should have tests done at regular intervals. Glaucoma is a disease that gradually increases tension of fluid within the eye. Symptoms are not that easy to recognize – one is inclined to notice just that vision is more blurred after reading or lights have halos around them; there may be pain around the eye and they can be more bloodshot than usual. You can finally lose your sight.

Sun glasses: good or bad for the eyes? As protectors, they are not necessary as the pupil regulates the amount of light entering the eye by contracting in bright light and dilating when it's dull. You don't damage eyes in bright sunlight, but you can put unnecessary strain on them. However, to wear dark glasses constantly even during continual sunshine is not a good idea as your eyes are denied the opportunity to adjust from dark to light, which is now thought to be an important nerve and muscle process that helps exercise the eye and preserve eyesight. It is interesting to note that in sunnier climates, fewer people need glasses and it's not simply because there are few pale eyes. The type of sun glass is important. There are many tints, but the best choices are brown, sage-green, khaki and grey. Stay away from the blue, rosy and orange shades. Also watch out for the cheaper plastic variety; check for lenses as well as looks because certain types can cause distortion and disturb vision particularly when going up and down steps. Glass lenses are superior; they are individually ground. Polarized glasses cut down on glare, so are good for sports. Photochromatic lenses are sun sensitive and their depth of colour adjusts to the surrounding light – darkening in bright light, lightening in dim.

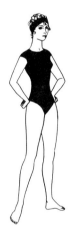

Swinging

If you consider glasses aging or unflattering – though they often look very good – there's always the alternative of contact lenses. The soft lens was first introduced in the 1950s and now has become so refined that almost everyone can wear them. They have a plus over glasses in that they provide a constant quality of vision. They must be fitted well and it is essential to go to a reputable specialist preferably recommended by your doctor. You will be shown how to put them in, take them out and the method of care. There are usually initial difficulties – either in the art of use or some sensitivity – but these are quickly overcome. There are choices of lenses: the first lenses were hard and many people still prefer them as they give a sharper vision than the soft lens; they can be repolished if surfaces are scratched and they can last for twelve years, sometimes longer. However, the hard lens is more difficult to adjust to and it can take up to a month before you are used to them. Soft lenses, on the other hand, are much more comfortable and it only takes a matter of minutes for eyes to adjust; they are also preferable in dusty and polluted environments. They wear out quicker than the hard lenses, lasting about eighteen months; they require special cleansing with chemicals which sometimes give an allergic reaction. There are also extended wear lenses which can stay in for one to three months, after which they are professionally cleaned; protein build-up on the lenses can be a problem and cause an infection – you need to watch out for any signs of redness, soreness or distorted vision.

It is not necessary to use a hard brush, in fact the flexibility of the softer bristles are invariably more effective. Place the brush against the outside surface of the teeth at an angle of 45°. Move it back and forth with short strokes, manipulating bristles so they splay along the gum line. Brush all outside areas. Now brush top teeth both inside and out from the gum downwards, then bottom teeth from gum line upwards. Finally use the dental floss – the new essential. Take about 45cm (18 inches) and wrapping the ends around one finger of each hand, coax the floss between the teeth with a slow sawing motion. Slide it a little way into the gum crevice and pull it back and forth. At first gums may bleed a little, but as they get healthier this will stop. Take floss between each tooth – it does take a little time but it's the only way to clean teeth thoroughly and prevent gum disease.

## TEETH

The way your teeth look makes a remarkable difference as to how old you look. Whatever you did in childhood is one thing, but neglect in adulthood can lead to the unnecessary loss of teeth because this is the time when a really disastrous condition can begin to cause tooth loss. The gums begin to recede and a space develops between the tooth and the gum. This leads to loss of teeth, as they can literally wobble and fall out, but more important – and more damaging – is that it also undermines the supporting bone. This is what causes that 'sunk-in' look that immediately stamps you as old. It can be completely avoided by thorough daily care and by going to the dentist for professional hygienic cleaning every six months. Even though teeth don't decay much after teenage years, eating over-refined sugar foods can continue to cause cavities. Everyone is at risk who doesn't take enough care.

The self-help answer is to spend more time cleaning the teeth. The quick brush, however regular, is simply not enough. Gum trouble is primarily caused by plaque, a substance that obstinately sticks on to the teeth and is a combination of food particles, micro-organisms, enzymes and saliva. It usually collects between the teeth at gum level. It is essential to use dental floss as well as a brush twice a day. Here's how:

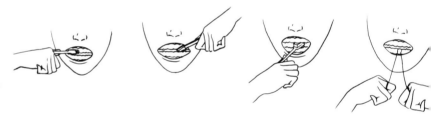

## HEARING

Hearing does deteriorate with age, and, by eighty, one in two people have a moderate to severe hearing problem. However, any problems up to sixty usually have to do with infections or a hereditary condition. Arthritis can be the cause at any time. Keeping your hearing at full capacity has a lot to do with the level of noise in your daily life. Recent studies have shown that if either your work or social conditions are at a continual pitch and intensity of sound you are at greater risk of impairing hearing. People who live in quiet country areas retain a sharp sense of hearing. Other than that there doesn't seem to be any other indications of how to prevent it. However, the less you interfere with your ears, the healthier they remain. They clean themselves and reject dirt and irritants. You may get a pile-up of wax and need periodic syringing by a doctor. Don't poke around on your own, as in this way you will push the wax further in and may actually puncture the eardrum.

## THE ENTIRE BODY

### The question of youth treatments

Is there such a thing as general rejuvenation? A medical therapy, that is, and not through a personal adjustment of lifestyle and habits? The medical community says absolutely not, and yet two treatments have been going on for some time and with considerable success: Professor Paul Niehans' cellular therapy and Professor Ana Aslan's procaine stimulation. Orthodoxy says there is no sound proof that either of them work to any degree, and that it is waiting for properly compiled scientific data. Yet there are thousands of patients who are living proof and there are detailed case histories giving before and after statistics on both metabolic and physical levels. I personally have met many enthusiastic recipients of both treatments, who claim they have a new lease on life. I have also met both Niehans and Aslan and their dedication to and belief in their work was obvious, their power of presentation persuasive and impressive. Neither treatment is going to miraculously turn back the clock, but both stress the fact that you will feel and look younger, you'll have more energy, more stamina to live a vital life and your entire metabolism will be given new impetus. Any treatment that provides benefit is surely valid, no matter how it is achieved and providing no harm is done. And even orthodox medicine can't always claim that.

### Cellular Therapy

It was in 1931 when Professor Paul Niehans of Switzerland startled the world with his claims that he could restore youth and vitality, boost glands and organs into renewed activity and help the memory. People rushed to Montreux, some in secret, including many famous personalities. Niehans died in 1971 (at the commendable age of eighty-nine) but his clinic of La Prairie still flourishes.

All his life Niehans had a bad time from the medical hierarchy, though early in his career – when he was on their side – he was considered a leading authority in endocrinology. It was through his work in this field that an accident led him to formulate his cellular therapy theories. A patient was dying of a parathyroid condition and there was no time for a gland implant, so on impulse he chopped up the parathyroid gland of an ox, suspended it in saline solution and injected it into the buttocks. The patient survived, tolerated the intrusion and lived for a quarter of a century in perfect health. From this incident Niehans reasoned that the body could probably benefit in many ways from animal cells. He decided to use embryonic cells because of their fast reproductive power and because the injection of animal parathyroid had healed the human parathyroid, he logically based treatment on the old medical principle of like heals like. He believed that the youth and strength of the body depended upon the vitality of the cell; in other words if you could bring the cell up to its optimum metabolic capacity, then the body would function

---

Has your doctor ever checked how your thyroid is functioning? Probably not, yet it can be responsible for many common problems – general fatigue, weight gain, menstrual and menopausal problems, skin disorders, headaches and a tendency to colds and infection. In fact, no organ system in the body escapes the effects of a thyroid excess or deficiency. The thyroid is the thermostat of the body – it regulates metabolic rate, the speed at which cells throughout the body use calories. Many diseases which are considered inevitable because the body is 'slowing-down' may be due to a mild form of hypothyroidism (low thyroid) and can be easily therapeutically corrected. So don't let your doctor overlook this important check – thyroid activity can be determined by measuring the quantity of the hormone in the blood and by temperature observation.

at optimum level too. Fresh cells are sometimes used, and these come from the foetus of a lamb. Niehans preferred to use them as fresh as possible, literally minutes after extraction. Today treatment can be with dried cells in solution or injections of the essential ribonucleic acids (RNA) which are now thought to be the stimulating elements.

Patients are first examined and clinically analysed by special tests to see what organs or glands are not functioning properly. The appropriate cellular matter is prepared – for example liver cells for an ailing liver – and then injected into the buttocks. Treatment may involve a dozen or more different cells and injections. Treatment lasts two or three days, but the stay at the clinic is usually a minimum of a week. A follow-up diet is prescribed, a list of rules given – such as no spirits, sun or saunas for several months. Results become evident after about three months and should last for years. Cellular therapy is particularly valid as a preventive measure to ward off age, though it is not a lifetime insurance – repeats every five years or so are recommended.

Cellular therapy is essentially a biological method of healing and it is possible to treat any part of the body where malfunction or slow metabolism is the problem. The best results are cited in glandular disturbances, degenerative and stress disorders – all part of the aging syndrome.

And the risks? Whatever the doubts and the general medical scepticism on cellular therapy, it has been proved extraordinarily safe. It is unfortunate that it was initially tagged as the miracle rejuvenator, which gave the wrong impression. Niehans never claimed his therapy could help keep anyone alive and years younger indefinitely, but always stressed that a more rewarding and more youthful life was possible at any age.

## Procaine Therapy

In 1957 Professor Ana Aslan of Romania announced that over the previous five years she had discovered a chemical compound that could diminish almost all the usual disorders of aging. She had treated thousands of patients in her clinic in Bucharest with a substance called 'gerovital', a white crystalline compound based on procaine hydrochloride, commonly used as a local anaesthetic (novocaine) in dentistry.

Akin to Niehans, she didn't set out to find a rejuvenating agent, but became aware of the possible powers of procaine when she was using it on patients suffering from rheumatism to help reduce the pain. She found it also helped them to become more active, sharpened mental ability and cleared up skin problems; metabolic rate and glandular function also improved. Backed by the government, she became head of a special geriatric clinic and large-scale experiments were initiated. How exactly it works is unclear, but there is now an impressive amount of data to show what it can do. The first change is in mental capacity, then physical improvements

*Sophia Loren*
'A woman becomes more attractive and self-assured as she gets older. I see myself at 80 – amusing, well-groomed, bright-eyed, a little shaky, but filled with good humour and warm memories.'

become obvious, notably in the skin – fewer wrinkles, better colouring. Important is its psychological effect, because once the mind becomes sharper it can help combat the deep depression so often associated with aging – and in itself the trigger point for many physical and metabolic disorders. It is essentially a body stimulant and is one case where it would appear that a chemical can spark the body's vital force into action. Patients at the Bucharest Clinic receive a series of twelve injections over a period from ten days to two weeks. Effects do wear off, so it is recommended to have repeat injections within a year – which is of course a snag.

It goes without saying that orthodox medics shrug off any claims of the value of gerovital, but surely a whole clinic cannot be based on a sham, particularly when it is under the auspices of the Romanian Ministry of Health. In 1957, the government registered Gerovital H-3 and certified its wide-scale use – mostly for the afflictions of middle and later years, ranging from circulation and digestive disorders, to bone, glandular and nervous conditions, and particularly to the whole spectrum of problems during menopausal years. Germany recognized the potential of gerovital and one company developed a drug that quickly became known as the youth pill (KH3). Its effectiveness has not been proved except subjectively, but it is said to have the same effect as a super-vitamin. This would seem to tie in with the value of megavitamin therapy (see page 71) in any stay younger programme and one instance where natural biological theories join hands with the chemical approach. This is but one of the many signs that the key to keeping the body as youthful as possible lies with the vitamins and minerals.

How valuable is a health check? There are definite advantages, but there is no need to be obsessive about it and feel that an annual physical and metabolic analysis is essential. Many diseases give off early warning signals in tests before physical symptoms are apparent. After thirty, it is prudent to have a check-up every three years to keep you in touch with the state of your health. Also reassurance is a vital health factor – you may very well have been worrying unduly about something, and worry itself could trigger off an illness. Measurement of blood pressure and blood analysis is important, so are urine checks and cancer screening. What you have to realize is that a health check is not a preventive tactic, but a diagnostic tool which a doctor can use to tell you where you are at risk and possible ways of counteracting the onset of a disorder.

# The bad bad news: Smoking

One would have thought by now there was no need to carry on anymore about the harmful effects of tobacco, but the point is that it remains the cause of many chronic diseases. As more women smoke more cigarettes, they are beginning to come through in the statistics as suffering increasingly from coronary thrombosis, chronic bronchitis and lung cancer. Furthermore, women are at even greater risk if they take the contraceptive pill because of the pill's effects on blood vessels and blood clotting. Smokers should not take the pill beyond thirty-five, but then you shouldn't be a smoker anyway.

The good news is that researchers feel once smoking stops, there is immediate benefit. Lung damage can be halted and in some cases reversed, while the bad effects on blood chemistry are quickly counteracted. The ill effects of smoking are mostly a result of inhalation. However, it is the nicotine in the tobacco that causes addiction. Smokers also have a much lower level of vitamin C in their bodies than non-smokers, which means that not only is resistance to disease lowered, but from a youth point of view the skin particularly suffers. This is because vitamin C is crucial in the formation of collagen fibres which help maintain the skin's firmness and suppleness. Skin ages more rapidly when you smoke.

There are three main dangerous substances in tobacco smoke:

**tar** – this is an irritant and primarily responsible for chronic bronchitis and lung cancer. It is now thought that cancer is more a result of irritation than the direct effect of carcinogens. Low tar cigarettes help the situation, but unfortunately they produce more carbon dioxide in the blood.

**nicotine** – the addictive part that has a range of subtle effects on the nervous and other systems. It is chemically a depressant and can calm you down, but it also raises blood pressure and liberates adrenalin, thus precipitating a stress-tension situation. The adrenalin causes blood sugar to be liberated from the liver. In this way, a cigarette can push up blood pressure and put too much sugar in the system.

**carbon dioxide** – this is a poisonous gas, in fact used to be a favourite method of suicide. What it does is displace oxygen in the red cells and if the blood then carries higher than forty per cent of carbon dioxide to the vital organs, it can lead to rapid death. Measurement of the carbon dioxide concentration in smokers reveals alarmingly dangerous levels. And unfortunately the concentration is higher with filter cigarettes than without.

## Breaking the habit: how to give it up

Most people who smoke would like to give it up, but like so many addictions it is easier said than done. Also the mere fact that it is socially acceptable makes it that much more difficult. Also despite the best will and effort in the world, the sad truth is that it is only five per cent of smokers in any one year that actually have success. Therapies do work and the smoker often stops, but rarely for ever, it is only a matter of time before the fatal first new puff. All the following can work, it's up to you whether they work forever or not; whichever you try there will be withdrawal symptoms making you bad tempered, neurotic, depressed and usually with a craving. Try to beat it, it's worth it for your health, your youth, your looks.

**will power** – we all think we've got it, but in reality few have. To be able to stop smoking on your own is the most difficult of tasks. Experts say it is better to cut it out completely, than attempt to cut down. However, if you think you can do it gradually, try to cut out your favourite cigarettes of the day first – the one after a meal, that first drag in the morning. Then whenever you feel the urge to smoke, postpone it for five minutes, then try ten, then twenty etc.

**hypnosis** – this involves a minimum of three sessions and at no point are you put into such a trance that you lose your self determination. Some people are more susceptible than others.

**aversion therapy** – therapy that is aimed to make you hate smoking. You need a minimum of three sessions, during which you are made to smoke – first one after the other until you feel ill, then with small electrodes attached to your wrists so that every movement to do with smoking gives you a disagreeable shock. The idea is that once on your own you will recall these unpleasant experiences when you reach for a cigarette and therefore abstain from lighting one.

**gum chewing** – based on the theory that it is nicotine addiction that's the real problem, a nicotine based chewing gum is given as a substitute. It certainly removes the hunger for nicotine, but smokers say it does not remove the desire and need for inhalation. The gum is available on prescription.

**acupuncture** – the channels of energy all meet in the ear, say acupuncturists (see page 179) and there are 150 of them in that small space. Treatment involves the insertion of a 'sleeper' in the right ear – this is a tiny needle with a rounded head which puts you in contact with the appropriate channel of energy. By twisting it, you can counteract your craving for nicotine. There is no pain, perhaps a slight discomfort. Craving may go, but withdrawal symptoms are still there. After ten days, the sleeper is put in the left ear. Like other stop-smoking methods, this odd-sounding system does work, but in the long run it is the individual's will that determines whether it's a short or long term result.

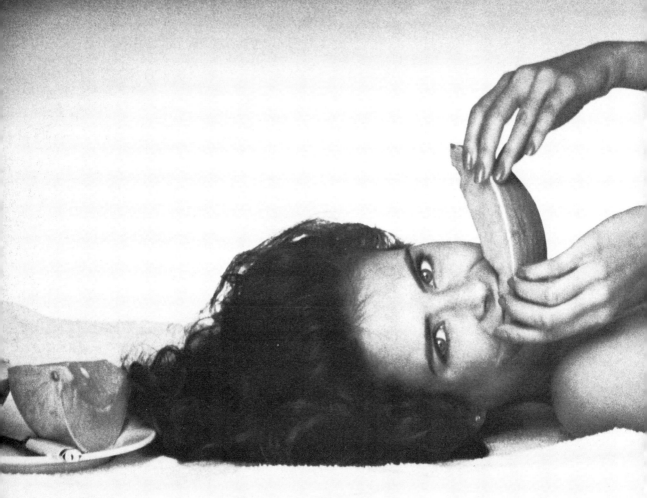

# FOOD
## The most basic thing to get right

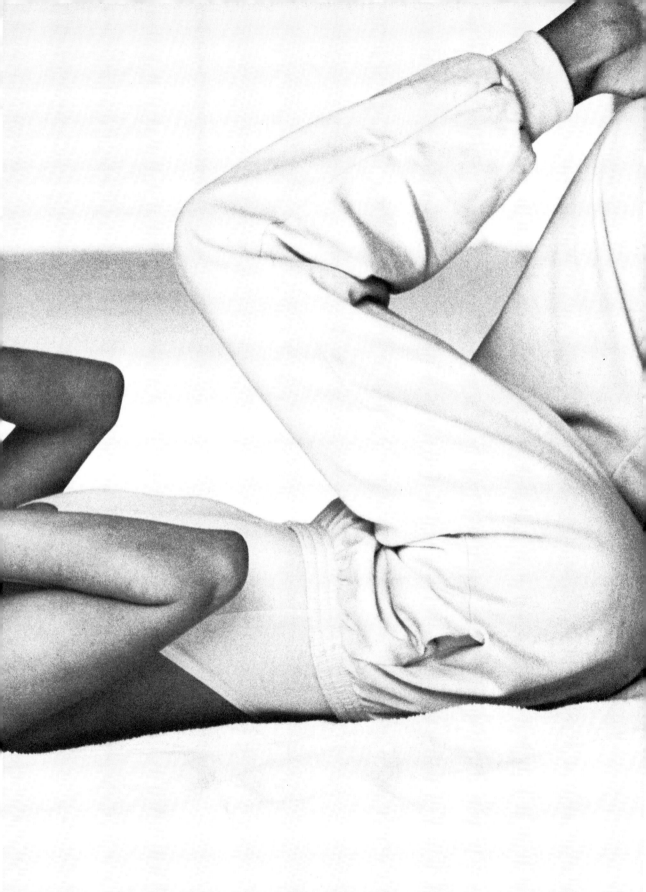

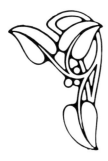

Good food is, of course, fundamental to feeling and looking younger. It is quite remarkable that, despite the reports that most of us are existing on a deathly diet, the facts just don't seem to sink in. We are warned about – indeed witness – the problems in middle years and later if we eat too much fat, too much sugar, too much salt, too many refined carbohydrates, too many convenience foods and not enough fibre. There's a slight swing to a little less fat (though fried foods are everywhere) and a new awareness that more fibre in the diet is important and that wholegrain bread is better nourishment than white. However, we are still consuming vast amounts of sugar, while packaged and tinned foods together with refined cereals are daily staples.

We can subsist on bad food but resistance to disease is impaired and the body's natural built-in therapeutic sources are depleted. Our affluent diet has resulted not only in an overweight society, but one where a high proportion of people suffer from one form or another of a diet-related disease. They are thought of as being inevitable diseases of middle age, though symptoms probably start in the thirties. Yet a preventive diet started early, could keep the body fit, strong and functioning at its optimum level way into old age. If you eat badly you are on the risk list for so many disorders including diabetes, high blood pressure, heart disease, stroke, constipation, diverticular disease, gallbladder trouble, cancer of the large bowel and colon: you may very well develop allergies and will certainly be deficient in vitamins and minerals.

If all this is at risk, why are most people indifferent? I believe it is due to the extremes of propaganda put forward by the two opposite camps: the natural food brigade and the establishment nutritionists. . Most of the recommended eating plans by those in favour of returning to a simple, natural way of eating often require such drastic rethinking and change of life-long habits, that most people don't even start. However, the basic natural food principle is extremely valid.

On the other hand, until recently even the majority of doctors considered diet of little significance – one only has to look at hospital food to realize that – and dismissed natural food as being faddist. They argued that in western societies it was almost impossible to be undernourished providing all the elements were there, albeit synthetically added. Nutritionists in mass production of food continue to take this attitude.

So who do you believe? Those who advocate a simple natural healthy diet are right when it comes to health and youth preservation – I have seen too many remarkable cures of disease, let alone signs of rejuvenation at various clinics, to think otherwise. The problem is that such a way of eating is not entirely right for life today. We no longer live in a simple society. Food is very much part of our social life. Food can and should be a joy, a pleasurable sensation, a rewarding one for your body as well as for your spirits, but one that is conducive to our lifestyle.

The answer is balance and compromise. Learn what the ideal diet is and stick to it when you can. We are all going to break rules from time to time – an over-rich restaurant meal, a plate of chips – but it doesn't matter providing you are not doing it all the time, and you know how to compensate for it. Plan your meals within the basic anti-aging diet rules and daily eating guide. Really get to know the value of vitamins and minerals (see pages 96–106). Be aware of the necessity of a periodic cleansing for your body, getting rid of toxic wastes by going on a juice fast or a raw food diet – it's not for life, it's just for a week (see page 109).

Food is talked about too much in terms of diet – how much weight can be lost. Food should be considered in terms of nutritional value, and if you are doing that right, chances are you will finally control your weight as well. Calories do count in weight control (see page 113) but it's important to be eating the right kind of calories. It is readjustment of eating habits to nutrient consciousness that wins both the weight and health stakes in the long run.

Rejuvenation through diet can be measured by definite changes in the body. Monitored regimens at clinics and health resorts show changes in skin texture and elasticity, improved functioning of the liver and digestive system, lowering of the levels of cholesterol and lippo-proteins in the blood, improved circulation, upgraded agility and general wellbeing. Established medicine is only just beginning to acknowledge what the right diet might be able to achieve – not to mention what the wrong diet has been and is still destroying.

Researchers studying longevity point out that the nutritional deficiencies are the main cause of premature aging. This doesn't mean not getting enough to eat, but not getting enough of the vital nutrients. We now have considerable knowledge about the chemical processes involved in food assimilation and many scientists feel that the secret of prolonging youth lies in the manipulative use of the nutritive chemicals – the vitamins and minerals (see pages 96–106). They are available in everyday fresh foods – if you eat the right ones – but it is recommended to take some in supplementary form because of current ecological imbalance.

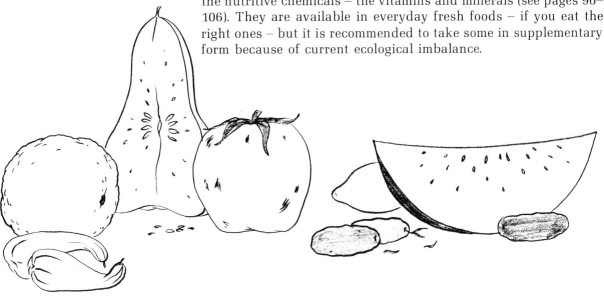

## THE BASIC ANTI-AGING FOOD RULES

Before you even begin to think about what foods are and what nutritional categories they come into, it is essential to get fixed in the mind the basic things that are good and bad, because this is what is at the core of youth extension eating; these are your guidelines for life.

### The Big Four Changes

- cut down on fats
- eat far, far less sugar produce
- use a minimum amount of salt
- eat much more fibre foods

### The Vital Health Guide

- concentrate on fresh foods
- cut convenience foods to a minimum, preferably out
- aim for fifty per cent of diet to be of raw foods
- check vitamin and mineral intake
- know the value of wholegrains, the cereals and the breads

### Revised Thoughts on Cooking

- stop frying in fat
- start grilling, roasting, poaching and steaming
- don't overcook vegetables
- baking pastries and cakes is time consuming and bad for health, start baking wholegrain bread instead

## FOOD CATEGORIES AND VALUES

It is not easy to find your way through the complicated vernacular of nutrition. There are three main types of food: proteins, carbohydrates and fats, all of which contain vitamins and minerals. But it's not that simple. Many proteins contain fats, many carbohydrates contain protein – and what is more there are many different types of carbohydrates, some beneficial, some not. So it is not as simple as it would appear at first. It is much more realistic to think of foods in relation to their specific value in a daily diet. Foods are usually categorized according to their major function, though they may dabble in other areas.

### Protein

These are essential for building and repairing body tissue. The amino acids in proteins are the significant part and not all proteins contain a full set. Fish, poultry, meat, game, milk, cheese, eggs and nuts are superior; wholegrains have a high ratio and so do some vegetables such as the legumes and avocado. In practice, a balanced diet provides all. The importance of protein was once considered the highest priority in a diet. The new thinking is that it is only necessary to make protein no more than twenty per cent of the daily diet and if possible to take that mostly from vegetable and grain sources.

## Carbohydrates

These provide energy for physical and mental activity and they assist in the assimilation and digestion of foods. The confusing thing is that there are three types of carbohydrates: sugars, starches and cellulose.

The sugars and starches are converted to glucose for immediate energy which if not used is stored as fat. Ideally, sugar should come from fresh fruits and honey, not from refined sugar or sweets, because the body has to process them in a different way which is ultimately harmful.

The starch carbohydrates are the grains and cereals, which are the most marvellous food if they are wholegrain (wheat, maize, corn, barley, oats, rice) and eaten as bread or as a cereal, but absolutely useless if refined. The reason why the natural grains are so good is not just because they contain a multitude of vitamins and minerals, plus being a good source of protein, but because they are a vital source of fibre which is essential for the efficient functioning of the digestive and the eliminating system.

The cellulose carbohydrates are good news on all sides. These are the fruits and vegetables which contain little energy value on their own (see how confusing the nutritional labels are) but are the main source of vitamins, minerals and fibre. The stringy cellulose threads of plant life provide most of the necessary bulk for the proper working of the bowels. It is really the connective tissue of plants and it passes almost unchanged through the intestine to be excreted as waste, yet its bulk is necessary to provide a smooth intestinal voyage for other nutrients, and as a sort of mattress to take away toxic matter. Also the cellulose matter in vegetables and fruits demands considerable chewing which produces saliva and gastric juices, aiding digestion. The three types of carbohydrates should together form from sixty-five to seventy per cent of your daily diet.

Fibre is very important. It is the rough part of your food that the body cannot digest, but it is essential to ease the passage of other foods through the body. Unfortunately the necessity of fibre has been ignored for the last thirty years, and only recently have doctors actually acknowledged its significance in retaining a healthy, well-functioning body. Be sure to take enough fibre every day. Good sources are: wholegrain breads and cereals, bran, artichokes, citrus fruits, all green vegetables, legumes such as beans, lentils, peas, apples.

## Fats

These provide a source of reserve energy and act as carriers for fat-soluble vitamins, so it is important to have a certain amount in the body to protect essential organs. Fats also prevent the skin from becoming dry and protect the body against cold. Although fat intake should be watched – and in most diets it is dangerously too high – it should not be cut out. Fat is not always obvious as in the dairy products, but it is also in meat, poultry, fish, grains, nuts and vegetables. It is virtually impossible to be without fat, which is why you have to watch and cut down on visible fat. There are two types: saturated fats which are solid at room temperature and come mostly from animal sources – and unsaturated fats, usually liquid, or at least very soft, and from vegetable sources. From a health point of view, it is considered better to limit animal fats and use vegetable oils (preferably cold-pressed) such as olive, sunflower, sesame. Beware of taking too much unsaturated fats (though many diets recommend this) because unless you have an adequate amount of vitamin E in your diet, they could oxidize to form toxic compounds which cause red cell damage. My choice is to carry on using butter in small amounts – it's so good on wholegrain bread and toast – and to stick to rich green olive oil for everything else. Fats should be a maximum of fifteen per cent of the daily diet, preferably lower.

## The Ideal Proportions

Working out an exact daily diet is not realistic on any specific terms, but if you can get the proportions within certain limits, then you are on the right way to an optimum long-living diet. As already mentioned, keep the following criteria in mind: the major part of your daily intake should be from the good carbohydrate group, around sixty-five to seventy-five per cent, then come the proteins at a maximum of twenty per cent, and finally the fats at a maximum of fifteen per cent. How you juggle to get to the full 100 per cent is up to you. Look at this table, which will help to give an indication as to the type of food and the quantity which would add up to the ideal balance of nutrients. A last important point: make an effort to take fifty per cent of your daily food raw – salads, vegetables, juices, fruits. In a warm climate it's easy, in a cold one it is extremely difficult, but reach the highest percentage you can because as far as health is concerned, it is well worth it.

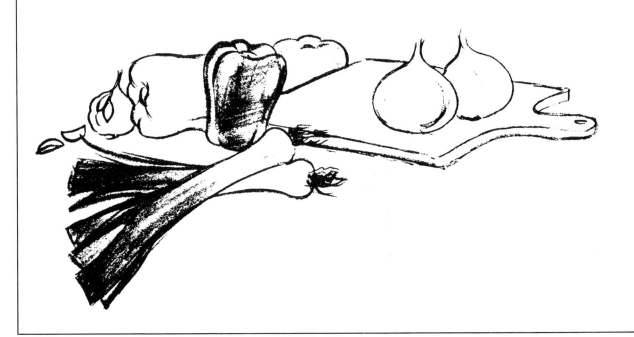

| FOOD TYPE | AMOUNT |
|---|---|
| **1. Vegetables and fruits** | **5 servings daily** |
| Vegetables: those with intense colour – bright greens and oranges are the most nutritious – broccoli, spinach, kale, sprouts, cabbage, green peppers, dark salad greens, alfalfa sprouts, turnips, carrots, potatoes with skin, tomatoes<br>Fruits: the berry group are excellent food value – strawberries, blackberries, blackcurrants – also apricots, the citrus fruits – orange, lemon, grapefruit – peaches, melon, pineapple | A serving is about 1 cup of vegetables. For fruits, one of medium size, a cup of berries, a quarter of a melon, 2 slices of pineapple |
| **2. Grains, cereals, beans and seeds** | **4 servings daily** |
| Grains: wholegrain breads, pasta, oats, brown rice<br>Beans and seeds: all seed beans, fresh or dried, lentils | A serving is about 1 cup of cooked grains, 2 slices bread, $\frac{1}{2}$ cup cooked beans or seeds |
| **3. Dairy products** | **2 servings daily** |
| Milk: preferably skimmed<br>Eggs: raw or cooked<br>Cheese: hard varieties are best, also cottage and goat cheese<br>Yogurt: natural low-fat | A serving is a glass of milk, one egg, 55g (2oz) cheese, 1 carton yogurt |
| **4. Meat, poultry, fish** | **1 serving daily** |
| Meat: liver, kidney, lean veal, lamb, beef<br>Poultry: chicken and turkey<br>Fish: number one choice in this group, all varieties, also shellfish | A serving is 125–150g (4–6oz) of fish, poultry or lean meat |
| **5. Fats** | **minimum amount** |
| You do need some. Take butter for bread; use olive or sesame oil for dressings; margarine in limited amounts for cooking | |
| **6. Sugars** | **minimum amount** |
| Honey and molasses for sweetening instead of refined sugar | |
| Flavourings: all the natural herbs, freshly ground pepper, limited salt and preferably sea salt, both fine and crude. | |
| Dressings: olive oil with cider vinegar or lemon juice for salads, plus added herbs and dry mustard; home-made mayonnaise. Avoid creamy synthetic dressings. | |
| Sauces: those without fat or sugar are fine, limit the others and only from time to time succumb to your own, which have a base of flour and butter. | |
| Sweeteners: avoid white sugar; use honey, molasses or natural brown. | |

Never give up bread, unless it's white. Wholegrain bread is one of the most nutritious things we can have in our diet. If it is full of the natural kernel, it will not add weight, but it will provide a great set of nutrients and a good amount of fibre which is essential to the diet.

## DAILY FORMULA FOR STAY YOUNGER EATING

Breakfast is more or less standard for everyone, but the lunch and dinner plan is interchangeable according to your lifestyle. From a health point of view, it is better to eat the most substantial meal in the middle of the day, but working and social habits invariably necessitate it being taken in the evening. It is not that important providing you are getting the essential nutrients during the course of the day – making sure that lunch is not a quick, convenient, unnutritious snack. Here is a general guide to a realistic, workable balance of foods.

### Breakfast: fresh fruit and wholegrains

Pull up your blood sugar level for energy with fresh fruits, provide protein through wholegrain cereals not through fat such as eggs and bacon.

- fresh fruit or unsweetened juice or dried fruits soaked overnight
- yogurt as a topping plus food supplements
- wholegrains in the form of cereal such as porridge or muesli, or bread, plus butter and honey or home-made preserves
- coffee or tea – preferably herbal

### Lunch: salads, vegetables or soups, wholegrains, cheese, eggs

It is good to have one meal a day mostly vegetables, whether raw or lightly cooked, with protein coming from the grains and dairy produce, and without fruit as this can cause an alkali-acid imbalance and disturb digestion.

- mixed salad of raw vegetables or lightly cooked greens
- eggs, cheese or wholegrains such as rice or pasta provide the protein
- wholegrain bread with butter
- yogurt if you need a dessert
- mineral water, glass of wine
- tea or coffee, if you must

### Dinner: fish, poultry or meat, vegetables, salads, fruit

This comes closest to the habitual meal though it's extended beyond the meat and two vegetables, and is minus the inevitable sweet dessert which is a lethal provider of harmful sugar. Protein is provided by the fish, poultry or meat (try and concentrate on the first two, unless it's liver); energy and vital nutrients come from the others.

- home-made vegetable soup
- salad and/or vegetables including potatoes
- fish, poultry or meat – or a vegetable protein dish such as bean casserole
- wine – more than one glass for pleasure – mineral water
- coffee or tea, if you must
- wholegrain bread or sticks as extras

What about condiments, flavourings for food? The main rule is to keep salt down, but you can add freshly ground pepper as you like, also all the herbs available. They are the best flavourings of all; spices are fine too, and hot chili pepper is particularly recommended as a rejuvenator for the body. Stay away from bottled sauces, they invariably contain too much fat, too much sugar and are full of chemicals and colourings. Make your own mayonnaise; for salads use olive oil plus lemon or cider vinegar.

## ALCOHOL: WHAT LIMITS

In this day and age, to say stop drinking is almost asking for the impossible, although in long-term health terms it is usually considered the ideal. I say 'usually' because there is evidence to support that a little bit of what you fancy in the form of intoxicating drinks can be a good thing, particularly as a buffer to stress. Even those tribes recorded as phenomenal long-livers had their moments of abandonment during drinking festivals. There are medical graphs showing that total abstinence can contribute more to circulation and heart diseases than the counteraction of relaxing alcohol. Again it's a question of balance and knowing your personal toleration. In excess, alcohol is, of course, a destroyer – of the liver, of metabolic functions and of the mind. It will affect your skin, your hair, your eyes, your all-over appearance.

Women have a lower tolerance of alcohol than men because our bodies contain five to ten per cent less water. Also response varies according to the menstrual cycle – there are higher alcohol levels during premenstrual and ovulatory phases. Excess alcohol can also upset the endocrine balance, thus affecting the menstrual cycle and causing problems during menopause.

A few drinks are fine, but what you have to realize is that contrary to popular belief, alcohol is not a stimulant at all, but ultimately a depressant. The initial lift is followed by a let-down, feelings of depression, anxiety and chronic fatigue. Alcohol is acceptable physiologically when used in moderation. It is measured in units – one unit equals a glass of wine, a measure of spirits, half a pint of beer. A light drinker consumes up to five units a week, a moderate drinker up to thirty-five units; over thirty-five units is considered heavy drinking.

Wine is the most acceptable form of alcohol, and is actually said to be beneficial to the digestion as it contains enzymes active in the metabolism of food. It provides Vitamins B-2, B-6, niacin, pantothenic acid and small quantities of the other B-complex elements. Minerals are present too. The more natural the wine the better, and better still if it is drunk in the area of production. To travel well, many wines have to be preserved with chemical additives.

Spirits and liqueurs are more concentrated alcohol and can rob the body of vitamins because like any other sugar carbohydrate they need the vitamin B-complex for assimilation. An important fact to remember is that alcohol contains many calories and it is often drinking that contributes to excess weight rather than food. Check the calorie chart on page 113.

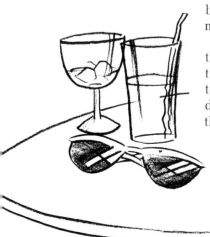

## WATER: THE STAFF OF LIFE

We may be able to live without food, but we can never live without water. Our bodies contain an incredibly high percentage of water and depend upon it. All foods contain some degree of water. We take it for granted, yet it rarely occurs to most of us to look into its value in relation to daily life. You should drink a minimum of a pint of water a day. Tap water is fine, if it is good, but you have to check on that. Most community water has been fortified with chlorine for purification and fluorine to help prevent tooth decay, but evidence of the toxic effects of both is causing concern.

You have to take to mineral water. On the continent this is normal. No meal, whether at home or in a restaurant, is complete without a bottle of mineral water. And quite right too, because natural water is the most marvellous source of untampered minerals, all of which can only be beneficial to your entire system. All water can be health-giving providing it is fresh, clear and uncontaminated. Running water exposed to the sun has special curative powers due to the absorption of solar energy which can be passed into the body. All of the great spas in Europe were based on the belief of the power of water, even just drinking a glass or two a day.

I am an absolute firm believer in the benefits of a pint of mineral water a day – more if you can take it. Don't worry about retaining it, because contrary to what may seem logical, if you drink mineral water in quantity it can reduce fluid retention because it is capable of swilling away the excess toxins that are actually holding water in the body. Also if you drink a sparkling water, it is not like drinking water at all. If it is added to lemon juice, which on its own is unpalatable to many, it fizzes up into what looks and tastes like a marvellous cocktail. And if you have drunk too much alcohol, glasses of mineral water the following morning will perk you up better than anything else. A fast on mineral water for one or two days can be very beneficial if you can take it, but it's not the only way of detoxifying your body (see page 109). However, do make an effort to include mineral water in your daily diet – drink it on its own, add it to juices, to your effervescent vitamin C tablets.

Water and weight: you may be overweight because you retain more water than you need. This is probably due to the fact that you eat too much salt – a lethal element in our daily diet. Cut it down, cut it to a minimum and use sea salt if possible. If too much salt is taken, water accumulates and the body swells up. You actually only need about a gramme of salt a day. Most of us eat twenty times as much. Watch it.

## HERBAL TEAS: THE BEST BEVERAGES

Tea and coffee are daily necessities for most people and although their harmful toxic effects are well publicized, to take them away completely is unrealistic. It is the caffeine that is the evil: it over-stimulates the heart, pushes the brain into pressured action and puts more and stronger acid into the stomach. Coffee contains much more caffeine than tea – and even cocoa has some – but it is prudent to cut down on both. It is often the habit of a hot drink every now and then that is responsible for the high daily intake of tea or coffee. It's a good idea to try and wean yourself off this caffeine dependency by gradually substituting herbal teas. At first, they may seem weak and ineffectual, but many have pleasant aromas and interesting tastes – add a little honey if they initially appear too bitter. Herbal teas are a health cure in themselves as they contain beneficial elements for many parts of the body and mind. These are the best:

**ginseng** – the great anti-aging tea with possibly the best record as an energizing and rejuvenating plant. It is an all round booster, helping mental efficiency and physical resistence; it is also said to purify blood, reduce accumulation of cholesterol and improve circulation. Orientals have sworn by it for years. Today most of the packaged teas come from China or Korea. Caution: don't overdo it.

**rose-hip** – this should become the standard substitute for regular Indian or China teas, as it is one of the best sources of vitamin C, which is vital for a longer, healthier life.

**sage** – the Chinese had and still have great faith in the overall benefits of drinking sage tea daily, while the Italians have always thought of it as a general preventive medicine. It is a stimulant for the nervous system and brain (hence the name) but it is also valuable as a digestive.

**camomile** – the great calmer; it is excellent for all nervous conditions as it has the capacity to adjust the entire metabolism to a lower, easier rate. It is therefore good to take before going to sleep, but in addition it can relieve indigestion and be a help for menstrual pains.

**comfrey** – for hundreds of years comfrey has been considered one of the most valuable natural healing plants, yet it is not commonly used as a tea, and you will have to make your own from the dried leaves (in all health centres). The most important element in comfrey is allantoin, which stimulates all growth and multiplication of cells – a very significant issue as you grow older.

**mint** – just about the best for the digestive system, but it has the added property of being able to stimulate the mind and is recommended for general listlessness, for counteracting the enervation of hot weather. It can help headaches and ward off colds.

**sarsaparilla** – if you can find this, it is certainly worthwhile, for it is a strong blood purifier and can help many skin problems. It is also claimed to be a good source of sex hormones. You may only be able to get the dried roots, in which case boil them for thirty minutes.

Many of the above mentioned herbal teas are now packaged for quick, convenient use, but if you use the dried herbs take one teaspoon per cup of water. Pour over boiling water and steep for ten to fifteen minutes; strain.

Sweeteners: the only ones allowed on a healthy diet are honey, molasses and natural sugar in small amounts. Natural, raw, unprocessed honey is a nutritional boost. It increases calcium retention in the system, aids circulation and improves the turgor of the skin; it is also useful in heart, kidney and liver disorders. Molasses, which is the by-product of sugar refining and has all the nutrients in it that sugar doesn't, is particularly valuable for anaemic women. It contains a host of minerals and vitamins, but is particularly rich in magnesium, vitamin E and copper. Use it to sweeten everything – fruits, yogurt, cereals, beverages. Brown sugar is dicy, because you cannot be sure if it is the real natural thing or simply coloured. Better stick to honey and molasses. Avoid white sugar altogether. It is quite possible to cook with honey.

# Know Your Vitamins

A comprehensive and full supply of vitamins is essential for a healthy body. They are not body builders or nutrients in themselves, but they regulate metabolism, in fact they indirectly control all body processes and help convert the carbohydrates and fats into energy.

Vitamins are manufactured by plants and are also available through certain animal and fish foods. If you are short on any vitamin, it could result in anything from a generally sluggish metabolism, depression or skin problems to glandular, bone or digestion disorders. However, the average diet in western societies – even if you are not yet eating in the healthiest way – rarely gives rise to such serious results as rickets or scurvy as it did years ago. But even mild deficiences can mean you are not feeling as good as you could be, not looking your best, not reaching your energy potential and not so mentally alert.

As you get older, it is particularly important to keep track of vitamin intake. If you are eating a balanced diet in the proportions indicated (see page 91) and taking most of it from fresh foods, you are most likely going to get what is necessary. As you grow older, however, I am all in favour of certain vitamin supplements (such as vitamins E, C and A) that are seriously becoming regarded as aids to staying and looking younger.

The idea of vitamins as a helping hand in rejuvenation is naturally one of considerable controversy. There is still the scepticism of the majority of medical practitioners to overcome. They say nothing is definitely proved along verified scientific pathways – and yet one hears reports all the time of people who claim remarkable results from vitamin supplements. Subjective reports cannot be dismissed lightly. I, for one, will swear to anybody about the value of taking vitamin E and vitamin C on a regular basis, despite the fact I've seen medical statements saying 'nothing yet satisfactorily proven.'

What should one do? You simply try for yourself, test your own reactions, listen to your body. Unless you are going to take huge amounts, there is little likelihood of harm. Commercial products indicate clearly on the package the recommended daily dose, which is usually very modest. Vitamins can be used as therapeutic doses (megavitamin therapy) and some extraordinary results have been claimed. It is not something you attempt on your own, but there are some doctors who are quite adamant that certain diseases and metabolic disturbances can be greatly helped by putting large doses of specific vitamins into the body. As you may well imagine, there's another group of medics who say it's nonsense. However, there are many case histories of very good results indeed. If you are interested, search out a doctor who has studied nutritional therapy – a different thing altogether to being a nutritionist. Many naturo-pathic (see page 189) doctors fall into this category.

The fact is that the extra dose of a vitamin here and there can make all the difference to your outward appearance (skin and hair

*Cyd Charisse*
'90 minutes each day of yoga and ballet exercise, a good healthy breakfast or orange juice, wholemeal bread, bacon and eggs; a glass of milk for lunch, and a light protein supper (no sugar or sweet things) and eight to ten hours sleep.'

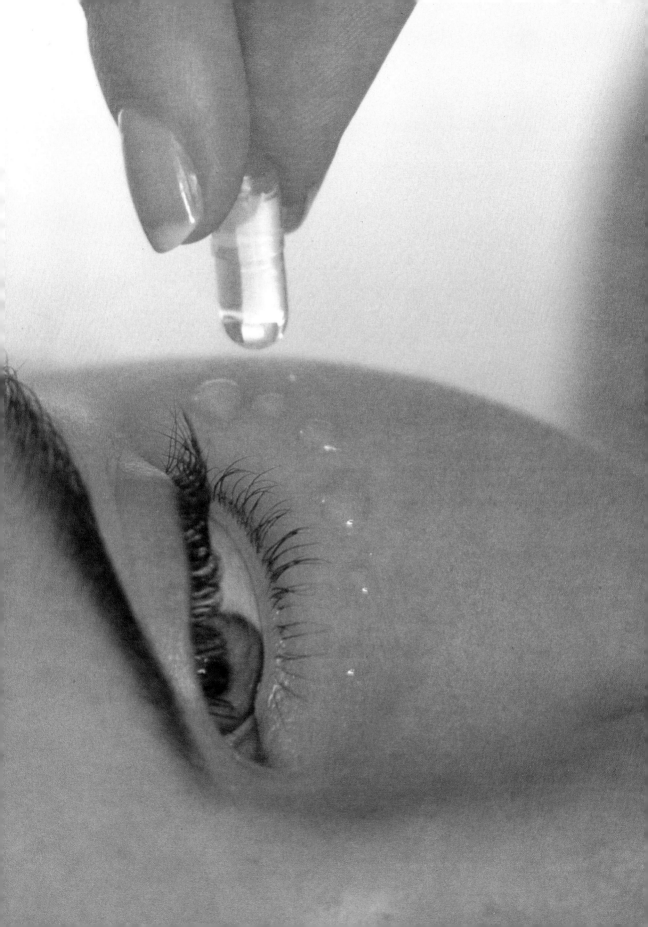

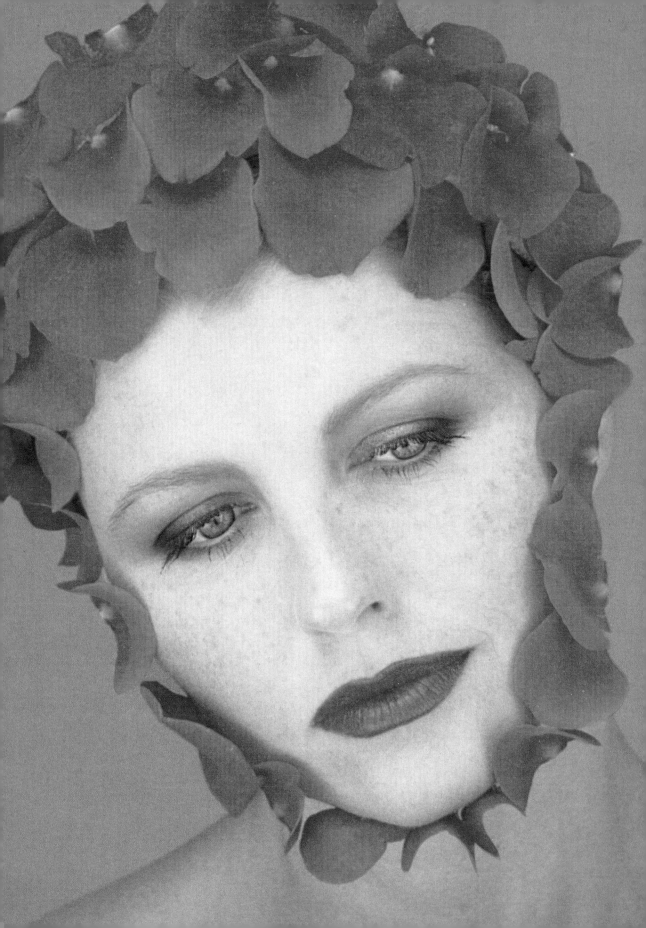

Have you ever eaten seaweed, ever had kelp? If not, start, because the two contain a beautifully balanced combination of minerals essential for a long living life. You can get kelp salt, which is a superb source of iodine. Both seaweed and kelp are rich in the B-complex vitamins, vitamins E, D and K. They help the skin, strengthen nails and give lustre to hair.

texture, for instance) as well as inward functioning. The first step is to be sure you are eating the right foods which will provide an adequate spectrum of vitamins, then you decide afterwards if you think any extras are necessary. From the charts, it is easy to work out the foods that repeatedly come up as good sources of more than one vitamin, and if you add these to your daily diet, you are well on the way.

There are two types of vitamins – those soluble in fat (A, D, E and K) and those soluble in water (C and B complex). The fat-soluble ones can be stored in the body, and they are the ones that could cause problems if taken in excess. However, the water-soluble vitamins are washed away in the urine if they are not used, and therefore have to be replaced in your daily diet.

You may wonder why vitamins are called by letters. There's a very simple answer: when they were discovered, no-one had any idea what their composition was – so letters seemed the obvious temporary means of identification, and they have stuck. Each vitamin performs a different function, but they all work together as a team, which means a deficiency in one can seriously affect the working of another.

Check out the chart which shows at a glance the rostrum of vitamins, their function and where you find them. Also included is the recommended daily need. This is an average estimate, because what a woman needs depends on age, state of health, individual metabolism, climate and environment. However, there is not that much variant to cause any concern. The older you get the more sure you must be of getting adequate amounts. Of course, I realize there is no way of knowing how much you are getting from food, which again depends on quality of produce and how it is prepared. As you can see there are so many variables to be taken into consideration that exact vitamin estimates are impossible. But do remember that the best nourishment comes from raw food though certain things like grains and animal and fish proteins need to be cooked – and if you are careless in cooking you can lose practically all the vitamin content. The body is very clever at working out the necessary amounts it requires. It is only when you are taking supplements in the form of capsules or concentrated juices that you need to watch the quantity. It is important to note that there are many vitamins in the B-complex group; in natural foods they occur together in varied ratios, but if you take supplements it is advisable to get a multiple-B formula, or go to a doctor for advice on specifics. The water-soluble vitamins are measured in milligrams (mg) and the fat-soluble in international units (iu).

| VITAMIN | FUNCTION | FOOD |
|---|---|---|
| **Vitamin A**<br>(Retinol)<br><br><br><br><br><br><br><br>Daily: 5,000iu | Helps repair body tissues and skeletal growth; promotes good eyesight; helps keep skin in good condition. Deficiency results in dryness and premature aging of the skin. Too much sunlight can cause loss of vitamin A | Deep yellow foods such as apricots, mangoes, papayas, carrots, cheese, eggs, liver, kidney, fish-liver oils; dark green vegetables like kale and broccoli, watercress, alfalfa, sprouts |
| **Vitamin B-1**<br>(Thiamine)<br><br><br><br><br><br><br>Daily: 1.5mg | Necessary for the conversion of carbohydrates into glucose for energy; important for nervous system, heart and liver. Lack of it reduces stamina and can make you tired and forgetful | Poultry, lamb's liver, sunflower seeds, wheatgerm and wholegrain cereals, green vegetables, brewer's yeast |
| **Vitamin B-2**<br>(Riboflavin)<br><br><br><br><br><br><br><br>Daily: 2mg | Vital to break down food for nutrition and energy; necessary for cell respiration and tissue repair. Any deficiency could cause dermatitis, cracks around the mouth, broken blood vessels, split fingernails, dandruff | Milk, cheese, eggs, brewer's yeast, wheatgerm, wild rice, poultry, liver, kidney, almonds, avocado, green vegetables |
| **Vitamin B-3**<br>(Niacin)<br><br><br><br><br><br><br>Daily: 15mg | Assists in the entire digestive process; important to mental health and the nervous system; most beneficial working with the other B vitamins. Without enough you can be lethargic, nervous, and depressed | Chicken, chicken liver, lamb's liver, kidneys, halibut, mackerel, sardines, peanuts, wholegrains |
| **Vitamin B-5**<br>(Pantothenic acid)<br><br><br><br><br><br><br><br><br><br>Daily: 5–10mg | Involved in the metabolism of fatty acids; helps free energy from foods essential for balanced functioning of the adrenal gland. Important for nerves, stress and digestion. Deficiency can lead to premature grey hair, and early onset of arthritis | Kidney, liver, egg yolk, bran, brewer's yeast, wholegrains |

Virtually all the vitamin C in diets comes from fruit and vegetables, but because it is readily lost during storage, preparation and cooking it is one of the nutrients that is frequently deficient in our diet. You can get an adequate daily supply if you include in your twenty-four hour diet the following: 1 orange, half a grapefruit, or the juice of 1 lemon; plus 1 large baked potato, a portion of green vegetables, lightly cooked. The best source by far is a bowl of blackcurrants, but they are not always available. A slice of liver is another marvellous source, which in itself could supply your entire daily requirement.

| VITAMIN | FUNCTION | FOOD |
| --- | --- | --- |
| **Vitamin B-6** (Pyridoxine)<br><br>Daily: 2mg | Connected with growth and important in regulation of the nervous system; aids in metabolic breakdown of foods; helps form antibodies and red blood cells. Because it helps to form collagen and elastin – important to keep skin smooth – it can keep you looking younger. Lack can cause anaemia. It can be destroyed by oral contraceptives, so watch that | Bananas, poultry, lamb's liver, mackerel, nuts, wheatgerm, wholegrains, peas, sunflower seeds, milk |
| **Vitamin B-12** (Cyano-cobalamin)<br><br>Daily: 0.005mg | Essential for normal functioning of body cells, particularly those of bone marrow and the nervous system. Important in the synthesis of the nucleic acids – the blueprint for continued efficient metabolism and vital in age prevention | Cheese, milk, poultry, fish, oysters, liver, kidneys, soya beans, wheatgerm, egg yolks (the white destroys the vitamin) |
| **Biotin** (Vitamin B complex)<br><br>Daily: 0.003mg | Helps to form fatty acids, burning them up with the carbohydrates for energy; necessary and needed more or less everywhere. Plays a vital part in healthy skin, glossy hair, sexual activity. Deficiency unlikely, but can cause fatigue, depression, greyish skin | Raw egg yolk (the raw white destroys vitamin) liver, kidney, black currants, molasses, wholegrains, brewer's yeast, fish, dried milk |
| **Choline** (Vitamin B complex)<br><br>Daily: negligible | Aids fat distribution from the liver; assists nerve transmission. Deficiency extremely unlikely but could result in hardening of arteries, high blood pressure and liver problems | Fish, liver, heart, lentils, wheatgerm, wholegrains, beans, lecithin |

| VITAMIN | FUNCTION | FOOD |
| --- | --- | --- |
| **Folic acid**<br>(Vitamin B complex)<br><br><br><br>Daily: 0.002mg | Helps form red blood cells and nucleic acids, essential for reproduction process. Thought to be very significant in age retardation | Liver, oysters, cabbage (raw), watercress, kale, asparagus, spinach, almonds, walnuts, brewer's yeast |
| **Inositol**<br>(Vitamin B complex)<br>Daily: negligible | Together with choline, inositol forms lecithin, which keeps the liver free of fats | Bran, nuts, sesame seeds, wholegrains, wheatgerm, lecithin granules, brewer's yeast |
| **PABA**<br>(Vitamin B complex)<br>Daily: negligible | Enables other vitamin B elements to function properly | Broccoli, cabbage, kale, kidneys, liver, meat, poultry |
| **Vitamin C**<br>(Ascorbic acid)<br><br><br><br><br><br><br><br><br><br><br>Daily: 50mg | Essential for preservation of health and beauty. Maintains level of collagen necessary for the formation of connective tissue, bone, skin and cartilage; helps virus infections, protects against pollution and counteracts stress. It is easily destroyed by light, heat and air | Potatoes, tomatoes, cabbage, cauliflower, broccoli, Brussels sprouts, green peppers, watercress, alfalfa sprouts, citrus fruits, blackcurrants, rosehips, strawberries |
| **Vitamin D**<br>(Calciferol)<br><br><br><br><br><br><br><br><br><br>Daily: 400iu | Essential for healthy teeth and bones as it helps take the calcium and phosphorus to the necessary building tissues. For older women it is important to get outside to get some sunlight, otherwise bones can become brittle, joints ache, arteries harden | Exposure to sunshine, egg yolks, cod-liver oil, mackerel, sardines, tuna, cheese |

Vitamin D is vital to maintain the level of calcium and phosphorus in the blood, and if deficient can lead to softening of the bones, particularly as you get older. It is obtained both from the action of sunlight on a substance in the skin and from the diet. Few foods contain vitamin D, but you can be sure of a plentiful supply if you eat herring or kipper once a week, eat a teaspoonful of dry ovaltine once a day and a teaspoon of cod liver oil.

| VITAMIN | FUNCTION | FOOD |
|---|---|---|
| **Vitamin E** (Tocopherol) | The most significant vitamin for prevention of aging (see below). Needed for normal metabolism, improves the entire circulatory system. It counteracts aging on many levels – skin, respiration, sexual system, circulation. It is a natural antioxidant (as is vitamin C) and so protects against irregular genetic activity | Carrots, cabbage, all green vegetables, eggs, olive oil, sunflower seeds, wheatgerm, wholegrains |
| Daily: 20iu | | |
| **Vitamin F** Daily: negligible | A group of unsaturated acids that help prevent heart disease and atherosclerosis, and help keep the skin in good condition | Wheatgerm, sesame and sunflower seeds, cod-liver oil and lecithin |
| **Vitamin K** Daily: negligible | Prevents haemorrhaging and aids the normal blood-clotting process; important for liver function | Broccoli, cabbage, potatoes, eggs, milk, yogurt |

How much vitamin E per day? The daily recommended amount is 20iu – but who can measure that? The more vitamin E the better, and large doses to date have not proved toxic. Try to eat two portions of green vegetables a day, a portion of wholegrain cereal, olive oil on salads and a sprinkling of ground sunflower seeds.

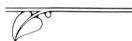

## THE SUPER ANTI-AGING VITAMINS

Many researchers believe that certain vitamins are particularly potent in their ability to reactivate the system as you get older and keep it metabolically at a younger level. Despite the fact that this theory is rejected by most traditional doctors, it should not be overlooked as an insurance for the future. Personally, I think it works, having seen positive results first hand when nutritional and megavitamin therapies have been used. The first thing is to check that you are taking all the foods that are high in these vitamins, then add supplements at your own discretion according to the guidelines below, or as indicated on commercial packages. Higher amounts should only be prescribed by a nutritional specialist. Vitamins are listed in order of importance.

### Vitamin E

This is number one, the vitamin every woman should take. Studies have shown that one of the main contributors to the aging process is the presence of certain chemicals in the cells (called 'free-radicals') due to a slowing down of metabolism. These substances affect normal cellular activity and it is now thought that vitamin E is a natural deterrent to their formation and if already present, is capable of counteracting their destructive power. Vitamin E is uniquely valuable in circulatory and heart diseases as it dilates the arteries and strengthens the action of the heart, thus improving the flow of blood. In this way it helps prevent and overcome varicose veins and phlebitis, and is one therapeutic answer to combatting angina pectoris. It's effective against arthritis, arterioschlerosis and diabetes, and is a strong stimulant for all sexual and reproductive functions. One of its most generally recognized uses is for regulation of periods, particularly when they are inclined to be heavy and erratic during the years prior to menopause. And during menopause, vitamin E alleviates hot flushes and headaches, helps itching and dryness of the external genitals. Best natural sources are wholegrains, sunflower and sesame seeds, olive oil and nuts. Vitamin E capsules are widely available, and the recommended dose for a boost is 600iu a day. If you have high blood pressure or a heart complaint, consult a doctor first.

## Vitamin C

The deterioration of skin during the aging process – dryness, wrinkles, appearance of veins – has a lot to do with the amount of vitamin C available to the body. If there is a deficiency, the collagen and elastin which 'cement' the cells together deteriorate, and the skin loses its elasticity, strength and smoothness. Vitamin C is vitally involved in all body functions and it is a potent anti-oxidant. It is of great help for arthritis, and is an important anti-stress vitamin. Older people also need larger amounts of vitamin C to provide adequate sex hormone production. Large doses of vitamin C are recommended to keep the body young and as a virus protection: 2,000 to 5,000mg a day. Natural sources are citrus fruits, rosehips, potatoes, broccoli, strawberries.

## Vitamin A

This vitamin together with vitamin E increases oxygenation of the tissues. It also makes the blood capillaries more permeable which helps prevent the skin from becoming dry or blemished. In addition it's a powerful anti-oxidant and disperser of 'free-radicals'; and it helps cut down cholesterol. Best sources are carrots, green leafy vegetables and tomatoes. Preventive doses are 25,000 to 30,000iu a day. Megadoses of vitamin A can be toxic when taken for a long time – so don't go above the 30,000 without having two or three weeks off every few months.

## Vitamin B-Complex

The combination of the many vitamins in this group are important to combat premature aging because they have something to do with practically every function of the body, giving a particular push to the brain and nervous system. It's essential you get an adequate supply. The best natural sources are brewer's yeast, wholegrains, wheatgerm, liver, green leafy vegetables. Supplementary recommended amount: one 50-strength tablet a day; it must be from natural sources, not synthetic.

*Gayle Hunnicutt*
'I have a regular massage by an acupuncture specialist, which is marvellous for toning up the muscles. If you travel a lot, as I do, a skipping rope is the most convenient form of exercise as it packs easily and gives a good work-out. Every morning I eat natural bran with live yogurt or acidopholous milk which cleans the system and is excellent if you have a cold. I also take a multivitamin pill, vitamin B and ginseng. I believe that appearance is all to do with health.'

# Know Your Minerals

Minerals are not as well known as vitamins but they are equally vital to general wellbeing and maintaining looks. They primarily act as catalysts, affecting function although they are not actually used – afterwards they are excreted in the urine and sweat, which means they must be replaced regularly. Although most of them are needed in minute amounts, they influence all life's processes: they control the water balance, the acid-alkali ratio, they influence the secretion of glands, they help draw chemical substances in and out of cells, they affect bone and muscle, they are important in transmitting messages through the nervous system and are vital for mental stability.

We obtain minerals through food, mostly plant life such as vegetables, fruits and herbs. The plants extract the minerals from the soil. The problem today is that with chemical interference in the soil and the wide use of insecticides, the natural balance of minerals has been upset. There is the possibility of getting too little of one and too much of another, and because the amounts are mostly so minuscule there's a very fine dividing line between too little and an overdose. This is the reason you don't hear so much about mineral supplements except in a few cases. It is perfectly possible to get an adequate supply from fresh foods, so don't be tempted to self-prescribe. Check with the chart and eat the right foods.

Calcium is a very important mineral in any anti-aging program and you may be surprised to learn that it is at one of its highest concentration levels in skimmed, dried milk: 100g yields 1,190mg of calcium. Cheddar cheese is another good source – you can get 800mg of calcium from 100g; canned sardines provide 550mg calcium per 100g. Watercress gives 220mg calcium for each 100g. If you can consume as much as 1,000mg of calcium a day, so much the better.

| MINERAL | FUNCTION | FOOD |
| --- | --- | --- |
| **Calcium**<br><br><br><br><br><br>Daily:<br>600–1,000mg | Necessary to build and maintain bones and teeth; important for heart regulation and nerve transmission. Helps offset aging. Deficiency weakens bones and could cause blood clotting. | Milk, cheese, almonds, olives, kelp and other seaweeds, sesame seeds, molasses, broccoli, wholegrains, yogurt |
| **Chlorine**<br><br><br>Daily: trace | In conjunction with sodium, is important in cell metabolism. Lack could be a cause of atherosclerosis | Celery, lettuce, spinach, tomatoes, kelp, salt |
| **Chromium**<br><br><br><br><br>Daily: trace | A trace mineral, helps regulate blood-sugar levels: believed to help keep the cholesterol level down. Deficiency might precipitate hardening of the arteries | Bran, brewer's yeast, poultry, fruits, green vegetables, nuts |

Lead poisoning, mainly from petrol fumes, can damage the heart, liver, kidneys and nervous system; it also replaces calcium in the bones and disrupts chemical processes in the brain. In all, lead can cause signs of early aging. Protection can come from a diet full of fresh vegetables, fruits, wholewheat breads and sesame seeds. Eat plenty of calcium rich foods and check mineral charts for produce also containing good supplies of zinc, manganese and chromium. Vitamin D is important for the absorption of these minerals – found in sunshine, egg yolks, cheese, cod-liver oil; and take that excellent all-rounder, vitamin C.

| MINERAL | FUNCTION | FOOD |
|---|---|---|
| **Cobalt**<br><br>Daily: trace | Necessary for function of vitamin B-12 and for red blood cells | Fruits, green vegetables, meat, wholegrains |
| **Copper**<br><br><br><br><br><br>Daily: 2–5mg | Significant in the production of red blood cells for the utilization of iron. Aids in forming hair pigment. Deficiency is rare but can lead to greying or loss of hair | Poultry, liver, kidney, shellfish, nuts, wholegrains, lettuce, cabbage |
| **Fluorine**<br><br><br>Daily: 1mg | Strengthens bones and teeth by helping to deposit calcium: counteracts tooth decay | Sea-food, fish, tea |
| **Iodine**<br><br><br><br><br>Daily: trace | Important for the proper functioning of the thyroid gland. Lack could lead to drying and wrinkling of skin, loss of hair | Shellfish, seafood, sea salt, seaweeds, kelp |
| **Iron**<br><br><br><br><br><br>Daily: 18mg | Very important mineral involved in oxidizing cells and forming haemoglobin. Most beneficial when plenty of vitamin C is available which aids absorption | Offal – kidney, liver – shellfish, egg yolk, dark green leafy vegetables, watercress, soya and sunflower seeds, wholegrains, molasses |
| **Magnesium**<br><br><br><br><br>Daily: 300mg | Important in cell metabolism; necessary as a catalytic agent for other minerals and vitamins and for the nerve and muscle systems | Almonds, wholegrains, molasses, nuts, sea foods and sea salt, olives, egg yolk, spinach |
| **Manganese**<br><br><br><br>Daily: trace | Activates enzymes; influences blood-sugar levels and helps maintain reproductive processes | Kidneys, parsley, watercress, spinach, cabbage, apricots, lentils, nuts, wheatgerm |
| **Phosphorus**<br><br><br><br><br><br><br><br>Daily: 1,000mg | The most active of all minerals, important for growth and maintenance; together with calcium provides hard structure for bones. Older people need more because their systems don't absorb it well | Meat, fish, egg yolk, cheese, wheatgerm, wholegrains |

| MINERAL | FUNCTION | FOOD |
|---|---|---|
| **Potassium**<br><br>Daily: 2,500mg | Often in partnership with sodium, maintaining a balance of fluids and important in muscle and nerve reactions. Involved in hormone activity, alleviates pre-menstrual tension | Sea food, potatoes, green leaf vegetables, bananas, citrus fruits, wholegrains |
| **Selenium**<br><br>Daily: trace | Works together with vitamin E in retarding the aging process. An important antioxidant it relieves high blood pressure. It is thought to be significant in protection against malignancies | Kidney, liver, nuts, sea food, wholegrains, brewer's yeast, eggs, garlic, onion, kelp |
| **Sodium**<br><br>Daily: 2–5mg | Works in combination with potassium and chloride: together they are often called electrolytes as they are significant in all cellular metabolism; protects the body against excess fluid loss, though too much sodium causes water retention, and aggravates high blood pressure | Poultry, green vegetables, kelp, sea salt, sea food, water and in many packaged foods |
| **Sulphur**<br><br>Daily: 850mg | Helps in the formation of body tissue; necessary for activity of vitamins thiamine and biotin; a trace mineral. It is essential for collagen synthesis therefore responsible for condition of skin, nails and hair | Eggs, poultry, beef, fish, beans, onions |
| **Zinc**<br><br>Daily: 10mg | Influences the enzyme and protein pattern in digestion. Necessary for collagen synthesis. Women on the pill and older women must be sure they have an adequate supply | Eggs, onions, fish, shellfish, wholegrains, beans, sesame seeds |

## THE SUPER ANTI-AGING MINERALS

### Selenium

An important antioxidant that works together with vitamin E as a major agent towards age-retardation. This is due in part to it being a powerful 'free-radical' disperser. Not all doctors would agree with this, of course, but researchers in nutritional therapeutics believe very strongly in its rejuvenating possibilities. Selenium, however, is a trace element – meaning it appears in only minute amounts in natural foods – but in large doses (which could only happen if taken in supplementary form) it is toxic. The best natural sources are: brewer's yeast, garlic, onions and wholegrains. In health shops you can find special yeasts that have a high selenium content.

### Zinc

Because of the tampering with soil and food, plus environmental pollutants, this is the mineral that is most likely to be deficient, particularly in women and even more so if you are on the pill or have been. It is involved in innumerable functions and lack can affect the skin and prematurely age it. Good natural sources are wholegrains, wheatgerm, eggs, garlic, sea food. This is one mineral that can be taken as a supplement – between 15 and 25mg a day.

### Calcium and Magnesium

These are two minerals where larger quantities are required than the trace elements. Calcium, of course, is a great aid to bones and teeth, but together with magnesium forms a team that helps reduce stress and keeps cholesterol levels down. They are both involved in almost every body function. Check the chart for the best natural resources, and in addition it is recommended to have 1,000mg calcium and 500mg magnesium per day.

Bones often become more brittle as the years go by because they lose both calcium and protein. This is much more prevalent in women than men, and is the main cause of a fractured hip. So check that you are getting enough calcium; consult the mineral chart.

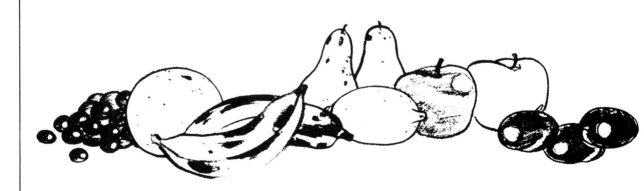

# The Super Anti-Aging Foods

Over the years a certain number of foods have been repeatedly mentioned as being 'miracle' ones for rejuvenation. The history of some go back to the earliest civilizations and their validity was based on empirical knowledge. Claims, however, have proved to be no accident, because now that scientific analysis is able to reveal exactly what is in these foods and what chemical reactions they cause in the body, it is established that they actually contain the highest concentration of the most important vitamins and minerals. They are miraculous in as much as you can get a fistful of vital nutrients in a single food. If you check back on the charts for vitamins and minerals, you'll see that some foods crop up time and time again as being the best source for the featured elements – such as brewer's yeast, sesame seeds, liver, etc., while the wholegrains are literally the most wholesome of all. Do more than make a note of them, go out and get them and start to add them to your diet every day. They are protectors and revitalizers; they will make a world of difference to your mental and physical health – and to your looks. Wholegrains of some sort – bread, rice, pasta, oatmeal, barley – should be a daily staple, then imaginatively incorporate the others.

The right diet can help stress. Certain foods excite and others can calm. If you stick to the recommended healthy diet you are almost there, but if you feel particularly stressful take supplements of vitamin C, lecithin, and vitamin E. Vitamin B complex is important, but take this in the form of liver rather than supplements.

### Brewer's Yeast

The most potent of the super foods, it is packed with vitamins and minerals (the richest natural source of all the B vitamins) and in addition has high quality proteins which provide essential amino acids. It is also a source of RNA and DNA nucleic acids which are the basis of cell rejuvenation. It is also one of the prime sources of zinc and selenium. Brewer's yeast comes in tablet and powder form (from all healthfood centres) but it is easier to use the powder – mix it in with yogurt, fruit or vegetable drinks, sprinkle on cereals and fruit. In this way you will get more brewer's yeast – and therefore more benefit – than if you swallowed a few tablets. And it's pleasanter.

### Lecithin

Not a food as we know it, nor a vitamin or mineral, lecithin is actually an organic fat substance very high in phosphorus. It is one of the main constituents of our brain and nerve tissues, and abundant in the endocrine glands. It is also present in some foods – eggs, for example – but it is recommended to take it in supplement form to make sure you are getting enough. It is a rich source of the vitamins E, D, K and choline and inositol from the B-group which are key factors in holding back the aging process. It plays a significant role in the breakdown of fat in the blood, thereby helping to guard against diseases related to hardening of the arteries – and because of this property, it is thought to help in weight control. Lecithin comes in granule and tablet form, but like brewer's yeast it is preferable to sprinkle it on salads or stir it into juices. Recommended dose is one dessertspoon a day.

### Sesame Seeds

Not exactly in everyone's daily diet, but they should be. These seeds contain more protein than meat and certain amino acids that are in short supply in most plant sources. They are richer in calcium than milk, and contain high amounts of vitamin E and B-vitamins – in particular niacin, inositol and choline. They are also marvellous sources of lecithin. Sesame seeds are available at all health-food centres and if you don't fancy eating them whole, a more palatable method is to grind them up for sprinkling over salads, fruits and vegetable dishes. Eat some every day – they are good on your breakfast muesli or yogurt.

### Yogurt

The western world was slow to recognize the benefits of yogurt, though in the Middle-East it has been used for thousands of years. Yogurt is fermented milk that contains bacteria helpful in keeping the intestine free from toxicity. It has gained a reputation for aiding diseases from allergies to arthritis, and is an antidote for acidity in the stomach because it is alkaline. It is rich in vitamins A and D and provides all the B-complex vitamins. Commercial yogurts invariably contain sugar, synthetic colouring and flavouring, and are too high in fat. It is best to make your own. Sterilize all equipment before use; bring one pint of milk to the boil, take it off the heat and allow to cool to the point where you can hold your finger in it. Put a dessertspoon of low-fat natural yogurt in a bowl and stir in the milk. Cover – it's best with a towel – and leave in a warm place for six to eight hours. If it is set properly, it should have layer of water on top. If not, put it back for a bit longer. Otherwise, drain off the water and chill. You can use your own yogurt as a starter for the next batch, but subsequent batches will get weaker and finally you need to start from scratch again. A healthier yogurt can be made by using skimmed, dried milk; mix the milk as instructed on the package.

### Garlic

This plant has long been synonymous with health, energy and longevity. It is one of the old country remedies – and for good reason. It is one of the best things for any circulatory problems, because it helps to clear the fatty substances from the blood vessels; it can prevent and greatly improve atherosclerosis. It's a great detoxicant, capable of clearing from the body waste matter that could hamper cellular activity. It is also a remarkable protector against bacterial and viral infections. Garlic can be added to salads, vegetable, fish and meat dishes. If you are worried about the after effects on the breath, chew some parsley – though it appears that the more garlic you eat, the more it becomes infused within your system and the less on your breath. Possibly one of the healthiest ways of eating garlic – and one of the most delicious – is how they use it on bread in Mediterranean country areas: rough local bread is covered with green olive oil, sprinkled with freshly chopped garlic and toasted on an open grill or barbecue. Don't be afraid to use garlic.

Play safe and avoid convenience, processed foods as much as possible. Work out a personal plan that is a compromise between your old habits and a new healthy regimen. Change is difficult. Gradually make yourself eat healthier. You don't have to change drastically from one day to the next, but set a goal for the future.

## THE SPECIAL POWER OF RAW FOOD

In the anti-aging diet, the recommendation is to try to eat fifty per cent of the daily quota in raw foods. This is not that easy, particularly in a cold climate, but the ultimate health rewards can be incredible. Vegetables and fruits are the natural therapeutics, and you get the best of the nutrients in their raw state. The most remarkable aspect of a raw food diet is the way in which it can completely clean out the body, get rid of toxins and all the sludge that is blocking up the normal working of the system. If you have been cheating, which of course we all do, the best way – in fact the only way – to compensate and give your body a chance to recuperate from excesses and almost start again from scratch, is to devote a week to a clean-out. This is actually the theory behind most health resorts, but if you are strong-willed you can do it at home. There are two ways: a fast on concentrated juices, which is the powerful approach – or you eat only raw foods. Whichever regime you choose, it is important never to mix fruit and vegetables. One meal for each, otherwise the digestive juices and processes get too mixed up. Going on to raw foods or juices is not only a health kick, but a very valid way to lose weight.

**juice fasting** – to be effective a fast should last for a minimum of four days, but not longer than a week unless under medical supervision. Fasting on juices is now considered much more beneficial than fasting on water alone, or water and lemon. During a fast, the body burns and digests unwanted substances. Although you will lose weight while fasting, the main benefit is the way the body is cleansed inside and out – improvement in skin tone, for instance, can be remarkable. During the process, the eliminating organs – lungs, liver, kidney and skin – are working hard getting rid of waste matter and toxins. Fasting gives a rest to the digestive organs and at the same time helps to stabilize the nerves. It also stimulates the glandular and hormone network, puts new life into the mind and because of the quality of the juice intake, it normalizes vitamin and mineral balance. At first, there may be some side effects, which is good news because this means that the toxins are being released from the body. You may find you have skin outbreaks, dark urine, bad breath, a dizzy feeling and some sweating. It is a temporary phase, so carry on as usual. Also don't take to your bed and rest too much; during a fast it is important to remain active. You'll feel a different woman at the end of it. You can drink any fruit or vegetable juice (you'll need to invest in a juice extractor, one of your best investments for health in fact) with a limit of four pints a day. Don't mix fruit and vegetables in one 'meal' and if you prefer to stick just to one, that's fine. When you break the fast, do so by slowly adding foods until you reach the daily anti-aging diet level. It is not good for the body to be plunged immediately into regular food intake – you'll need about three or four days to get back to normal healthy eating.

*Olivia Newton-John*
'I eat home-made muesli for breakfast, yogurt and juice for lunch and have a proper dinner. I weigh myself every day and won't allow a variation of more than 2lb. At home I ride every day and play a lot of tennis. In the morning I splash cold water on my face then get into the fresh air for 10 minutes.'

**raw fruit diet** – a marvellous way to rejuvenate the body and for many women more acceptable than subsisting on just juices. It is very simple: you eat the usual three meals a day, but everything you take must be uncooked. There is a wide choice of food available – fresh fruits and vegetables with yogurt included to use as a dressing. You are allowed herbs and seasonings (but only the merest hint of salt) plus a maximum of a tablespoon of olive oil a day if you need it for a dressing. You can drink herb teas, mineral water, fruit or vegetable juices, but nothing else.

It is important to remember not to mix the fruit and vegetables in the same meal; it is also better to start the day with fruit and this will provide immediate energy and raise your blood sugar level. A raw food diet should be undertaken for a minimum of a week, if you can continue for an additional week, so much the better.

## The Super Fruits and Vegetables

All fruits and vegetables that are fresh are healthy, but some have particularly beneficial properties, so include these in your normal daily diet, not only when doing a juice or raw food clean-out.

**apple** – traditionally the great health provider, both on a preventive and curative level. It is particularly high in mineral salts – a larger quantity of phosphates than any other fruit or vegetable – and rich in vitamins. It also provides pectin, amino acids and natural sugars. Some doctors advise apples to combat excess cholesterol in the blood.

**blackberry** – this fruit is rich in mineral salts and known to help anaemia; it's a tonic and a restorative treatment for the mucous membranes.

**grapefruit** – although not the slimming miracle some diets proclaim, it is very beneficial because of the high vitamin C content, and it provides good amounts of potassium, magnesium and calcium.

**lemon** – just about the most valuable of all fruits for preserving health. It is full of vitamin C; it can neutralize harmful and infectious bacteria, which is why in many hot climates the juice of a lemon is a last-minute addition to meat and fish dishes. Lemons, together with limes, are digestion-promoting foods and a great stimulant to the liver; lemon juice should be diluted with mineral water if drunk on its own and in this way helps to dissolve uric acid crystals in the tissues – these could cause gout. Lemon juice is a remarkable counter remedy for excess drinking because of its capacity to rejuvenate the liver. A day should not go by without a glass, and if you are watching weight, lemon juice first thing in the morning is ideal.

**orange** – as high as lemon in vitamin C but even better in its calcium content, with levels of phosphorus and potassium very good too. Although oranges are usually consumed as a juice, try to eat some raw for the cellulose fibre.

*Raquel Welch*
'I never, ever have salt or sugar. I don't drink and I alternate between grilled meat, boiled fish and steamed green vegetables. I have an apple at 4 o'clock every day. I do an hour of yoga. With yoga I don't need to make myself up or dress sexily anymore. I am sexy.'

**papaya** – also known as paw-paw, this tropical fruit is an amazing health restorer and its reputation as a rejuvenator is due to its ability to keep the digestive system in peak condition. It is extremely rich in the enzymes that make the digestion of protein possible. Papaya is also extremely rich in vitamins, in particular vitamin C and has the highest calcium content of any fruit. It is used in clinics as a cleansing and therapeutic food.

**pineapple** – another fruit that is hailed for its cleansing powers and also as an aid to the dieter. Both claims are true because of its high mineral salt content, especially potassium.

**strawberry** – here you'll find a rich supply of salicylic acid which aids the functions of the liver, kidneys and joints; it is a good detoxifying agent and large quantities have been known to cure gout. Because it is very high in iron, the strawberry is often used in the treatment of anaemia; it also helps to lower blood pressure.

**artichoke** – one of the few vegetables that contain therapeutically valuable oils which have a stabilizing effect on the metabolism. It is very beneficial for the liver and acts as a diuretic if you suffer from water retention.

**avocado** – a nutritious source of vegetable protein, it is also high in vitamin C and a potent way to get therapeutic amounts of magnesium and potassium.

**beetroot** – amino acids here are good in both quality and quantity and so this vegetable is always used by naturopathic practitioners on a curative basis. It is a general body tonic, and when combined with carrot and cucumber juice it can help liver and kidney problems – or on the other hand, prevent them.

**cabbage** – a humble vegetable, ignored by many, but it should be taken up in a big way, because the cabbage offers many aids to health. It is tops in vitamin C, and has generous amounts of calcium, magnesium and potassium. As a juice it has proved valuable for cirrhosis of the liver, especially when caused by alcoholism, so logically it is a good preventive. It also helps protect against arthritis and gout.

**carrot** – one of the best aids for the liver because carrots increase the number of red blood corpuscles. The high vitamin A content is the benefactor, but don't take more than a glass of concentrated juice a day. It is true that carrots help eyes, because they aid night-sight and also act as a restorer for eyes strained by bright lights – incidentally, vitamin A is destroyed by harsh lighting.

**celery** – a good source of chlorides, potassium and sodium; one of the few vegetables high in essential oils that have a calming effect on the nervous system. Celery also has strong diuretic powers, which makes it useful for slimming but also as a help to control arthritis, rheumatism and gout.

**cucumber** – the most important property of cucumber is its ability to draw water out of tissues and with it any toxic matter. It is therefore a prime interest to those who retain fluid, and also for all rheumatic conditions. This water-lure aspect of cucumber is the reason why it is recommended for the face, for puffy eyes.

**lettuce** – all the minerals are present, including iodine, phosphorus, iron, copper, cobalt, zinc, calcium, manganese and potassium. It could be your most important restorer of mineral balance. The outer green leaves are the most beneficial and make sure the lettuce is very fresh. Lettuce also has the ability to calm the nervous system and is actually prescribed for palpitations and a glass of juice is helpful for insomniacs.

**onion** – the oils that give the onion its pungency are therapeutic agents which have a great cleansing and purifying effect. The onion has the same powers, but to a lesser degree, as garlic. It stimulates the growth of beneficial bacteria in the intestines, normalizes the nervous system, lowers blood pressure and aids digestion and secretion of bile.

**potato** – like the cabbage, this common vegetable should be eaten every day. First of all, it is not fattening – sugars and fats are far worse – and it contains masses of vitamin C plus the valuable B vitamins and a rich supply of potassium. It is a staple food and should be used as such – the raw juice is very potent and even if you drink the water in which potatoes have been boiled you will reap some benefit. The essential nutrients lie just under the skin, so the healthy way to eat potatoes is scrubbed, baked or boiled but never peeled.

**spinach** – when you actually look at the vitamin and mineral content of spinach, it is perfectly reasonable to accept that Popeye could do incredible things after eating it. It is remarkably high in magnesium, potassium and sodium; its calcium content is way ahead of any other vegetable; it's the only one with a high folic acid content – a very important anti-aging vitamin in the B group – and it has a lot of vitamin C. Eat spinach raw, it makes a great salad, because if you cook it too long and in too much water you will destroy all the valuable vitamins.

**watercress** – rich in sulphur, nitrogen and iodine. It is one of the finest blood purifiers and is an excellent source of vitamins A and C. It is known as a tonic for liver and kidney troubles.

Potatoes are good for you – eat them every day because they are a great source of vitamins and minerals. Leave on the skin as that is where most of the nutrients are focused. Potatoes will not make you fat. Sugar and fat will. Potatoes should be our staple food.

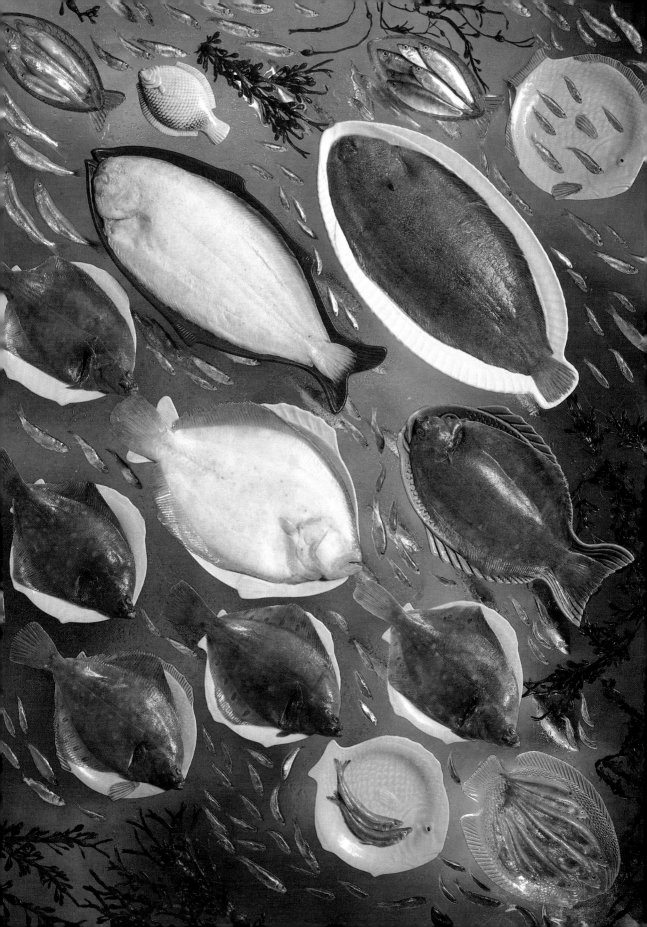

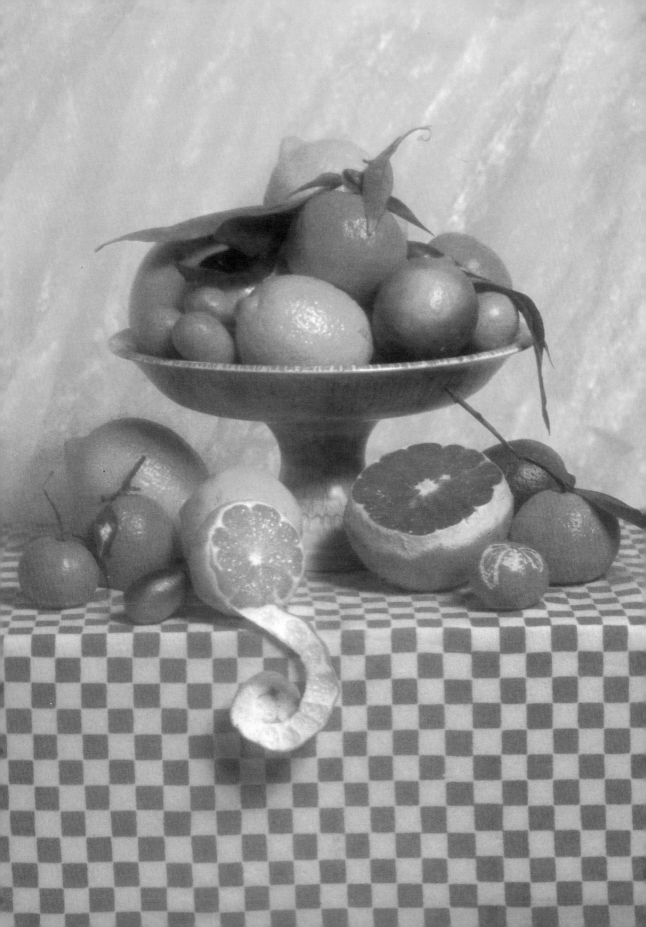

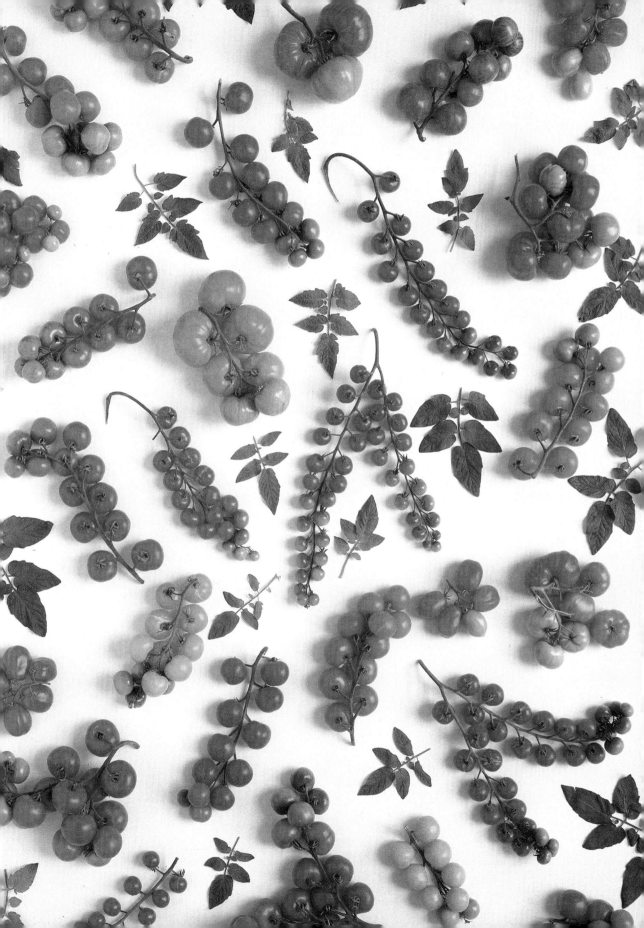

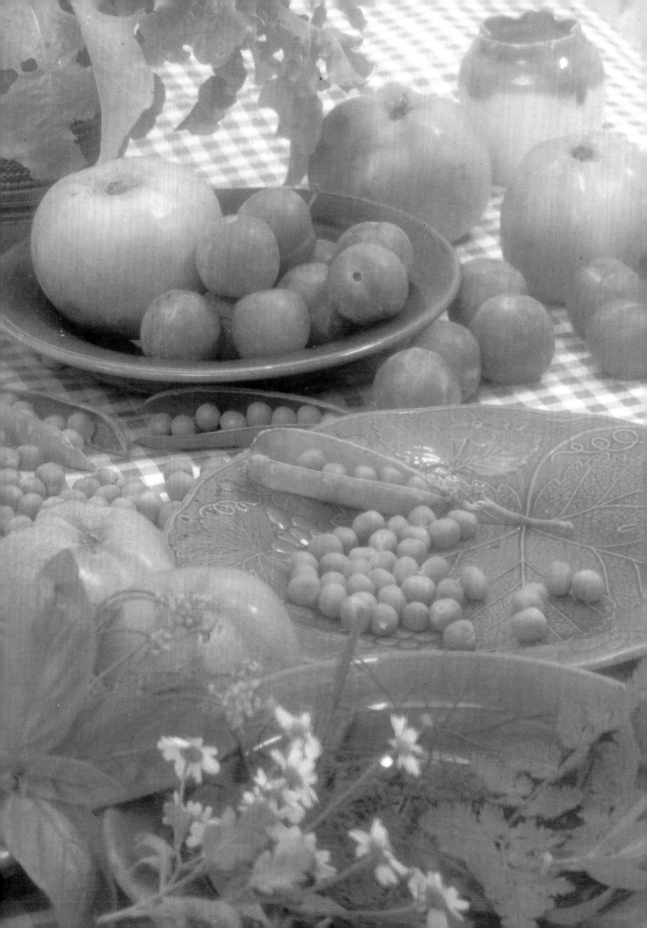

# Calorie Chart

Even on a healthy diet you need to watch the calories in order to balance your food intake with your energy output during activities. It is not necessary to know the exact calorie count, but gradually to familiarize yourself with the energy units each type of food has. In time it will become second nature and you won't have to consult the charts at all. It is, in fact, impossible to estimate exact calorie figures because there are so many dependent factors – time of year, place produce was grown, lapse between harvesting and measuring, and in the case of meat, fish and poultry there is always a variant in fat content. This is why you can check food on different calorie charts and find considerable differences in the figures. All calorie charts have to be taken as a guide only. This one features the healthy, natural foods – there's no mention of tinned or convenience foods of any kind, nor biscuits, cakes, desserts, because you shouldn't be eating them.

| DAIRY PRODUCE | | | Calories |
|---|---|---|---|
| butter | | 1oz (30g) | 220 |
| cheese | Brie | 1oz (30g) | 85 |
| | Camembert | 1oz (30g) | 85 |
| | cottage cheese | 1oz (30g) | 20 |
| | Cheddar | 1oz (30g) | 110 |
| | cream cheese | 1oz (30g) | 120 |
| | Danish Blue | 1oz (30g) | 100 |
| | Edam | 1oz (30g) | 85 |
| | Gouda | 1oz (30g) | 85 |
| | Parmesan | 1oz (30g) | 120 |
| | Stilton | 1oz (30g) | 130 |
| cream | single | tablespoon | 45 |
| | double | tablespoon | 110 |
| | clotted | tablespoon | 140 |
| eggs | small | | 75 |
| | medium | | 80 |
| | large | | 85 |
| | yolk | | 65–70 |
| | white | | 10–15 |
| | boiled | | 75–85 |
| | fried | | 130–150 |
| milk | whole milk | 1 fl oz (30ml) | 20 |
| | long life | 1 fl oz (30ml) | 20 |
| | goat's milk | 1 fl oz (30ml) | 20 |
| | skim | 1 fl oz (30ml) | 10 |
| | powdered | 1oz (30g) | 140 |
| yogurt | natural | 1oz (30g) | 20 |
| | | 5oz (140g) | 100 |
| | fruit | 1oz (30g) | 30 |
| | low-fat | 1oz (30g) | 15 |

| SWEETENERS | | | Calories |
|---|---|---|---|
| honey | | 1oz (30g) | 80 |
| sugar | brown | 1oz (30g) | 110 |

| FRUIT AND NUTS | | | Calories |
|---|---|---|---|
| almonds | | 1oz (30g) | 170 |
| apple | raw | | 50 |
| | stewed, no sugar | 1oz (30g) | 10 |
| apricot | fresh | 1 | 10 |
| | dried | 1oz (30g) | 65 |
| banana | | medium | 65 |
| blackberries | | 1oz (30g) | 8 |
| blackcurrants | | 1oz (30g) | 12 |
| cherries | | 1oz (30g) | 10 |
| figs | stewed, no sugar | 1oz (30g) | 35 |
| | dried | $\frac{3}{4}$oz (20g) | 45 |
| gooseberries | | 1oz (30g) | 10 |
| grapefruit | | $\frac{1}{2}$ | 30 |
| grapes | | 1oz (30g) | 15 |
| lemon | | medium | 15 |
| loganberries | | 1oz (30g) | 5 |
| lychees | | 1oz (30g) | 20 |
| melon | | 4oz (115g) | 16 |
| orange | | medium | 50 |
| peach | | medium | 40 |
| peanuts | shelled | 1oz (30g) | 160 |
| pear | | medium | 60 |
| pineapple | | 1oz (30g) | 15 |
| plums | | large | 20 |
| | stewed, no sugar | 1oz (30g) | 6 |
| prunes | stewed, no sugar | 1oz (30g) | 20 |
| raisins | | 1oz (30g) | 80 |
| raspberries | | 1oz (30g) | 12 |
| rhubarb | | 1oz (30g) | 2 |
| strawberries | | 1oz (30g) | 10 |
| tangerine | | 1 | 20 |
| walnuts | | 1oz (30g) | 150 |

| MEAT | | | Calories |
|---|---|---|---|
| bacon | grilled | 1oz (30g) | 115 |
| beef | steak, grilled | 1oz (30g) | 55 |
| | | 4½oz (130g) | 250 |
| | roast | 1oz (30g) | 65 |
| | minced | 1oz (30g) | 65 |
| | hamburger | 1oz (30g) | 75 |
| | | 4oz (115g) | 300 |
| brains | calf or lamb | 1oz (30g) | 31 |
| chicken | roast | 1oz (30g) | 45 |
| | portion | 7oz (200g) | 315 |
| | poached | 1oz (30g) | 40 |
| duck | roast | 1oz (30g) | 90 |
| | portion | 7oz (200g) | 630 |
| gammon | baked | 1oz (30g) | 65 |
| goose | roast | 1oz (30g) | 90 |
| grouse | on bone, roast | 12oz (340g) | 290 |
| guinea fowl | on bone, roast | 12oz (340g) | 370 |
| ham | boiled | 1oz (30g) | 75 |
| kidney | grilled | 1oz (30g) | 40 |
| lamb | chop, grilled | 3oz (85g) | 200 |
| | roast | 1oz (30g) | 75 |
| | portion | 3oz (85g) | 225 |
| liver | grilled | 1oz (30g) | 70 |
| | pâté | 1oz (30g) | 100 |
| pheasant | roast | 1oz (30g) | 60 |
| pork | chop, grilled | 3oz (85g) | 300 |
| | roast | 1oz (30g) | 100 |
| sausages | grilled beef | 1oz (30g) | 60 |
| | grilled pork | 1oz (30g) | 90 |
| sweetbreads | braised | 1oz (30g) | 66 |
| tongue | boiled | 1oz (30g) | 85 |
| tripe | stewed | 1oz (30g) | 28 |
| turkey | roast | 1oz (30g) | 40 |
| | portion | 4oz (115g) | 160 |
| veal | roast | 1oz (30g) | 65 |
| | portion | 4oz (115g) | 260 |

| CEREALS | | | Calories |
|---|---|---|---|
| All Bran | | 1oz (30g) | 75 |
| bread | French | 1oz (30g) | 75 |
| | wholegrain | 1oz (30g) | 60 |
| barley | boiled | 1oz (30g) | 102 |
| cornflakes | | 1oz (30g) | 110 |
| cripsbread | | 1 slice | 20–30 |
| flour | wholemeal | 1oz (30g) | 95 |
| melba toast | | 1 slice | 30 |
| muesli | | 1oz (30g) | 120 |
| pasta | cooked | 1oz (30g) | 35 |
| porridge | with water | 4oz (115g) | 50 |
| rice | boiled | 1oz (30g) | 35 |
| wheatgerm | | 1oz (30g) | 100 |
| yeast | | 1oz (30g) | 100 |
| yeast extract | | 1oz (30g) | 35 |

| FISH | | | Calories |
|---|---|---|---|
| anchovies | | 1oz (30g) | 40 |
| caviar | | 1oz (30g) | 75 |
| clams | | 1oz (30g) | 20 |
| cod | grilled | 1oz (30g) | 35 |
| | on the bone | 7oz (200g) | 140 |
| cod's roe | | 1oz (30g) | 60 |
| crab | | 1oz (30g) | 30 |
| fish-cakes | | 1oz (30g) | 45 |
| fish fingers | | 1oz (30g) | 60 |
| haddock | grilled | 1oz (30g) | 35 |
| | poached | 1oz (30g) | 25 |
| | smoked | 1oz (30g) | 30 |
| hake | | 1oz (30g) | 30 |
| halibut | | 1oz (30g) | 40 |
| kedgeree | | 4oz (115g) | 240 |
| kipper | | 1oz (30g) | 45 |
| lobster | | 1oz (30g) | 30 |
| mackerel | grilled | 1oz (30g) | 45 |
| | smoked | 1oz (30g) | 70 |
| mussels | shelled | 1oz (30g) | 25 |
| oysters | 6 | 3oz (85g) | 45 |
| plaice | | 1oz (30g) | 20 |
| prawns | shelled | 1oz (30g) | 30 |
| red mullet | | 1oz (30g) | 40 |
| salmon | boiled | 1oz (30g) | 50 |
| | smoked | 1oz (30g) | 45 |
| | tinned | 1oz (30g) | 45 |
| sardines | tinned in oil | 1oz (30g) | 75 |
| scampi | boiled | 1oz (30g) | 30 |
| | fried in breadcrumbs | 1oz (30g) | 90 |
| sea bass | | 1oz (30g) | 30 |
| shrimps | | 1oz (30g) | 30 |
| sole | poached | 1oz (30g) | 25 |
| trout | grilled | 1oz (30g) | 30 |
| | smoked | 1oz (30g) | 30 |
| tuna | tinned | 1oz (30g) | 80 |

| DRESSING, OILS, SAUCES | | Calories |
|---|---|---|
| French dressing | 1oz (30g) | 125 |
| horseradish sauce | ½oz (15g) | 30 |
| low-down dressing | 1oz (30g) | 30 |
| mayonnaise | 1oz (30g) | 200 |
| mustard | 1oz (30g) | 5 |
| olive oil | 1 fl oz (30ml) | 270 |
| sunflower oil | 1 fl oz (30ml) | 270 |
| vinegar | 1 fl oz (30ml) | 1 |
| Worcestershire sauce | 1oz (30g) | 50 |

## VEGETABLES

| | | | Calories |
|---|---|---|---|
| artichoke | globe, boiled | 8oz (225g) | 15 |
| | heart, boiled | 4oz (115g) | 15 |
| asparagus | | 3 stalks | 10 |
| aubergine | boiled | 2oz (55g) | 10 |
| | fried | 2oz (55g) | 70 |
| avocado | | $\frac{1}{2}$ medium | 100 |
| bamboo shoots | | 2oz (55g) | 15 |
| beans | broad | 2oz (55g) | 30 |
| | butter | 2oz (55g) | 50 |
| | runner | 2oz (55g) | 10 |
| | kidney | 2oz (55g) | 185 |
| | lima | 2oz (55g) | 70 |
| | soya | 2oz (55g) | 250 |
| | bean sprouts | 2oz (55g) | 16 |
| brussel sprouts | | 2oz (55g) | 10 |
| cabbage | boiled | 2oz (55g) | 16 |
| carrots | raw | 1 medium | 10 |
| | boiled | 2oz (55g) | 20 |
| cauliflower | raw | 1oz (30g) | 6 |
| | boiled | 2oz (55g) | 15 |
| celeriac | | 1oz (30g) | 4 |
| celery | raw | 1 stick | 2 |
| | boiled | 2oz (55g) | 5 |
| chicory | raw | 1oz (30g) | 3 |
| corn on the cob | boiled | 5oz (140g) | 170 |
| courgette | raw | 1oz (30g) | 3 |
| | boiled | 2oz (55g) | 6 |
| cucumber | raw | 1oz (30g) | 3 |
| endive | raw | 1oz (30g) | 3 |
| garlic | raw | 1 clove | 1 |
| leeks | boiled | 2oz (55g) | 15 |
| lentils | boiled | 1oz (30g) | 30 |
| lettuce | raw | 1oz (30g) | 3 |
| marrow | boiled | 2oz (30g) | 4 |
| mushrooms | raw | 1oz (30g) | 7 |
| | boiled | 2oz (55g) | 6 |
| | fried | 2oz (55g) | 100 |
| olives | with stones | 1oz (55g) | 23 |
| onions | raw | 1oz (30g) | 8 |
| | boiled | 2oz (55g) | 16 |
| parsnips | boiled | 2oz (55g) | 35 |
| peas | boiled | 2oz (55g) | 35 |
| peppers | raw | 1oz (30g) | 4 |
| potatoes | boiled | 2oz (55g) | 45 |
| | new | 2oz (55g) | 42 |
| | chips | 2oz (55g) | 180 |
| radishes | raw | 1oz (30g) | 4 |
| spinach | raw | 1oz (30g) | 10 |
| | boiled | 2oz (55g) | 18 |
| tomato | raw | 1oz (30g) | 4 |
| turnips | boiled | 2oz (55g) | 10 |
| water chestnuts | tinned | 1oz (30g) | 15 |
| watercress | raw | 1oz (30g) | 10 |

## SOUPS – home-made

| | | Calories |
|---|---|---|
| chicken | $\frac{1}{4}$pt (1.4dl) | 50 |
| consommé | $\frac{1}{4}$pt (1.4dl) | 25 |
| cucumber | $\frac{1}{4}$pt (1.4dl) | 50 |
| fish | $\frac{1}{4}$pt (1.4dl) | 75 |
| mushroom | $\frac{1}{4}$pt (1.4dl) | 50 |

## ALCOHOLIC DRINKS

| | | | Calories |
|---|---|---|---|
| beer | | $\frac{1}{2}$pt (2.8dl) | 90 |
| Champagne | | $\frac{1}{4}$pt (1.4dl) | 110 |
| cider | dry | $\frac{1}{2}$pt (2.8dl) | 100 |
| | sweet | $\frac{1}{2}$pt (2.8dl) | 120 |
| cognac | | 1 fl oz (30ml) | 65 |
| gin | | 1 fl oz (30ml) | 65 |
| liqueurs | average | 1 fl oz (30ml) | 110 |
| port | | 1 fl oz (30ml) | 45 |
| rum | | 1 fl oz (30ml) | 65 |
| sherry | dry and medium | 1 fl oz (30ml) | 35 |
| vermouth | dry | $2\frac{1}{2}$ fl oz (70ml) | 140 |
| | sweet | $2\frac{1}{2}$ fl oz (70ml) | 150 |
| vodka | | 1 fl oz (30ml) | 65 |
| whisky | | 1 fl oz (30ml) | 65 |
| wine | red, dry | 1 fl oz (30ml) | 20 |
| | red, sweet | 1 fl oz (30ml) | 25 |
| | white, dry | 1 fl oz (30ml) | 20 |
| | white, sweet | 1 fl oz (30ml) | 25 |

## NON-ALCOHOLIC DRINKS

| | | | Calories |
|---|---|---|---|
| apple juice | natural | $\frac{1}{4}$pt (1.4ml) | 50 |
| bitter lemon | | 4 fl oz (1.1dl) | 40 |
| carrot juice | natural | $\frac{1}{4}$pt (1.4dl) | 32 |
| coffee | black | 1 cup | 4 |
| | white | 1 cup | 20 |
| | white with sugar | 1 cup | 50 |
| Cola types | | $\frac{1}{4}$pt (1.4dl) | 60 |
| ginger ale | | $\frac{1}{4}$pt (1.4dl) | 35 |
| grapefruit juice | | $\frac{1}{4}$pt (1.4dl) | 45 |
| lemon juice | | 1 fl oz (30ml) | 2 |
| orange juice | natural | $\frac{1}{4}$pt (1.4dl) | 50 |
| pineapple juice | | $\frac{1}{4}$pt (1.4dl) | 75 |
| tea | with lemon | 1 cup | 2 |
| | with milk | 1 cup | 20 |
| | with milk/ sugar | 1 cup | 50 |
| tomato juice | | 1 fl oz (30ml) | 5 |
| tonic water | | $\frac{1}{4}$pt (1.4dl) | 30 |

# Check on weight: What is ideal?

Most women, it seems, whatever their age, worry about their weight. Whether twenty or fifty the battle to stay slim rages unabated – witness the enormous numbers of slimming books and products sold. But as you grow older the sad news is that chances are you will put on weight. Underweight women are in the minority and usually it has to do with some basic metabolic disorder which needs to have medical control. Too thin can be as potentially hazardous as too fat. However, if you are a normal, healthy woman in reasonable health you are going to have to watch your weight, simply because the risk of so many diseases is in direct ratio to the number of pounds you are overweight. Also, and I don't care what doctors say – and they all do – about there being no reason for you to be fatter at forty than twenty, it is that much more difficult to keep the weight down even if you are eating the same amount and exercising as usual. Clearly something happens to the metabolism which has yet to be established, possibly a lowered metabolic rate, that necessitates your keeping an eagle eye on food intake, energy expenditure and fat accumulation. It is a bore, but it is important.

The ideal weight is an enigma. Charts originated with insurance companies who wanted to work out weights in relation to life expectancy. They came up with average figures, which work very well, but they are just that: average. If you are within the limits for your height, then you are doing all right in general terms. Only you can personally assess if you are fat or not – and all of us can do that if we are honest. There is no point in pursuing the thin-thin image if you are by nature a big woman. Dieting to be thin is pointless. Thin is not all that attractive anyway. Dieting to be in the peak of health is another matter. If you follow a healthy eating pattern, do some exercise, learn to be conscious of your body and its demands, you will quickly recognize at what weight you look and feel your best. That is the most important thing. So check the chart below to get a general idea, then check your body yourself to get the exact record. If you need to lose weight do it gradually. Calories do count and count them you must. Follow the anti-aging eating guide and check the calorie charts (page 113) to see how much energy-producing food you are taking in. The equation of weight control is very simple: calories-in minus calories-out in energy should equal nil. That is to keep your weight constant. If you want to lose weight you have to expend more calories in energy than you take in as food. As you get older you usually need fewer calories, but that is only because you may slow down on activity. If you keep active, you can continue to eat as usual. Calorie needs for a woman from twenty-five to forty-five are between 2,200 and 2,700 a day, from the ages of forty-five to fifty-five, between 2,200 and 2,500 a day and from fifty-five onwards around 2,000. If you want to lose weight, you must go lower.

You can easily work out your daily need by checking the calorie charts against the recommended anti-aging diet. If you want to try a specific regimen, refer to pages 234–252 where I have listed the

Overeating and in particular a high intake of animal protein is potentially dangerous to older people who are not active and have a slow metabolism.

weekly regimens undertaken at health resorts. They are actually a combination of the diet recommended in this chapter, plus watching your calories. If you are on a diet, don't weigh yourself every day, it can be discouraging. Do so every three or four days and then you get a pleasant surprise. Even if you are on a strict diet, it really only works for two weeks and then your weight reaches a plateau and will refuse to budge for days. Hang on, eat moderately, then go back on the diet regimen in a week's time, and you'll probably start losing again.

Weight can fluctuate from day to day and the menstrual cycle also can cause an increase during ovulation and the premenstrual phases. However, if you are not on a diet, I do recommend weighing-in every day, because if you can correct weight on a daily basis so much the better. The quickest way to take off weight for a day or two, if you have indulged too much, is to go on a one-fruit or one-vegetable only regimen: all strawberries, all pineapple, all courgettes, all string beans. It works. In this way you can continually balance excesses. If you do it only for a day, it is beneficial.

*Susan George*
'I went through a stage of eating everything, then at last I regulated myself. I lost weight gradually by eating the right foods. I never go without breakfast – cereal and fruit then boiled eggs and always brown bread. Today I am an active, outdoor person, although I never do anything to excess.'

| HEIGHT (BAREFOOT) | | SMALL FRAME kg | lb | MEDIUM FRAME kg | lb | LARGE FRAME kg | lb |
|---|---|---|---|---|---|---|---|
| 1.42m | 4'8" | 39–42 | 86–92 | 41–46 | 90–101 | 44–51 | 98–113 |
| 1.45m | 4'9" | 40–43 | 88–95 | 42–47 | 92–104 | 45–53 | 100–116 |
| 1.47m | 4'10" | 41–44 | 91–98 | 44–49 | 96–107 | 47–54 | 104–120 |
| 1.50m | 4'11" | 43–46 | 95–102 | 44–50 | 98–111 | 49–56 | 107–123 |
| 1.52m | 5'0" | 44–47 | 96–104 | 46–52 | 102–114 | 50–57 | 110–126 |
| 1.55m | 5'1" | 45–49 | 99–107 | 48–53 | 105–117 | 51–59 | 113–129 |
| 1.57m | 5'2" | 46–50 | 102–110 | 49–55 | 108–121 | 53–60 | 116–133 |
| 1.60m | 5'3" | 48–51 | 105–113 | 50–57 | 111–125 | 54–62 | 120–137 |
| 1.62m | 5'4" | 49–53 | 108–116 | 52–57 | 114–128 | 56–64 | 123–140 |
| 1.65m | 5'5" | 50–54 | 111–119 | 53–60 | 116–131 | 57–65 | 126–143 |
| 1.68m | 5'6" | 52–56 | 114–123 | 54–62 | 120–136 | 59–67 | 130–147 |
| 1.70m | 5'7" | 54–58 | 118–127 | 57–64 | 125–140 | 61–69 | 134–151 |
| 1.73m | 5'8" | 56–60 | 122–131 | 59–65 | 129–144 | 63–70 | 138–155 |
| 1.76m | 5'9" | 57–61 | 126–135 | 60–68 | 133–149 | 65–73 | 143–160 |
| 1.78m | 5'10" | 59–64 | 130–140 | 62–69 | 137–152 | 67–75 | 147–165 |
| 1.81m | 5'11" | 61–65 | 134–144 | 64–71 | 141–156 | 68–77 | 150–169 |
| 1.83m | 6'0" | 63–67 | 138–148 | 66–73 | 145–160 | 70–79 | 154–174 |

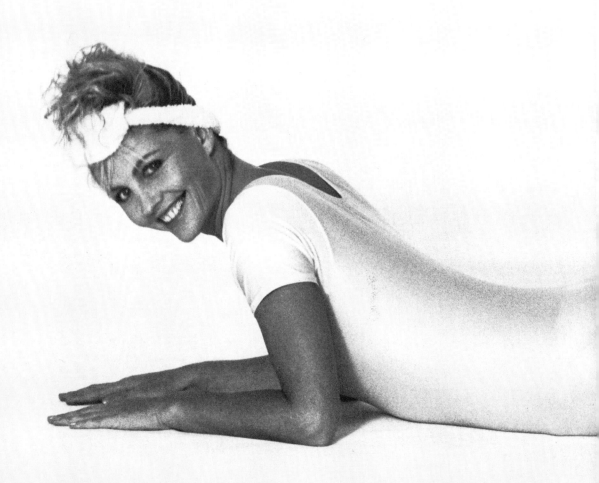

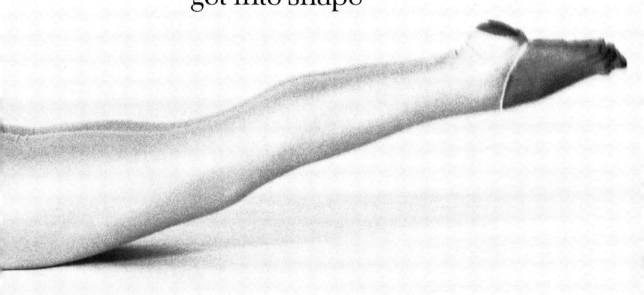

# FITNESS
## It's never too late to get into shape

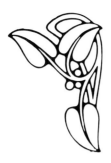

Exercise is definitely an antidote for age and you can start at any point in your life, and at any level of fitness. What you do and how you approach it depends on your age and inclination. All activities are great, but if you don't do them regularly they are meaningless. However, if you've never exercised before, it is extremely important to realize from the start that you must get into it gradually, particularly if you're older. It's all very well to be inspired to supreme effort, but if you do too much too soon you can seriously damage your body and health.

Exercising regularly in your twenties and establishing the habit for life will be of enormous benefit in keeping you looking and feeling young and healthy but there's no reason why an older woman can't do as much as a younger one once the body has been trained. There are examples of marathon runners in their seventies. It's a question of building up stamina and disciplining muscles. Bodywork taken step by step on a daily basis can result in your having a better body at forty or fifty than you had at twenty.

Exercise along with the right food is the basis of fitness and good health. It gets the circulation going, keeps the body supple and tones the muscles. It puts a jaunty spring in your step, bolsters your energy level and can help hold depression at bay. All these qualities are associated with youth, and if you have them you immediately look younger, modern, vital. Exercise prevents the body from taking on an older aura. If you feel fit and are in control of your moving systems, you will never get that stooped look, never drag your feet, never walk rigidly.

Exercise is so significant in establishing your level of wellbeing that even if you eat an inadequate diet, the benefits of recharged metabolism compensate for dietary inadequacies. The healthiest diet in the world can be to no avail if you are sedentary because the body cannot properly digest, utilize or eliminate the food. Of all the nutrients you require, oxygen is the most important.

The old attitude to exercise was to work at specific areas to whittle away inches, shape and firm. Most women are, of course, in search of a better body and while that end result of exercise still holds good, the new attitude and methods go further. Now exercise is geared to put you on a new level of fitness, both physically and mentally. The exercise plans worked out on the following pages will help you live longer and look younger as well as improve shape because their principle is to promote good health and clockwork metabolism. They also provide high energy levels and a new freedom of body and spirit that is fundamental to true health and beauty.

A word on shape and size. Every woman has her own perfect individual shape which is primarily dependent on body type and the skeletal proportions. This doesn't necessarily mean slender. Some women look and feel better when they are big. By big, I don't include huge or obese. But it is possible to be a naturally big woman and be in good condition. You can be big without carrying excess fat. Big can mean firmness and controlled curves. It can also look very good particularly in middle age. If you aim to be too skinny it can actually be aging.

It is a good idea to think for a moment about your shape in relation to your character, fitness level and lifestyle. You know without having to check guidelines whether you are too fat or too flabby. You know if it's affecting your daily activities and your health. Don't be cajoled into believing that it is only the lean body that's ideal. Think of your body as an expression of yourself, not as something to be assessed by others and judged by model standards.

Exercise is the best way to get in touch with your body. By all means look at your shape and decide what should be done to improve it, but the main thing is to think about how fit it is, how flexible, how mobile, how it functions, how comfortable you feel about it.

If you start looking at your body from within, you'll think of it differently. You'll come to realize that exercise is not something to just trim down the surface. Throughout the following pages I want to convince you that exercise is essential for healthy living. Motion is life. Exercise can be a joy and not a chore. It is possible to follow a simple, planned programme with ease and without taking up too much time.

Women who regularly do bodywork in some form – and that could include walking, cycling, a sport, calisthenics or Yoga – find that it has a definite, positive effect on their attitude towards themselves. Confidence is restored through such disciplines. Achievement on a physical level is quickly transferred to the mind. Competence is catching and can spread to encompass all aspects of life.

There's another side benefit and one that is very significant in relation to hectic modern living. Exercise helps you to recover more quickly from stress. This is because it disperses and uses up any excess adrenalin in the body. Adrenalin is the hormone that the body unconsciously summons in an emergency in preparation for a fight or flight situation. Nowadays it is invariably emotional or mental harassment that causes the adrenalin to flow and because this rarely leads to physical flight or action, the adrenalin is stored, adversely affecting moods, bringing on tiredness and straining the heart. A quick bout of exercise can alleviate it.

The first rule: start slowly. Don't be too ambitious, don't attempt a programme that doesn't stand a chance of being kept up. There are an awful lot of degrees between being unfit and superfit. What's wrong with aiming to be just fit? There's a vast difference between doing and overdoing. Moderation is the key and don't let anyone or any article convince you that a certain number of hours and effort to the point of agony are essential. Some fitness freaks have ended up with sprained ankles, wobbly knees, prolapsed organs, spine injuries and strained hearts.

The truth is you can get yourself fit by exercising for half an hour three times a week. It's as easy as that. But exercises have to be done at a certain pace in order to increase intake of oxygen and get the

Exercise during menstruation: forget the old idea usually handed down from mothers, even from grandmothers, that you should have no physical activity during your period. Most doctors now agree that not only is it all right, but that there are positive benefits. A fit body is better able to cope with any stress, and any exercise continued during menstruation can help relieve back pain and stomach cramps. Routines may have to be calmed down to a degree, but that's better than eliminating them altogether. You may have a heavy flow on the first or second day which makes any vigorous activity impractical, but try to do a little, and on subsequent days any moderate activity can only but be positive. Bear in mind that many Olympic athletes have performed magnificently during menstrual periods.

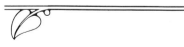

heart pumping faster. They should, however, be done within your capabilities at that time. If you expect more of yourself than is possible or even reasonable, guilt due to non-achievement can convince you there's no point in carrying on.

And don't force it. Making yourself work harder is a gradual process. The ideal is to work up to doing something every day which should be developed over a period of four to six weeks. It doesn't have to be the same routine every day, which many exercise programmes recommend. If you are working on a crash course, fine, but if your plan is now to start thinking of exercise as a life-long project, I cannot stress too strongly the need to diversify for continued enjoyment. Walking can be alternated with swimming, cycling or a sport; an exercise workout can be balanced with aerobic dancing; Yoga can be practised at intervals. Monotony leads to boredom and that leads to evasion and finally to giving up completely.

The single most important aspect is regularity. Exercise benefits cannot be stored. It is far better to do a little every day than an energetic bout once in a while. If you are serious about elevating your fitness level, changing the shape of your body and boosting morale, you have to make a commitment. And it certainly isn't easy. There are only a small minority of women who actually look forward to it, though oddly enough the thought and the mechanics of getting organized are more of a hassle than the actual action. I, for example, have to really push myself to achieve that daily minimum, despite the fact that I am the first to preach the rewards. It can be a nuisance and interfere with seemingly more important matters, but once you make yourself get into the habit, you'll be more eager to keep it up, simply because you begin to realize what good it does.

It helps to remind yourself that no matter what age you are, you can start to reverse the body clock by moving more. Remind yourself that youth and beauty have everything to do with energy – and that comes from physical activity more than from any other source. However, commonsense will tell you that everyone has lapses of inertia. It would be unrealistic to expect otherwise. But because you give up for a day, a week, a month or more, don't give up for ever. Your body has amazing recuperative powers, and even after a lapse you can once again bring it back into better condition. Of course, this is not as beneficial in the long run as continuous activity, but it is still streaks ahead of doing nothing.

It may sound as though I'm harping, but I must repeat that the best approach is moderate sustained activity throughout life regardless at what age you begin. It is interesting to note that when top level athletes stop their rigorous training, their bodies start to go downhill just like anyone else's despite earlier excessive activity and optimum fitness. There is no savings plan for fitness. It has to be an on-going investment.

Exercise and the menopause: no pause at all, please. In fact, just the opposite. With hormone production ebbing, it is even more important that the major contributory factors to health are out in full force. Now is the time you really need to draw on the beneficial resources of daily activity in order to maintain and further health levels. Exercise need not be strenuous, but should be a continuous moderate programme, so planned that you can keep it going at various levels of energy output for the rest of your life. Plan a feasible regime, an enjoyable and socially rewarding one. But keep it up.

## Exercise and weight loss

The connection between exercise and weight loss has no equation unless diet is taken into consideration. Exercise is something that gets you fitter and in better body form, but no matter how much you do or how energetically, weight loss is never to the degree you may imagine or hope for. In itself, exercise doesn't shed pounds quickly. For example, you would need to walk around thirty-five miles a day to get rid of just one pound if you kept your diet at a constant. Other more energetic activities do provide greater calorie expenditure but still not to the extent of making a significant contribution to weight loss.

Exercise combined with calorie control does make a difference. If you are on a diet and undertaking an exercise program of moderate intensity, you will most likely lose weight at a much speedier rate. More important is the fact that you will lose fat only, without depleting muscle tissue. The snag about going on a strict diet without exercise is that about a quarter of the weight loss is in the muscle mass. You end up with a higher ratio of fat than muscle which tends to make you feel inert, sluggish and look flabby. Also if you return to old eating habits, you'll regain weight in fatty areas not in muscle, which only exaggerates the problem and results can be worse than when you started.

Diet alone will never reshape your body. You may have a comfortingly lower reading on the scales, but it's a false achievement. Reshaping works only when exercise is involved and pounds lost this way are usually lost forever. However, when diet and exercise are combined you probably won't lose so quickly at the beginning. In fact, you may well gain weight. But don't panic, this is actually a good sign that pays dividends in the end.

Muscle tissue weighs more than fat, so if you are exercising well, you will be building up your muscles faster than you are shedding fat. The good news is that you'll be losing inches. This can happen very quickly and can often be more startlingly obvious in relation to your body image than a loss of pounds. Surely what you and others see, the pleasure that comes from clothes feeling loose, is more of a boost than a number on the scales?

But doesn't exercise create an appetite? One would think so, possibly based on memories of youth when after energetic sport one was starving. Probably you were fit and fairly lean in those days and you needed more food to replace the calories burned up, because you had little fat to supply the need. When you exercise, the body requires carbohydrates for energy. This comes directly from food, but when this is not readily available, the muscles begin to use fat for fuel. If you are low on fat, you will definitely feel hungry – and an extra bite or two will make no difference to your shape. If you are high on fat, you won't have an urge to eat, because fat is immediately at hand to be turned into energy for activity. Once active, you will find your appetite depressed. There's another factor involved: when you exercise your blood sugar level remains stable since the muscles are using more fat than sugar for fuel. It is a sudden drop in blood sugar level which makes you feel hungry.

## Exercise in relation to heart and lung performance

The two most crucial systems in the body are those of the lungs and the heart. They are interdependent – one cannot function effectively without the other. The oxygen in the air is our force of life. The more of it that gets into the lungs, the greater volume in the blood and the harder the heart needs to work. This results in more oxygenized blood being pumped around the body to benefit individual cells and revitalize the entire metabolism.

Genetically we are programmed to work on a level of oxygen determined by a mobile lifestyle. Modern life has reduced motion to about ten to fifteen per cent of what it was. Studies conducted in areas where people live long healthy lives have revealed that in all cases, lifestyle involved constant movement in the course of daily work.

Today, aside from a few exceptions, the only way to bring more oxygen into the system is to deliberately go out and get it – and that means going outdoors to breathe in fresh air by doing some form of activity. Even brisk walking is worthwhile – it was once known as the 'daily constitutional' but is now categorized as an 'aerobic activity'.

I'm often asked what exactly are 'aerobics'. It is simply today's somewhat technical term for getting air into your lungs at a certain level of exertion. Our ancestors were hardly aware of it because it was part of life. Now aerobic specialists are recommending programmes that are often too ambitious and I would imagine beyond the comprehension of former generations. It's important to look at the whole aerobic syndrome in sensible, practical terms.

Sports medics agree that we definitely do need to get more oxygen into our lungs and push our breathing and heart rate to higher levels of effort, but within certain safe limits, for a controlled time – usually twenty to thirty minutes. Why? Because most of us have got to the point of doing nothing, and because deeper conscious breathing will first of all strengthen the chest walls and empty the lungs of stale possibly toxic air, particularly if you are still smoking. In addition, if oxygen is passed through the lungs at a faster rate, it makes the heart work harder as it is forced to take care of the increase of oxygen in the blood. The heart is a muscle and like any other muscle, it needs to be exercised to be in optimum condition and perform at a peak. The stronger it gets, the fewer beats it needs to pump oxygen-carrying blood through the vascular system. In this way, you are finally able to reduce the overall effort of your heart, thereby preserving it.

Do you think you get enough exercise by pacing around the office or doing household chores all day? You may be exercising some muscles, though only to a degree, but you have done little for your heart, lungs and circulatory system. If you feel tired it has probably more to do with mental pressure or the boredom of doing routine things. Real physical exercise makes you feel relaxed in mind and body.

## AEROBICS: activities that step-up breathing and condition the heart

All exercise that calls for continuous movement and demands efficient use of oxygen is classified as aerobic. This includes everything from walking and cycling to sports and dancing. Jogging is not the only aerobic activity, as many women think. It is but one of many and if you don't like the idea of jogging, you can do equally well with any of the other activities.

All aerobics involve large muscle groups, primarily those of hips and legs. Ideally aerobics should be done outdoors in order to get the full value and exhilaration from fresh air – needless to say, that should be country air – but even when done indoors, the basic benefits remain the same. The duration period is recommended to be between twenty and thirty minutes; the frequency is a minimum of three times a week, preferably not on consecutive days.

The crux of effectiveness is effort. You may think you are exercising well, but you may not be appreciably increasing your heart beat. It is essential to work out your training level – that is the rate at which your heart should be beating during exercise in order to have a beneficial effect. Your heart should be beating from approximately seventy to eighty per cent of its safe maximum. Check the chart below to ascertain levels. However, if you have not exercised for a long time, begin by aiming for a sixty per cent of the maximum and gradually work upwards. Never, never push yourself too hard at first, it could be extremely harmful.

You need to take your pulse after you have been exercising hard for a few minutes. Put the ends of the first three fingers of your right hand on the artery on the inside of your left wrist. Count the number of beats in ten seconds and multiply by six to get the heartbeat rate per minute.

Taking your pulse can be tricky at first, but it is the only way to find out if you are making too little or too much effort. Adjust your effort accordingly. In time you will be completely in touch with your body and effort level and you won't need to check constantly.

After your forties, and if you have not exercised for ages, don't extend yourself beyond a count of 120 heartbeats per minute. If it is too high, check your pulse again after ten minutes and regulate activity. When you have finished exercising, wait for ten minutes and check your pulse. It should be down below 100, if not it's a sign to cut back on your exercise.

### What's best as you grow older?

Age isn't really a barrier, because all aerobics are possible if you are trained into them. What you undertake depends on your fitness level. Social sports – tennis, golf, riding etc – should be considered purely for enjoyment and not as a programmed work-out. To build up fitness you should work at one of the following: walking, jogging, swimming, skipping, cycling, dancing (see page 130 for the routine). Before embarking on any, it is good to do the warm-up sequence on

Exercise in relation to increased cell metabolism is under particular discussion at the moment. It is known that lean bodies have stepped-up metabolism, but now it is thought that if you exercise regularly – that is doing a continuous aerobic exercise three times a week – your metabolic rate will rise, thus food is assimilated and converted into energy much more quickly. It is not likely you will lose weight by exercising and still eating the same amount, but you will more easily be able to keep your weight and shape constant without repeatedly resorting to diets.

page 128. Commitment should be for twenty to thirty minutes three times a week.

The most important point: get to know your own capacity. Never get ahead of yourself, work gradually to the ideal effort level. Rushing not only invites trouble, it invariably causes it. If you are overdoing it, you'll have some or all of the following symptoms: severe breathlessness, tightness or pain in the chest, dizziness, lightheadedness, a feeling of nausea, cramp in muscles. Calm down, Rome wasn't built in a day and neither is your fitness. All healthy bodies are perfectly capable of getting into better condition, but it must be done in stages. If at first you don't succeed, it doesn't mean you never can. Listen to your body. Go along with its tempo and capabilities.

**walking** – the simplest way to exercise and maintain health. It may take up more time per session, but it has the great advantage of being feasible anytime and anywhere. For those of you who are self-conscious, it doesn't even look like exercise. You can actually walk your way to aerobic fitness if you do it properly. The most important thing is to walk briskly, a stroll will do nothing for fitness. Aim for a continuous easy movement at a consistent speed. You don't have to walk fast, but train yourself to be able to walk at a certain momentum for a specific length of time. Take good strides, swing arms, hold head high, breathe in deeply, look around you and enjoy the sights. Start by trying to walk 2.5 kilometres (one-and-a-half miles) in thirty minutes. Do this for the first week, then on the second week push yourself to do 3.5 kilometres (two miles) in thirty-five minutes. It is enough to continue at this level, but if you are more ambitious you should be able to cover 4 kilometres (two-and-a-half miles) in forty-five minutes. If you can do this, great. However, the minimum to get results is the second level – but the point is to try to get yourself into the habit of a daily stint at the moderate or maximum stage.

**jogging** – fast becoming very popular, but it is certainly not for everyone, and should be considered with caution as you grow older. Aim for fifteen minutes at first, three times a week. To begin with jog until you are tired, which may not be very far, then walk until you feel like jogging again. It is all a matter of personal capacity, judgement and enjoyment. Some people get a thrill out of it, others put it in the category of agony. Only you can decide if you like it – and then you gradually build up to your capacity. You may end up by jogging five miles every day or just two miles in thirty minutes three times a week. It doesn't matter, providing you work within the framework of your individual fitness programme. Style and technique are important because they could make the difference between accomplishment and frustration. Get the right footgear and watch foot movement. The heel of your foot should hit the ground a little ahead of the rest, then ease gently to the ball, finally move to the toes which will give you the spring to go into the next step.

## Working out a Lifetime Fitness Programme

It is essential to be realistic and plan a total fitness programme that can easily be integrated into your lifestyle. You need to consider three major things: your temperament, facilities and enjoyment. There is no benefit in planning a super regimen if it is not practical. But whatever you do, it should include the four essentials.

**flexibility exercises** – a quick series of movements to warm you up before a more intense aerobic session or a general work-out. (See page 128.)

**aerobics** – an activity or sport that forces you into continuous effort making heart and lungs work to capacity. (See page 130.)

**muscle workouts** – an exercise regimen that tones muscles, takes off inches and reshapes the body. (See page 132.)

**hatha yoga** – controlled precise movements that can be done at any pace, at any age. (See page 138.)

The more varied your bodywork the more likely you are to enjoy it – and stick to it. Try doing aerobics and muscle workouts on alternate days, then slip in a couple of sessions of yoga every week. You'll soon discover what you like doing most – then concentrate on it.

**stationary jogging** – for those who don't really want to expose themselves outdoors, running on the spot inside can provide aerobic benefits. It is, however, not recommended for women after menopause. For others, there is the chance of foot and ankle problems unless you do it properly. Don't jog barefoot unless on a special spring stand (see page 137). Otherwise wear sports shoes and do it on a resilient surface, rather than on bare boards. It is also not so easy to reach the required effort level. You need to raise the foot well and do sixty steps per minute. It can be very boring to keep this up for twenty minutes – possibly the only way is to have your favourite music playing.

**swimming** – this is really the best all round exercise but it has to be energetic swimming. You can build up beautiful muscles if you go about it seriously – this means every other day making yourself do a certain number of lengths. Breast stroke may not be the most sporty, but it is the most beneficial. Start by doing as many lengths as you can in twenty minutes. Keep to that for the first week, then aim for two lengths more in the same time, then go for those number of lengths in less time. Check your effort level constantly. You'll be amazed how quickly you can add up the lengths and reduce the time. On the last length, give an extra push to see what store of energy you now have.

**cycling** – this is a good endurance sport and could easily become part of your everyday life. Don't just pedal, make yourself go faster, go up hill. Check your effort. Start by cycling at a certain continuous speed for fifteen minutes and work up to half-an-hour, three times a week.

**skipping** – this may hardly sound serious, but it is actually a very effective aerobic exercise. Jump with both feet together or step over the rope with alternating feet. Start with a rate of seventy to eighty steps a minute and work up to 100.

No matter what enthusiasts say about woman's physical equality to man, the scientific fact is that the two glandular systems work differently and react differently to stress. Women should not take up too strenuous forms of exercise and this is even more significant as they grow older. It could cause hormonal imbalances and menstrual disturbances. Women benefit most from aerobic activities such as walking, mild jogging, swimming, cycling and dancing, stretching exercises, specific muscle work-outs and Hatha Yoga.

## HEARTBEAT AND EFFORT LEVELS

| Age | Safe maximum heartbeat per minute | Maximum Training level per minute | Beginner's goal |
|---|---|---|---|
| 35–40 | 180–185 | 130–145 | |
| 40–45 | 175–180 | 125–130 | 60% |
| 45–50 | 170–175 | 120–125 | of |
| 50–55 | 165–170 | 115–120 | safe |
| 55–60 | 160–165 | 110–115 | maximum |
| 60 upwards | 155–160 | 105–110 | heartbeat |

# First Steps to Fitness: warm-up movements to increase flexibility

A body that is not used to regular exercise cannot be plunged into frenzied activity without first gently coaxing the muscles into working order. Here is an easy series of stretches to get you moving. Do them as your first exercise routine, and then use them as a warm-up sequence before attempting the more precise body work-outs, before Yoga poses (see page 138) and before aerobics such as the dancing routine (see page 130), jogging, swimming etc.

**1** Start by standing at ease, legs apart. Stretch arms above head, really pushing the fingers upwards; hold for a moment, then using arms to force the body forwards, bend over pushing bottom out and finally thrust arms through the legs; hold to the count of three. Swing arms upwards and repeat the sequence ten times.

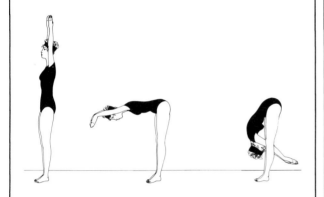

**2** Stand straight, legs apart. Clasp hands behind back and arch back as far as possible, making sure elbows are straight and arms really stretched. Bend forward bringing arms up high, hold to the count of five. Move slowly back, hold to the count of five. Repeat five times.

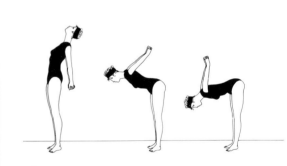

**3** Stand with feet well apart, clasp hands over head, elbows relaxed. Keeping the torso vertical, slowly bend to the right from the waist, hold to the count of three; then bend to the left, hold to the count of three. Do ten bends on either side.

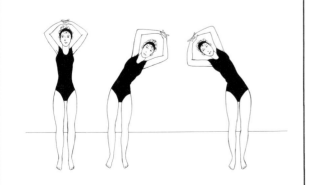

**4** Sit with legs bent and the soles of your feet together. Hold on to the feet, drop and relax the head and slowly bend forwards aiming to touch feet with the forehead. Feel the stretch in the back, hold to the count of ten. Relax. Repeat five times.

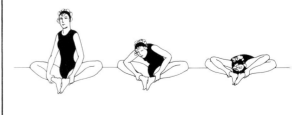

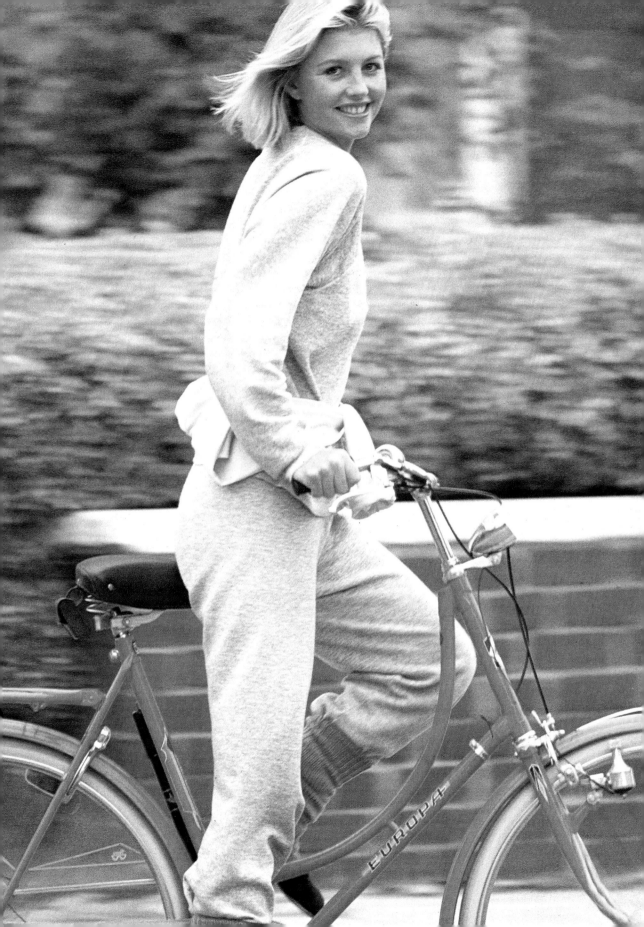

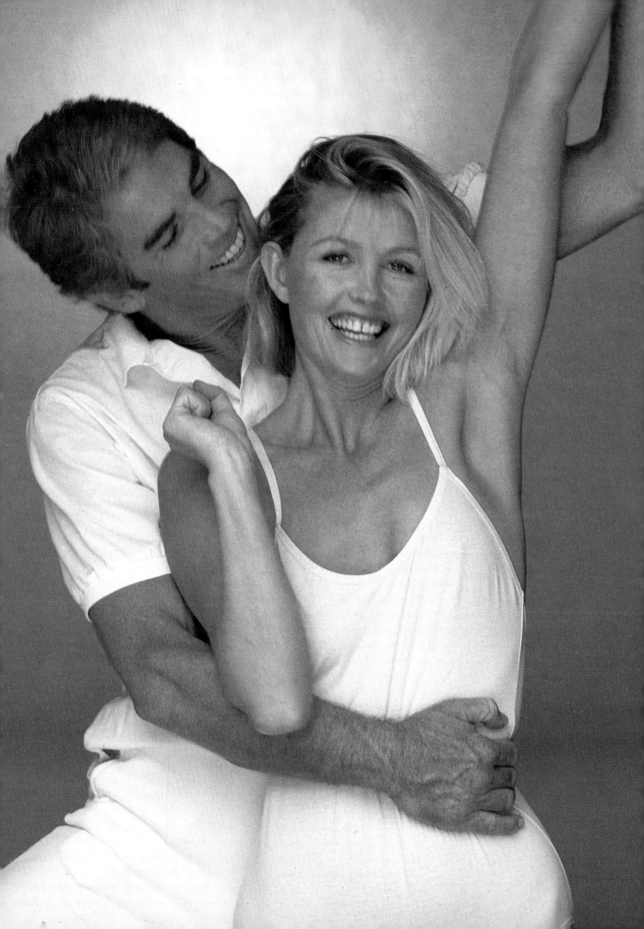

**5** Sit on the floor with your right leg straight and the left one bent with the heel firmly pushed against the bottom. Clasp the ankle with both hands, then straighten the leg pulling it as high as possible without relaxing the grip on the ankle; hold to the count of three. Return to the bent position. Do three times with each leg.

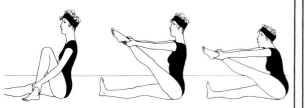

**7** Lie flat on back, arms at sides, palms flat on the floor. Using stomach muscles, slowly raise legs over the torso. Use arms and hands to balance the body and prevent wobbling. Raise legs high and support body on hands, hold to the count of three, then bend knees and lower to the forehead. Hold to the count of three. Slowly lower the back, unfurl the legs. Relax for a second, then repeat three times.

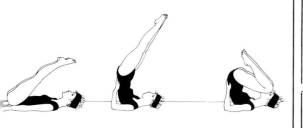

**Caution:** It is advisable for anyone over forty, who has not exercised for years to have a medical check-up before embarking on a serious exercise programme. You need to check physical fitness level and blood pressure. This may involve tests to evaluate your heart recovery level after exercise as well as your safe level of effort.

**6** Lie relaxed on your back, legs together, arms at sides. Bend knees, bringing heels as close to the bottom as possible. Slowly bring the knees to the chest using stomach and back muscles. Clasp hands around knees and really pull them close to the torso. Hold to the count of ten. Relax and return to starting position. Repeat five times.

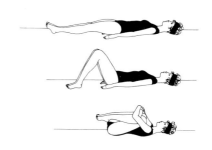

**8** Kneel on all fours, bring arms up to clasp behind shoulders, keeping elbows straight and arms stretched to their limit. Curve forward until head touches the floor, hold to the count of five. Repeat ten times.

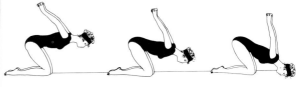

**9** Stand with legs apart, reach up high over the head with outstretched arms and hands, raise the body on tip toes; hold to the count of three, then completely relax by first curving the spine, then bending the knees, lowering the toes and finally sagging to the floor. Hold to the count of five, then stretch upwards again. Repeat five times.

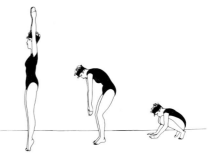

# Aerobic Dancing: 10 Minutes a Day

## A fun way to fitness

The whole idea of aerobic exercise is to get more air pumping into your lungs and to get your heart to work harder. This can be achieved by any outdoor sports, but if you want to do something in the privacy of home, this is a very effective routine. Do it to music and keep the body in constant movement. Start slowly, if you take it too fast at first you'll be puffing after a couple of minutes. As you build up stamina you can push yourself to rigorous steps. Do the flexibility movements (page 128) to tune-up the body; then start the series in a gentle way building up to a crescendo so that when you get to the high kicks you are really working hard. Taper off energy during the last movements, so your heart rate slows down gradually. An abrupt stop is equally bad as an abrupt start. Afterwards relax in the Yoga Pose of a Child (page 140).

**1** Jog on the spot to the count twenty, each foot hitting the floor is one count; use your arm as though you were really running.

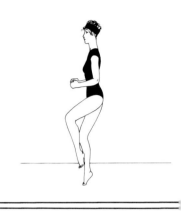

**4** Put hands on hips, keep legs and feet together and swing hips from side to side by moving balance and weight from one foot to the other. Keep the top half of the body facing to the front. Swing briskly to the count of twenty.

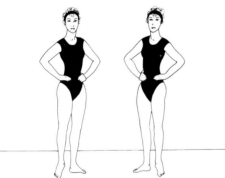

**5** Keeping legs together and knees relaxed, adjust hands so that the right palm is on your stomach and the back of the other hand is on the hips. Now rock back and forth pushing out the bottom and then tucking it in by pushing hips forward. Do twenty counts – each thrust is one count.

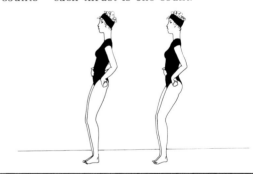

**8** The kick now goes higher, real Can-Can movements doing five counts with each leg. Put hands on hips to help lift and balance. This is when your effort should be at its peak.

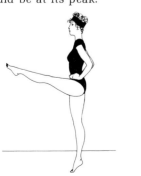

**9** Calm down a little and run on the spot bringing knees up as high as possible. Do five counts with each leg.

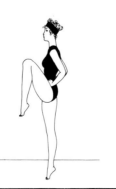

**10** Now kick the legs backward and forwards with knees bent; rocking movement – first bound on the left foot with the right k up then the right foot down an the left knee back. Do five counts, reverse legs, do five cou

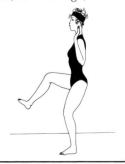

**2** Move into jumping jacks for fifteen counts; jump up, open legs and at the same time raise arms and clap overhead; land on open legs, jump again bringing legs together and arms down to sides. The two movements make one count.

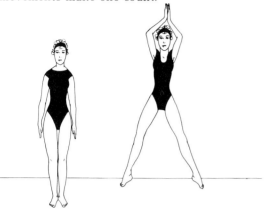

**3** Pretend you are holding a skipping rope and do thirty skipping steps, moving hands and arms as if you were directing the rope.

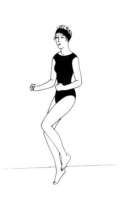

**6** The legs and feet are still together, but now move into body twists by bending the knees and swinging arms at shoulder level in the opposite direction; then jump to the other side, swinging arms across the body. Do twenty counts – that means ten each side.

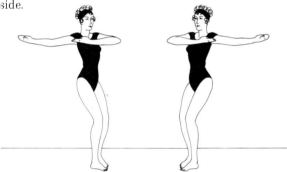

**7** Get the legs really on the move by starting with low scissor kicks to the count of thirty; try to point the toes and move the arms for balance.

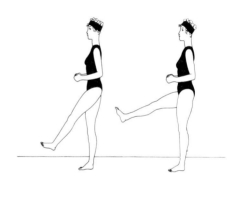

**11** Easy leg swing; jumping on the left foot swing your right leg and arms out to the right side, then back across the body. Swing for ten counts. Repeat by jumping on the right foot and swinging to the left, ten counts.

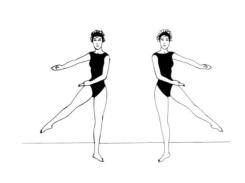

**12** Gradually come to a halt by jogging on the spot to the count of twenty, consciously slowing down your speed until your body is only just moving.

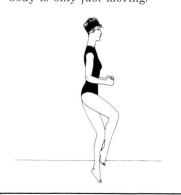

# Work-Out: Stage One

Many work-out routines can be too strenuous for those just beginning to take to exercise. It is important to start gently, doing these movements slowly at first, and then gradually building up to putting more force and punch into them. Follow this series for a few weeks and when you feel confident you are performing them well and with ease, move on to Stage Two on the following pages.

**When not to take exercise unless with medical permission or under supervision**

There are certain medical conditions that restrict exercise particularly of the aerobic kind. A doctor or physiotherapist can recommend more gentle forms of movement, including using special equipment and therapeutic water activity. Check this list before embarking on your own plan. If any of the problems listed below apply to you, get in touch with your doctor for personal advice on what is possible in the way of exercise.

- a recent heart attack
- any degree of heart disease that causes chest pain
- irregular heartbeat
- high blood pressure
- diseases of the heart valves
- previous bout of rheumatic fever
- sugar diabetes
- kidney disease
- lung problems
- circulatory problems in the legs, including varicose veins
- anaemia
- during convalescence from any infectious disease
- obesity – if you are more than thirty pounds overweight

If you have a tendency to fat, an exercise programme can eliminate the need to be on and off diet all your life. Once you've reached your desired weight and shape, moderate sustained activity will keep you trim.

**1** To help upper arms, stand with legs together, feet flat on floor. Raise bent elbows sideways, firmly clench the fis and hold around bosom level. Unbend arms and stretch out shoulder level, hold to the cou of three; bend and hold to the count of three. Repeat ten time

**5** To firm thighs, particularly the inner upper leg, lie on one side supporting head with the arm and balancing the body with the other arm. Slowly raise the upper leg as high as possible, keeping knees straight and toes pointed; hold to the count of five, lower very very slowly. Repeat ten times with each leg.

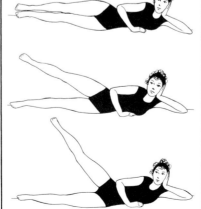

**6** Another good movement for firming thighs and toning calf muscles: stand with feet slight apart, arms straight with palm on thighs. Raise feet to balanc on toes, then slowly go down into a crouch position, remaining on toes; hold to the count of three; straighten legs. Repeat ten times at first and build up to twenty or more.

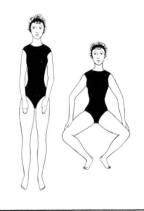

For a firmer bosom, stand and
old arms by grasping each
orearm below the elbow with
he opposite hand. Now push
ard towards the elbows
ithout moving the hand up the
m; you should feel a pull
nder the bosom. Do twenty
mes.

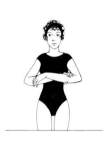

**3** To make the waist area work,
stand with legs a little apart
and raise arms above the head,
interlacing fingers. Keeping
elbows slightly bent, bend
alternately to the left and to the
right, making sure the torso
doesn't come forward. Repeat
ten times to each side.

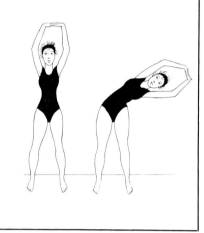

**4** An easy stomach exercise – lie
flat on your back, as shown.
Raise one leg off the ground, raise
at an angle and hold to the count
of five, now raise as high as
possible and hold to the count of
five; then lower very very slowly.
Repeat eight times with each leg.

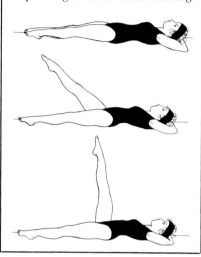

For thighs and stomach, kneel
n floor, back straight, arms
eld out in front at shoulder
vel; tighten and pull in bottom,
en slowly lean backwards as
r as possible, feeling the pull
thighs; hold to the count of
ve, return to vertical position.
epeat ten times.

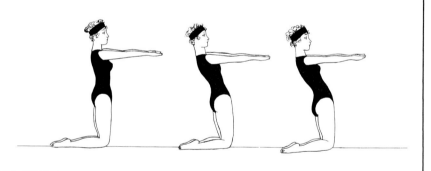

A good way to end any
xercise session. Lie on back,
end knees and pull towards
est; now lift hips off the floor,
pporting back with hands;
ext straighten legs and push
ck so that toes touch the floor,
old to the count of ten; bring
ees towards the head and
old for a few seconds. Uncurl
lowering hips. Repeat once
ore.

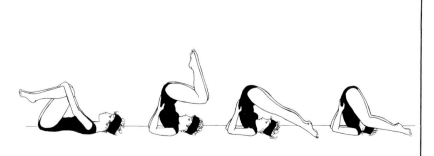

# Work-Out: Stage Two

This is a more demanding routine than on the previous page and is one that you can continue on a regular basis, working up to doing more repeats of each movement, putting more effort into it and making your body work hard. However, a word of caution: don't push your body beyond its capacity, there is no benefit from exercise that causes stress and strain – regularity at a sensible level brings the best results.

**1** Keeping arms trim – stand with feet apart, arms in fron fists clenched; throw arms a on the diagonal and stretch hard, pulling in opposite directions, return to starting position, then fling arms in t reverse direction; repeat five times in each direction, holdi to the count of four when outstretched.

**3** Get the waist going to trim it – sit with legs as far apart as possible, feet flexed, back straight and arms held high. Twist to one side and push as far to the feet as you can, hold to the count of five. Return and bend to the other side. Repeat five times each side.

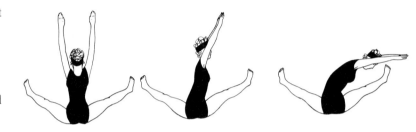

**4** To strengthen stomach muscles – sit on floor with knees bent, back at a leaning angle and arms folded in front; push arms forward and straight, slowly move backwards brining arms over the head, relax for a second; now pull the torso up, bringing arms forward, hold to the count of three, fold arms and hold to the count of three. Repeat ten times.

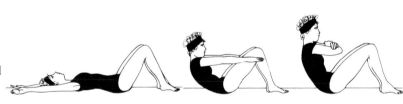

**5** Excellent for thighs and legs: lie on back, hands on stomach, legs up but with bent knees and held slightly apart; open knees, pressing soles of your feet together; straighten legs and spread into a wide V, feet flexed and hold to the count of three. Very, very slowly draw legs together, keeping knees straight and feet flexed; hold to the count of three. Repeat ten times.

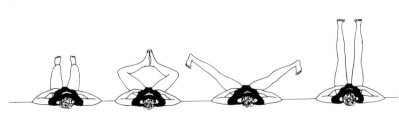

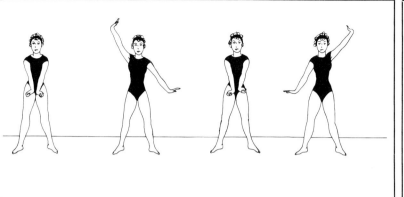

**2** An aid to chest muscles for bosom support – sit cross-legged, raise arms and place palms together over the head, keeping elbows bent; now push the palms tightly together, hold to the count of five, relax. Repeat ten times.

For the buttocks: lie on your back, knees bent, arms at sides with palms down; raise your buttocks off the floor and try to raise your heels as well; hold to the count of five keeping buttock muscles taut; lower slowly. Repeat ten times.

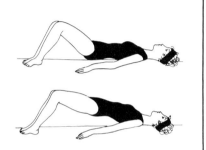

For innter thighs and stomach: lie on back, raise torso supporting back with your hands, heels also off the floor; raise legs vertically and alternately straighten and bend legs, keeping toes pointed. Make twenty leg movements.

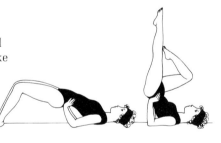

Doesn't exercise build up muscles? No, because women do not have enough of the male hormones to make it possible. Exercise tones and strengthens muscle to provide bodies with firmness and better shape. Only if you really go in for muscle power and body building in a big way can you develop muscles to a noticeable degree.

The wind-down exercise: stand with feet slightly apart, slowly bend over to touch toes, keeping legs straight; now bend elbows putting fists under arms, hold to the count of three, straighten arms behind head, hold to the count of three; bring arms forward, allow to swing relaxed for a second and gradually unfurl the body to a standing position. Repeat once more.

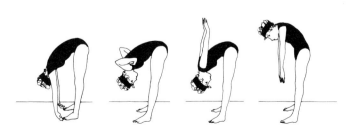

# Exercise Equipment

Gymnasiums offer a wide variety of equipment to encourage physical activity, and if you need this kind of motivation to fitness, it is possible to purchase various items for use at home – here's a selection of the most useful.

**Exercise Mat:** it is bad for your back to exercise on a hard floor, and although a carpet, blanket or towel will suffice, there is a lot to be said in favour of a special mat. The mere act of getting it out and putting it down motivates you to exercise consciously for a certain time.

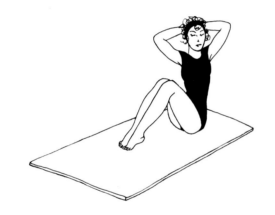

**Body Exercising Bench:** this is a versatile piece of equipment for those who find it difficult to get the body going without some kind of mechanical aid. It is good for all kinds of abdominal exercise, for waist, for the bust and for leg precision work. The body is balanced over the main cushioned curve, legs can go under or over the smaller roller, while the body can be reversed so that the hands hang on to the roller.

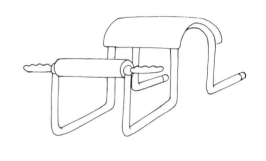

Exercise and brain power: research has shown that an efficient circulatory system delivers more oxygen to the brain, resulting in a higher level of mental alertness. This has been tracked down to the presence of certain chemicals and hormones, which appear to be in greater abundance after physical exertion. No-one is quite sure why this should be so, but for the moment it is yet another reason for getting moving.

**All equipment is from the Olympic Way at Harrod's**

**Weighted Bands:** these make your muscles work that much harder, giving leg, arm, shoulder and chest exercises that much more clout. Bands wrap around wrists or ankles, are self-adhesive and can be used with any work-out routine – but never use them for warm-up sessions.

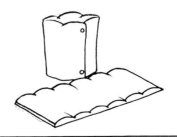

**Dumbbells:** these come in various weights and are primarily for building up and firming the arms, shoulders and chest area – but not to the point of bulging muscles, unless you want them and do specific daily exercises.

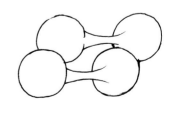

**ipping Rope:** the simplest way
 fitness, take it with you
erywhere whether away for
e weekend or on long distance
 wel. Try to skip outdoors,
en though it may only be on a
rrace. Oxygen intake matters
 much as body activity.

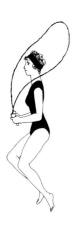

**Exercise Bicycle:** probably the
most popular of all the indoor
equipment, the bicycle makes
you do at home what you may
be reluctant to do outside. The
exercise benefit is great, the
problem is the intake of fresh
air – so open windows, take the
bike into the garden or
somehow get it on to a terrace.
There's a wide selection of
stationary cycles on the market,
many of which come with
accessories to establish speed,
distance and level of
physical exertion.

**Vibrating Wooden Rollers:** one
of the classic mechanical aids in
all slimming salons; it helps
thighs and buttocks – you can
sit as illustrated or astride. It
really batters the flesh quite
hard, which helps to break down
fatty tissue, but as stressed
elsewhere, the best results are
attained when its action is
combined with work-out
routines.

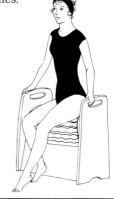

**bration Belt:** not quite the
 me as bullying your own
uscles into action, but
 brating belts do have the effect
 jolting unwanted flab into
mmer and firmer lines. The
 lt can be used on thighs,
ttocks, stomach and waist –
 t it is recommended to
mbine this with regular work-
ts.

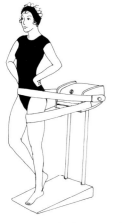

**Indoor Circular Jogger:** if you
are too timid to jog outdoors, a
worthy substitute is to jog on
the spot indoors. However,
jogging on a hard surface can
harm feet, ankles and calf
muscles, so consider investing in
a resilient floor jogger, rather
like a miniature trampoline.

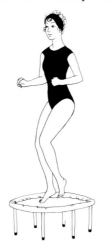

**Door Bar:** a very unobtrusive
device that can easily fit into
any doorframe and remains firm
because of special safety screws.
Pulling up on the arms is not
just a shoulder and upper arm
developer, but because the body
is elongated, the spine is
beneficially stretched, the
stomach forced into more control.

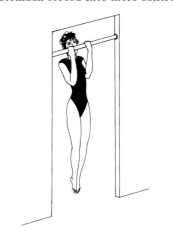

# YOGA: youth-giving poses and movements for any age

Yoga, although one of the oldest self-improvement concepts, remains the best body discipline. It can be undertaken at any age, because you simply go your own pace – listen to your body, never force it. On the following pages are details of the simpler postures (called asanas). At first you will find it difficult to achieve the poses, let alone hold them for more than a minute, but you will gradually become accomplished. If you can find a teacher, it is a good idea to take classes initially. However, you can quite easily start doing it on your own from the following detailed sketches and instructions. You can learn to breathe properly, to bring energy to mental and physical processes, to become more flexible and supple. The practice of yoga is youth-giving because it stimulates the circulatory, endocrine and nervous systems, it relaxes the mind and eases tension. On top of that, yoga can improve the shape, grace and beauty of a body.

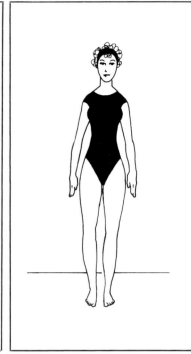

### The Traditional Sitting Poses

You are probably familiar with the cross-legged Lotus position which is the pose most used when meditation is the aim. However, for beginners, it is often difficult to attain and even more so to retain balance. Also for simple exercises and basic breathing techniques, it is not necessary and there are two alternatives familiar to everyone. The first is simply kneeling on your legs – knees should be together, while the feet should be apart but so positioned that your body rests comfortably on your legs. Keep the back straight, head balanced and hands relaxed on the thighs with palms upward. The second pose is the common cross-legged position, each foot under the opposite thigh. Hands should rest on the knees, palms upward, back straight and shoulders down.

The most accomplished pose is the Lotus. Sit straight with legs outstretched, then first bring the right foot up into the left groin – you will probably need to use your hands to coax it into position. Now bring the left foot into the right groin. If you can't achieve this, try the Half Lotus, which is sitting in the usual cross-legged position and then bringing just one foot into the groin. Apart from being the ideal positions for meditation which helps alleviate stress (see page 168) and for deep breathing, all three help to slow down circulation in the legs and thereby increase the blood supply in other areas. This can have a refreshing and rejuvenating effect. However, a word of caution: if you have varicose veins, do not sit in any of these positions for long – five minutes will bring adequate benefits.

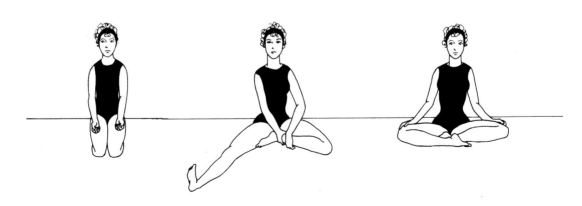

## The Basic Standing Pose

Learning to relax is one of the essentials of Yoga and because the aim is to re-energize and exercise the body without straining it, the first move is to learn how to hold it properly. Stand in front of a mirror and check your body, not only with your eyes but consciously with your mind. Stand with feet together and with weight evenly distributed on heels and toes. Think of pulling your body upwards, elongating it to the maximum by stretching the spine and the neck. Pull up the knees as well, using thigh muscles. Keep the shoulders back, but in a relaxed manner and allow the arms to hang loose. The stomach should be pulled in. Balance the head by holding it high and slightly tucking in the chin. Keep the pose for a couple of minutes, concentrating on what you are doing with your body, how you are stretching it, how you are holding it in a well-aligned position.

## Balancing Poses

These poses develop both physical balance and mental equilibrium. First stand on the left foot with left hand on the hip. Bend right knee and rest the sole of the foot against the left knee. Hold to the count of ten. Repeat reversing leg positions. Now bring the right foot up high into the groin, raise arms above head, palms together. Hold to the count of ten. Repeat reversing leg positions. The next step is the Tree Pose. Bend the right leg back, holding the foot and raising the right arm. Try to push the heel close to the buttocks; keep the head balanced high. Hold to the count of ten. Repeat reversing leg positions.

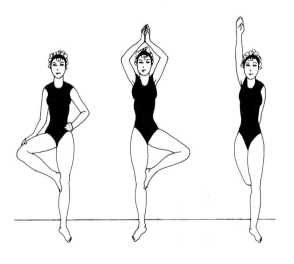

## The Importance of Proper Breathing

Correct and regular breathing is fundamental to all Yoga practices. You may think you breathe properly, but chances are you do not. Most people do not breathe deeply enough. It is not just a matter of getting enough air into the lungs – more significant is getting the stale air out. In Yoga breathing, the lungs are completely filled and completely emptied. Breathing is done through the nostrils which should be relaxed. You have to be conscious of the movement of the diaphragm and stomach. Most of us are taught to breathe, or rather automatically breathe, in the reverse way to the Yoga teaching. As you inhale, allow your stomach to expand as this lowers the diaphragm and brings air to the bottom of the lungs. As you exhale, draw in the stomach so the diaphragm lifts and the ribs relax. It can be a problem adjusting to this type of breathing, but if you lightly place your fingers on the ribcage you'll feel it opening and closing. Breathe in and out slowly and rhythmically for five minutes. Mentally be aware of the deepness and slowness of breathing. Get used to and be comfortable with the pace because it should be consistent during all the Yoga exercises.

### Getting rid of tension

The neck and shoulders are areas of concentrated tension and these simple exercises help relieve tautness and put your body and mind in a more relaxing mood for the asanas.

Sit in any of the sitting poses, hands on knees, shoulders down. Roll head to the left, around to the back stretching the neck, then to the right. You'll probably feel your neck creak. Do five rolls first going to the left then five rolling first to the right.

Turn face to look over right shoulder, holding the chin up high. Return to front and drop to chest. Hold to the count of five feeling the stretch in the back of the neck. Repeat turning to the left. Do three times either side.

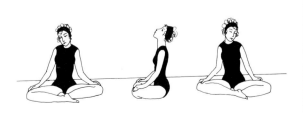

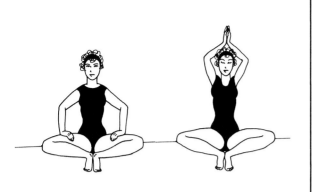

## Pose of a Frog

Sit with knees wide apart, buttocks on heels, toes together, hands on thighs. Raise the arms and place palms together over the head. Close the eyes and concentrate on deep breathing. Inhale through the nostrils and inflate the stomach like a frog, hold to the count of five. Slowly exhale deflating the stomach. Repeat ten times.

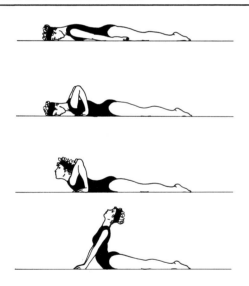

## The Cobra

Lie on stomach, face down with forehead touching the floor. Elbows are bent and raised, palms flat on floor, Legs are stretched straight, toes pointed. Slowly raise the head as high as possible pushing the chin forward. Now lift the shoulders and chest up, throwing back the head. It is only the front part of the torso that is raised – everything from the navel back must be kept straight and take care not to relax the knees. Hold to the count of three to begin with. Build up to a minute. Slowly return to the supine position.

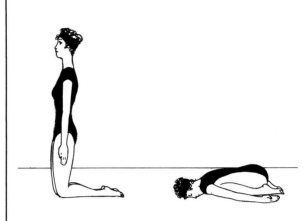

## Pose of a Child

Start from a kneeling position with both knees and feet together, arms at sides. Slowly bend over to curve into a relaxed position, bringing the head down to the ground and as close as possible to the knees. Arms are limp at sides. Breathe calmly and stay in the position for two minutes. This is a restful and recuperative pose and is the perfect way to relax the body after stretching or strenuous movements.

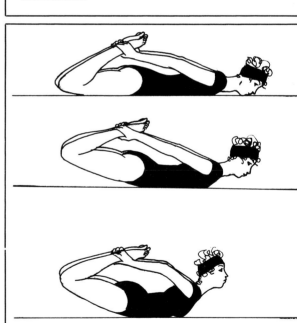

## The Bow

A strenuous pose only recommended for the experienced. Lie face downward, bend knees back and keeping head down, grasp heels with hands. Slowly raise your head, then pulling on your legs raise thighs and shoulders from the floor. Try to hold to the count of five.

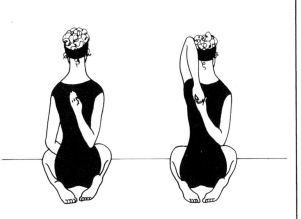

## The Grip

Also called the Head of a Cow. Kneel with buttocks resting on heels, back straight. Bend right arm behind the back, hand resting between shoulder blades with the palm facing outwards. Raise left arm over the head, bend it backwards and try to clasp the right hand, interlacing fingers and pulling gently in opposite directions. When final extension is reached, hold to the count of five. Relax. Repeat three times. Then do the same bending left arm and raising the right one.

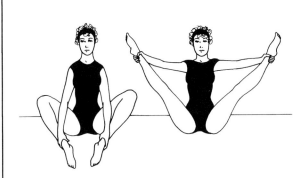

## Angular Pose

Sit with knees bent. Grasp toes and slowly stretch out your legs like scissors, trying to get your knees perfectly straight without letting go of the toes. The body should be balanced on the buttocks – the inclination is to fall backwards. Try to hold for five deep breaths.

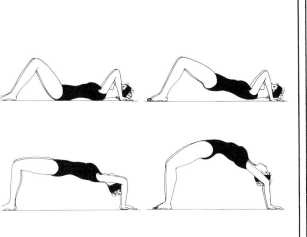

## The Back Bend

Lie on back with knees bent, raise arms and place palms on either side of your head. Push up your body into the highest possible arch. Hold to the count of ten. Slowly lower yourself to the starting position. Repeat three times.

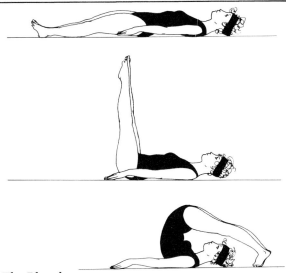

## The Plough

Lie flat on your back, legs outstretched, knees straight, arms by sides, palms face down. Using hands for support and push, lift the legs keeping them straight until in a vertical position. Hold to the count of three, then slowly swing the legs over the head aiming to touch the floor with your toes. Try not to relax or bend the knees, and slide the toes as far away from the head as is possible. Hold to the count of ten concentrating on deep, regular breathing. Return by first bending the knees and unfurling the trunk. When the buttocks reach the floor, finally straighten legs.

**Twenty reasons why you should start to exercise moderately and continue to do so for life**

1. heart muscle becomes stronger
2. resting heartbeat is lowered
3. lowers blood pressure
4. more efficient circulatory system
5. more oxygen means more energy
6. strengthens chest walls
7. better and deeper breathing patterns
8. makes bones and joints stronger
9. less fatigue for skeletal muscles
10. better digestion
11. a higher proportion of muscle to fat
12. lower concentration of blood fats
13. glucose requirements reduced
14. improved skin tone
15. better balance
16. calming effect on stress and moods
17. better weight distribution
18. helps to lose inches
19. higher level of self-esteem
20. heightened sexual response

### But a word of warning

Although moderate activity is marvellous, excess can be as destructive as none at all. There is a controversy regarding the balance between effort and benefits, but many scientists believe that excessive athletic activity can cause stress with all its chemical and psychological effects. So don't get too carried away and overdo it.

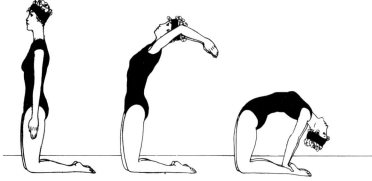

### Pose of a Camel

Kneel with legs a little apart, thighs in line with the torso, arms at sides. Raise your arms and pull them back around shoulder level. Arch the back and stretch the arms so that hands clasp the heels. Allow the head to fall back. Hold to the count of ten, inhaling and exhaling rhythmically. Relax. Repeat once more.

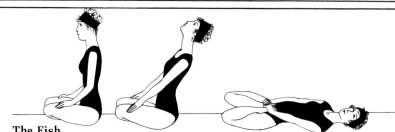

### The Fish

Start by sitting cross-legged, preferably in the Lotus position if you can achieve it. Stretch the spine, balance the head and place hands on knees. Slowly lean backwards, using arms for balance. Arch the back and rest head on the floor. Hold to the count of five. Now lift hands from knees and grasp the toes; stretch arms and further stretch the spine. Hold to the count of five.

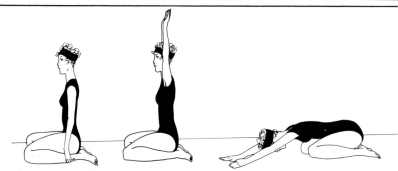

### The Cat Stretch

Kneel down, feet together and knees a little apart, buttocks on heels, back straight, arms at sides. Raise arms above head and at the same time, bend over bringing head to the knees. Aim to push as far forward as possible, sliding the hands on the floor and making a greater distance between hands and knees. The stretch starts at the hips and goes through the spine. At the fullest stretch, hold to the count of five. Relax. Repeat. Now roll slowly to the right so that the shoulder touches the floor; continue to stretch, hold to the count of five. Roll to the left side, stretch, hold to the count of five.

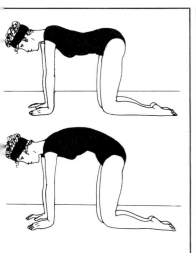

### ose of a Cat

neel on all fours with adequate
istance between the knees and
ands to allow the spine to be
traight but not stretched. Drop
he head and hump the back. Then
ring the head up and arch the
ack. Move the spine up and down
o the torso is alternately raised
nd lowered just like the move-
lent of a cat. Breathe deeply. Keep
loving for two minutes.

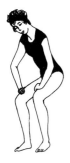

### Stomach Movements

Stand with legs apart, knees bent;
ean the torso over the thighs
supporting it by placing hands on
he thighs, fingers inward. Start
by breathing deeply and regularly,
out independently of the breath-
ng rhythm start to contract and
expand stomach muscles; you
should clearly see the stomach
being pushed out and pulled in.
Do ten movements, relax. Do
another ten.

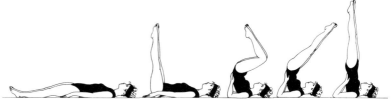

### Shoulder Stand

Start by lying flat on your back, legs outstretched, arms at sides, palms
down. Raise the legs slowly, keeping the knees straight and close
together, toes pointing. Elevate legs until vertical, stretch them, pause.
Then pressing hands and elbows on the floor, also lift the torso, back,
stomach and finally chest and slide your hands under the small of the
back to help balance the body. Hold to the count of ten. Slowly bend
your knees, keeping head tucked in, hold to the count of five. Straighten
legs and lower them slowly to the floor returning arms to sides as torso
contacts the floor.

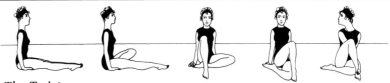

### The Twist

Sit on the floor with legs outstretched, arms at sides for balance, palms
on floor. Bend the right leg, tucking foot under left thigh. Draw up the
left leg, bending the knee until it rests against your torso; now lift the
left foot over the right thigh and place the sole flat on the floor. Balance
the body with the left arm, grasp the toes of the left foot with the right
hand. Twist torso to the left from the waistline, trying to look behind
you. Hold for three deep breaths. Relax. Reverse sides and repeat.

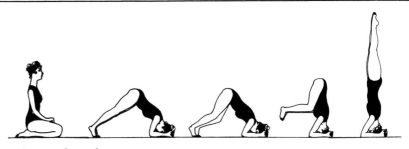

### The Headstand

This is the ultimate of all Yoga positions for it helps rejuvenate the
whole body. However, if you are over forty and overweight, go with
caution. If you have high blood pressure don't do it at all. Initially never
practise it alone and use a wall for support. Kneel down, link fingers
together and using elbows and hands form a circle on the floor. Put your
head in this protective enclosure, keeping elbows as close together as
you can. Now straighten out legs and walk towards your elbows, then
bend the knees and try to raise feet from the floor, gradually lifting and
straightening the legs until the body is in one line. Hold for a few
seconds this first time. Return slowly, first bending the knees into the
stomach and folding yourself up until feet touch the floor. At first you
will probably have to kick your legs up, or get someone to pull them up.
Also it is important to abide by the rule of only a few seconds at first,
and a gradual build up to holding the pose for several minutes.

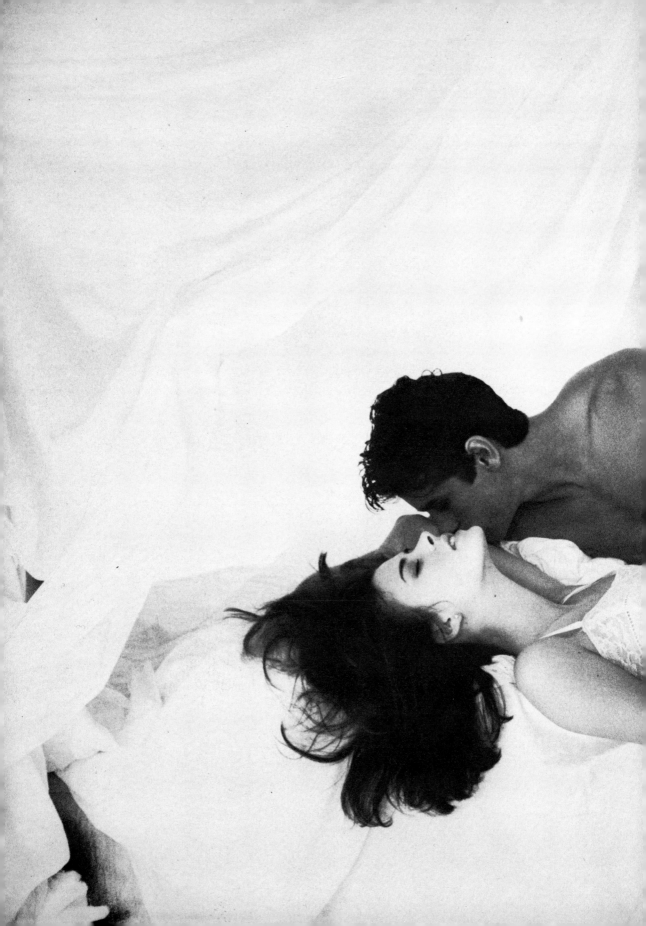

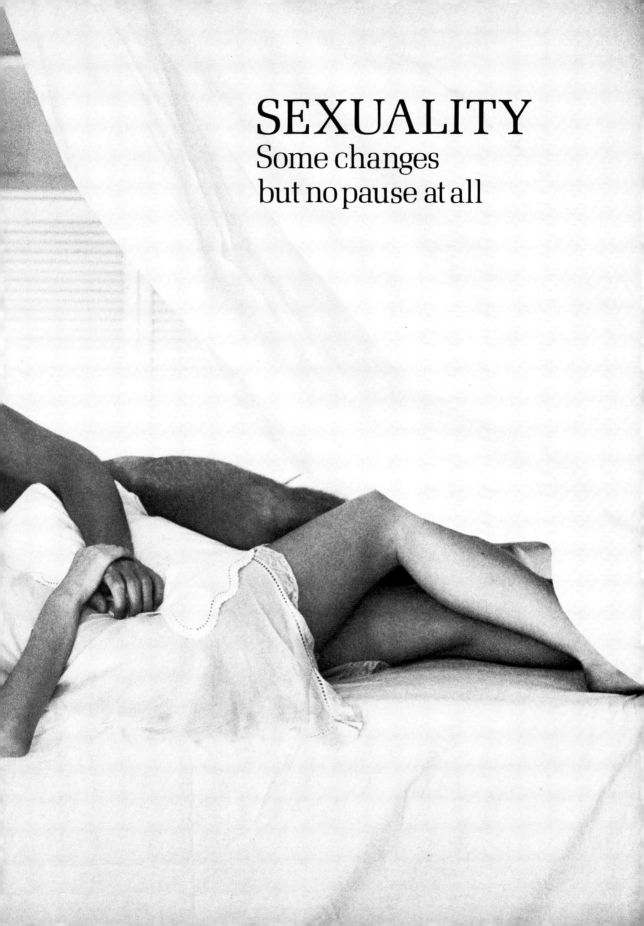

# SEXUALITY
## Some changes
## but no pause at all

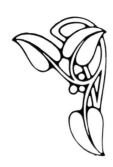

Young women who are enjoying a full sex life may be surprised to learn that there may be even better times ahead of them. Sex can become more enjoyable as you grow older and the extra years can give positive advantages which will considerably enhance your pleasure and appreciation. Nor does it all have to come to a grinding halt with the menopause. Although society is still reluctant to associate sex with age, many older women are now willing to come out in the open and say that everything to do with sexuality is still very much part of their lives. It is no more a question of whether there is sex after forty, fifty, sixty, etc. but on what terms. Women who are enjoying sex more are those whose maturity has brought new positive plateaus of self-awareness and self-esteem, both of which bring confidence to all things – including intimate relationships.

Until in their late twenties or thirties, few women really come to terms with who they are emotionally and how this can be expressed and nurtured in a sensuous, rewarding way. There's a build-up of wisdom through intimacy over the years, which is a mature woman's main asset. She has learned to balance love and sex rather than equate them. She has learned to relax about the importance and pressures of both and put them into perspective within the wide boundaries of a modern woman's life, rather than considering them the beginning and end of everything. She has also learned how to give and receive sexual pleasure.

All this means that as you get older chances are that you will enjoy sex more because you are more comfortable with yourself and more at ease with a partner. You know what sexuality is all about – for you and for him. Add to this, the fact that a woman doesn't really reach a sexual peak until middle thirties – a level, needless to say, that can be maintained for many, many years – and you must conclude that the old idea of only a young woman being capable of participating in and enjoying sex is rubbish.

Actual age doesn't play such an important role as many women believe. What is old anyway? As far as sex is concerned, if you are well, healthy and in good shape, you simply don't feel old. The basics of sexual attraction operate the same way all your life. Desire doesn't diminish until very late in life, but it has always been considered not quite nice for an older woman to show sexual interest – and some women stop sex altogether because they think it's ridiculous. Don't believe that it's the priority of the young and lovely to claim sexuality. Times are changing, not because women are looking and feeling so much younger than their mothers did in middle years, but because they feel it's their right to have just as extended a sex life as a man. Bear in mind that most men over forty are hardly the answer to a maiden's prayer.

Despite all the good news and positive signs of change towards female sexuality, many women around the age of forty are still influenced by past standards and start to panic, thinking that time is running out. The tendency is either to fall victim to depression or to make a last desperate stand and try to make up for lost time.

---

Sexuality is more than just having sex, it is the embodiment of all the physical and mental aspects of being a woman. It enters into all phases of life. It has always been said that men want an orgasm and women want romance. True to a degree, because men find it relatively easier than women to participate in sex with little or no involvement. A mature woman has few illusions about romance as such, but what she looks for is friendship on an affectionate and intimate level.

Women who have never thought of having an extra-marital affair, often do so at this point. Boredom and frustration with life in general can also trigger it off. An affair can be exciting, thrilling and absorbing; it can also reveal that you've previously never really known what sexuality was all about. This may come as quite a shock, but it is not the grounds for breaking with the past, whether it be a marriage or a steady partner, nor is it the basis for bitterly regretting all that's gone before. It is part of sexual maturity and as such should be put into context with the rest of your life. It is only after a certain age that you can judge what is a sexual encounter and what is or could be more.

Sex for the mature woman is not just an orgasm. It is everything before and after; it is contact, skin, sensuality. Sexual intimacy is a splendid thing, but it's not always the most enduring. Sex is many things. It is passion, it's giving and receiving pleasure, it's communication, it's mutual care and regard and at its best it's love and total, affectionate intimacy. Sexuality is an integral part of our lives and is on our minds no matter what our age, but it takes age to judge its level and value.

Sex keeps you young, so keep at it, say the experts. That's all very well and doubtless true, but there's one major problem for many women – opportunity. First of all, there are more women than men, while the number of homosexuals is increasing. Then, although the divorce rate is high, men who remarry or take new lovers usually choose younger women. It is not easy for a single, divorced or widowed woman to find a partner. Ironically enough it is usually easier for a married woman to find a lover – maybe men feel this is safer and there will be fewer demands. However, women of achievement, power and influence have fewer problems and these days are often taking younger lovers or husbands, which is very sound, physiologically. This is a new phenomenon and is not entirely due to prestige and position, but is influenced by the fact that these are the women who are out and about, doing things, meeting people, getting caught up in the business world – and because of this they are interesting, vital and full of energy, and make a point of taking care of their looks and appearance as well.

A woman's opportunity for sexual or romantic experiences is limited to the environment she moves in. Sitting alone at home is going to get you nowhere, and although a woman still can't move about as easily and as freely as a man, there are ways to get yourself involved with others, if not through work, through clubs, societies, community service and travel. There are a lot of people out there. However, even given the opportunity and feeling the desire, many women stall right there. Complexes come to the fore: will I measure up, is my body too old, too fat, too wrinkled? Surely he'd really rather be with someone younger? If you think about it, these concerns are connected purely with the physical and as such stem from old standards, and although they shouldn't apply today, it is very difficult to shake them off. Your personality and vitality are also of great importance. Also you must judge yourself by your

Sexuality and femininity cannot be separated and together they can be a woman's great asset – not to be used as a weapon, but as a way to soften and round off the rough edges in any relationship. We may value our new found independence and assertiveness, but most women are content to give it up momentarily during an intimate encounter. Giving way to a natural gentleness is not a weakness; it can be a pleasure to both.

standards of today's woman, not his. Try not to think if you are what he wants; ask yourself is he what you want. There are two sides to the sexual coin and it's no longer heads the man wins and tails the woman loses. The stakes are now equal. There's no need for age to give you complexes about your sexuality; you require but two things: good health and the right attitude.

As far as sex is concerned, capacity does not diminish with age (a commonly held belief) and unlike men, women can continue with an active sex life indefinitely. It is often social factors which contribute to abstinence rather than physical ones. Men do slow down and are unable to perform completed sexual intercourse as frequently, but women can retain a level of intensity and participation until they finally reach the age of disinterest. Many women take years to learn how to experience orgasm and it is usually the mature woman who has worked out how to have multiple orgasms. It may appear that an older woman is not interested in sex because she is simply not enthusiastic about sex per se. When you are older, you expect more and are not so tolerant of a brief encounter as you were in your youth. A mature woman wants more attention, more foreplay, more mutual response and she is not likely to be eager or willing about entry until she is ready for it psychologically – otherwise she'd just as soon do without. This has led to the misconception that a woman's response slows down as she gets older. What has happened, in fact, is that she is more honest about her feelings and her reactions.

However, as one approaches the menopause – any time from early forties to late fifties – there are some physical changes, which although they have no direct effect on libido, capacity or enjoyment, can be troublesome if you don't know how to cope with them. I am talking here about those directly connected with sexual intercourse, not overall symptoms and psychological aspects, which are discussed in detail on pages 157–161. There can be a general drying up of the vagina, which means a reduction in lubrication both inside and on the surface areas. This may cause shrinkage of the fold which protects the clitoris and leaves it exposed to irritation – even from clothing – and infection. If this happens, genital stimulation can be very painful. In addition, because of lack of lubrication inside, the vagina becomes less distensible and so it is more difficult for the man to penetrate; not only can this be sore, but if intercourse takes place, friction could cause small slits or little scars in the vaginal lining. Dryness stems from a diminished supply of the hormone oestrogen and can be corrected by using special oestrogen creams available on prescription. In many instances, the use of a normal vaginal lubricant is sufficient. Dryness occurs to some degree in every woman as she ages, but it is not something you have to put up with, and no reason for ceasing sex completely.

During and after the menopause some women experience abdominal pain during orgasm. This is due to shrinkage of the uterus and instead of contracting regularly and then relaxing gradually, it can go into a spasm for a minute or two. There is treatment to both avoid or relieve this condition. Any problems such as dryness and pain should never be meekly accepted, but should be discussed with your doctor and a treatment worked out. Don't be shy about it.

The condition of dryness is often caused and frequently aggravated by lack of sex. A woman over forty who is participating in regular sexual activity is unlikely to have this problem, but women with infrequent sexual contact are usually unaware that anything may be going wrong until they actually engage in sex, and the resulting lack of lubrication can be very embarrassing. Like any other part of the body, limited use leads to limited function; if organs are not used, they rest, and if they rest they rust. It is prudent to keep your body in good working condition. This is an accepted fact when it comes to muscles, for example, but when it comes to the parts of your body that are involved in sexuality, it is invariably overlooked either through ignorance or modesty.

On your own, what can you do to keep yourself in top sexual condition? Apart from general checks on hygiene, there are two things: masturbation for continued lubrication and relief from tension, and exercise of the vaginal muscles. Both of these are rarely written about simply because of the taboos that still surround what is considered self-indulgence and gratification. However, in this day and age, there are many doctors who say that such activities can be a practical and sensible way to keep your sexuality in good healthy order on both the physical and psychological levels. Why? Masturbation is a good thing because it may help postpone genital atrophy. This is the medical term for the general drying-up and shrinkage of the genital organs, and any stimulation will help to counteract the thinning of the mucous membranes of the vagina and go a long way to retaining the elasticity of the walls.

Masturbation creates lubrication, which is good for you. It is also a pleasurable source of orgasm for most women, bringing release from emotional tension. Although it is a natural instinct, a cloud of guilt surrounds masturbation and there are strong overtones of shame and fear. Most women have grown up with the unspoken rule that they were not to touch their female parts. It was implied that it was all right for men to masturbate, but women – no. Actually many women do, but it's something you probably wouldn't even mention to your best friend. Apart from encouraging lubrication, another health benefit is the exercise given to the uterus and vagina because of the contractions. It has also been said that the uninhibited masturbator makes the best lover – and research has shown that a clitorally induced orgasm is the most intense.

On the other hand, you can exercise the muscular walls of the vagina without having an orgasm. If you concentrate, you can draw inwards and upwards the whole genital area. At first, there will be a negligible pull and contraction, but with practice you should be able to brace and hold the vaginal muscles for a count of six, then relax and repeat six times. Do it a few times each day.

Sex is better when you are older if you feel freer than you did in your youth. Sexual inhibitions tend to ease away, and mature women enjoy masturbation because they finally lose their guilt about it.

## Contraception

As you grow older it is very important to take a new look at your contraceptive methods. If you have been on the pill, and using it more or less constantly for fifteen years, you should be aware of the risks involved if you continue to do so. On the pill, unwanted effects can exist at any age, but they become more significant after thirty-five, because most of them are concerned with circulation which is a frequent disorder – with or without the pill. Research has shown that circulatory diseases are about four times more common among pill takers. At its most serious, circulation failure can result in heart attacks, strokes and venous thrombosis. Risks are even greater for smokers, and at any age. Most women do not realize the health damaging effects of combining the pill and smoking. If you smoke a packet of cigarettes a day, you are aging yourself by five to ten years, so if you are also on the pill, you have to think about changing your contraception method five to ten years earlier than a non-smoker – that is, around thirty. A non-smoker is considered to be relatively safe up to forty, but personally I feel that the sooner you make the change, the better.

How can you tell that something could be going amiss? Firstly, it is extremely important to have blood pressure monitored regularly when you are on the pill, even if you are taking low dosage of both oestrogen and progesterone. A change in blood pressure is the first sign of a problem – then there are warning symptoms which you should recognize as being pill-related and not pass them over as middle age inevitables; watch out for:

- breathlessness, aggravated breathing, heart palpitations
- pain in the chest, centrally located and severe
- acute abdomen pain
- prolonged headaches, or the onset of headaches if you have never had them before
- numbness or weakness in any limb, tingling of fingers
- a fainting attack
- blotchy skin rashes
- jaundice – yellow skin and eyes

These may not be serious or due to the culmination of risk years on the pill, but they are all signs of a disorder of the circulation or liver (the clearing house for everything that goes into your body). Should you be affected by any of these symptoms, stop taking the pill until you have had a thorough health check and the green light from your doctor.

## Alternative Methods

If you've been used to the convenience of the pill, you naturally feel reluctant to change but there are acceptable alternatives. You should never put your health at risk for the sake of convenience, nor should you delay the change over through laziness. Consider one of these:

**Progestogen only Pill** – because this is oestrogen free, and contains but a minimal dose of progestogen it has little or no effect on the circulatory system. It is a good choice for older women, but you can't afford to be forgetful, as this pill must be taken regularly, preferably at the same time each day and if possible a few hours prior to sexual contact – work out what you consider the most common time.

**IUD – Intrauterine Device** – primarily a method for older women, because complications such as expulsion and pelvic infection are less common in a mature woman. The IUD is very effective, though slightly less so than the pill. There are two main types for long term use, both are of plastic; a well-known one is the Lippes Loop and then there are medicated versions with copper wire around them. They need to be replaced every two or three years. Insertion is a simple procedure, but there can be side effects of cramps, lower back pain and heavier bleeding during menstruation – the latter particularly applies to women whose periods become more copious as they approach the menopause. However, these symptoms usually die down after the first few menstrual cycles, but if they don't you should consult your doctor – sometimes one type of IUD gives trouble, and another doesn't.

**Barrier Methods** – the original contraceptives, the diaphragm and the cervical cap, are still extremely effective (particularly when combined with a spermicide) but many women regard them as cumbersome and messy compared with modern alternatives. They are, however, absolutely safe, and strangely enough they are recommended and favoured by many doctors. The problem is to persuade women to return to a method they abandoned many years ago. Near the menopause, there can be difficulty in retaining the cap or diaphragm due to a prolapse of the vaginal walls or uterus.

**Sterilization** – the ultimate contraceptive method, but not one that many women are willing to undergo even when they are sure they do not want any more children. It involves an operation on the fallopian tubes which stops eggs passing from the ovaries into the womb. The normal menstrual cycle continues. The operation is hardly ever reversible.

**Future Possibilities** – interest will centre on a variety of long-acting implants, improved cervical caps and better spermicides. There's much talk about the convenience and value of the vaginal sponge, which is impregnated with spermicide and left in the vagina for up to forty-eight hours. It does not, of course, interfere with the hormone output. It can be rinsed and re-used; it is being cited as the future effective barrier for mature women, as it has many advantages over conventional diaphragms, which some women have trouble keeping in place as they grow older.

## Late Pregnancy

In theory, a woman can conceive right up until the time her periods finally stop, however the chance of it happening decreases with age due to diminishing ovulation. Many more women are now having babies – often their first – in their late thirties and forties and do so with little trouble either during pregnancy or delivery. It's a trend of the Eighties to have children later, so as to reap the benefits of a career first, instead of doing things vice versa. It can be very satisfying to be a late mother and I believe in many ways it helps to keep you young. The old idea was that such a woman had neither the physical stamina nor the necessary patience and tolerance to cope with a baby or young child. That's not true. Firstly, older women can be as strong and as healthy as a twenty-five year old. Secondly, mentally, a woman who's had experience from life and satisfaction in a career, is usually quite content to devote time to motherhood with none of those youthful thoughts that she is missing out on something. Then, the fact of having a baby or young child forces you to be younger because you have to find the energy to cope. A late mother is more likely to keep checks on her health, eat properly, take exercise (if only pushing the pram or rushing around to get things done) and keep her mind and attitude attuned to new ideas in order to associate with the other, younger mothers and to finally keep abreast of the times for the sake of her child. It is because a late mother is still influenced by the negative thoughts about her position that she is even more determined to keep herself up to scratch in every way. It all helps to keep you younger, longer.

Never be put off starting a pregnancy because of your age, but you do have to take very special care of yourself. Constant health and progress checks are essential and you must be meticulous about ante-natal disciplines and guidelines (see below). One very important factor to be aware of is the increased risk of mongolism (Down's Syndrome) if either parent is over forty. It used to be thought that the age of the woman was the significant factor, but recent studies have revealed that some babies are affected because of defective sperm. The higher the combination of ages, the greater the risk. A younger partner would obviously be preferable (another plus point for the newly emerging younger man-older woman combination) but most women have older partners. There is a very efficient test to determine any malformation. This is called amniocentesis and can only be done after the fourteenth or sixteenth week of pregnancy. If your doctor doesn't suggest it, ask for it to be done as it means you can go through pregnancy with peace of mind and avoid any distress at birth.

Amniocentesis detects spina bifida as well as mongolism. Under

A woman's fertility begins to decrease after the age of thirty and ovulation can become less frequent. There's always the chance of conception though, so if you don't want a child, you need to continue contraception right up until after the menopause. It is advisable to continue until a year has passed without having a period, and if you are under fifty at this stage, it's better to continue for two years.

local anaesthetic a hollow needle is inserted through the abdominal wall into the uterus to draw off a sample of the amniotic fluid surrounding the baby. This fluid contains cells from the foetus and on analysis the presence of abnormalities can be determined. There is an extremely slight chance that amniocentesis would cause an abortion, as today ultra sound techniques are used to locate the baby's exact position. Results also reveal the sex of the child, which some mothers don't always want to know, but it is a significant factor if there are any sex-linked disorders within the family.

Medical checks should be planned on a regular basis with your doctor. On a day to day level, you are responsible for your health and that of your child. Make a note of the following:

**Diet** – more than at any other time of your life, it is vital to watch what you eat. Check basic diet rules (see page 88) and work within the suggested plan, eating a lot of fresh foods. Keep track of your weight; over nine months you must not exceed an increase of more than 20lb (9.2kg). Your doctor may not even want you to gain that much, because being a late mother, chances are that you were a little bit overweight to begin with, plus the additional risk of circulation problems. You may need iron, calcium and folic acid supplements, but that is something for your doctor to establish.

**Alcohol** – if you drink excessive quantities, there is definitely the increased risk of the baby being born abnormally. Recent research has shown that moderate drinking can also cause defects, particularly to heart, limbs and face. Two to three whiskies a day, or the equivalent, could lead to mental retardation as well as malformation. Also it is wise to cut down on the intake of caffeine; limit your coffee and tea to three cups a day – substitute with herbal teas.

**Smoking** – of all the hazards, this is the most dangerous. There is a stack of medical evidence to support the link between cigarettes and a roster of foetal problems. Foetal death alone rises by thirty-five per cent in women who smoke more than twenty cigarettes a day. Other risks: higher rate of miscarriage, lower birthweight, inability to breathe properly, low resistance to and an increased risk of infection for many years, respiratory disease and a high mortality rate within the first few months. Smoking passes on chemical toxins to the foetus and also reduces the supply of essential oxygen.

**Drugs** – all should be avoided, even mild ones such as aspirin, unless they are absolutely necessary for a medical condition. And it goes without saying that hard drugs are absolutely lethal.


### Vaginal Health

The health of the vaginal area depends on its level of acidity. This is a very fine balance and maintained by bacteria which are present in every healthy vagina. They produce lactic acid, but if the numbers or types of bacteria are disturbed, vaginal infections can develop. These infections are different to those transmitted sexually. Personal hygiene plays an important part in keeping the area healthy, but during the menopause, diminished oestrogen can contribute to infection. The vagina is self-cleansing, so there is no necessity under normal conditions to overdo it by trying to soap the inner surfaces, or by overuse of douches or vaginal deodorants. Gentle lathering with a mild soap of the anal and outer vaginal area, once or twice a day, is sufficient. Over enthusiastic cleansing could interfere with the physiology of the vagina and in itself cause problems.

Every healthy vagina has a certain amount of discharge; this is quite normal and varies according to the time in the menstrual cycle. It is thin, clear and a bit gluey before ovulation; afterwards it is thicker, whiter and much stiffer. A normal discharge doesn't make you sore or itchy, and it doesn't have an unpleasant smell. A discharge that stems from infection can be irritating, cause redness and smells strange. The following are the most common infections; all need medical attention but can be successfully treated. Each type is a distinct disease caused by one or more micro-organism and it is necessary to analyse a sample of the discharge to accurately diagnose the problem. All-purpose creams may give temporary relief, but they do not cure the infections. Because warmth and dampness encourage growth, check that you are wearing cotton underwear as synthetics can trap moisture.

---

From the aesthetic point of view, there are two changes which take place in the vaginal area which could affect your attitude towards your sexuality. The colour of the outer and inner linings changes as we age – from maroon to a lighter red and finally to pink. Pubic hair does go grey – the odd hair or the whole lot – and it can thin out a little. If the grey bothers you, particularly if it is premature, it can be tinted in the same way as hair on the head, but a great deal of care must be taken so as not to infect the vaginal area. A precaution is to first insert a tampon, and be sure to select a tint that only colours or darkens and doesn't contain a bleaching agent.

**Non-specific Vaginitis** – here the vagina is inflamed, dry, sore and itchy. It is particularly prone to flaring up around the menopause because of the drop in oestrogen. Oestrogen stimulates the secretion of vaginal fluid, which keeps the walls moist and provides a healthy acidic environment for the bacteria. Lack of oestrogen means lack of fluid and an imbalance in the acidic level. The external area of the vagina can also dry out, crack and become itchy, reaching a chronic condition at times. Local application of hormone creams can help, also the insertion of oestrogen-containing pessaries bring relief internally. A natural remedy is a douche with an infusion of equal parts of marsh-mallow, plantain and yarrow – check with a herbalist.

Sexuality for a woman is a whole range of experiences. The beginning is to enjoy one's own body, be happy about it as a whole and not think of it as bits and pieces to please a man. Your efforts against fat and sag should be for your own personal pride. After all, your body is yours all the time, and only temporarily for someone else. Think of your sexuality as being something for you, not just in relation to him.

**Moniliasis** – also known as candidiasis, yeast infection or referred to as 'the whites'. Discharge is white, thick and curdy. It is caused by the excessive growth of a normal inhabitant of the vagina. Other symptoms are vaginal and vulva itching, the vaginal lips may become dry and red, intercourse could be painful. It is prudent to stop sexual intercourse until treatment is complete – which could be two weeks.

**Trichomoniasis** – this is usually the result of an imbalance in body chemistry, but it is sometimes spread by sexual activity. It produces an abundant, malodorous, yellow or greenish-white discharge. It can cause inflammation, itching, soreness and bleeding of the vagina. Because it can be passed back and forth, both partners require treatment; men, however, have few symptoms.

## Sexually Transmitted Diseases

Women in their twenties and early thirties are far more prone to contacting a sexually transmitted disease than those over thirty-five, when the figures begin to drop considerably. Many doctors consider this is due to less sexual contact and less promiscuity than in youth, but others cite the possibility of the body building up a certain amount of immunity. The chances against being infected with genital herpes, for example, improve with age. However, if the other diseases have not been detected, diagnosed or treated, this could be crisis time. And in the case of a much younger partner, there is a greater possibility of infection, which could be passed on to you. If you suspect you have had intercourse with someone who has venereal disease, see a doctor or go to a special clinic immediately. Women often have no symptoms until infection is quite far gone, but any kind of sore on the genital area that doesn't heal within a few days needs to be checked. Your sexual partner is more likely to show earlier signs by discharge from his penis or sores on his genital area. These are the most prevalent infections:

**Gonorrhoea** – a small percentage of women have symptoms; in the early stages there's an inflammation of the urethral lining, causing discharge and frequent burning urination. Later there's an abundant yellow discharge. The danger point is when the virus invades the fallopian tubes and causes a chronic inflammation of the pelvic organs, known as pelvic inflammatory disease, which is extremely hard to eradicate even with strong antibiotics. Sometimes total hysterectomy is the only solution. Penicillin is used to treat gonorrhoea, but during the Seventies, a penicillin-resistant strain became very prevalent. Scientists are still working on alternative methods of treatment, not always with success.

**Syphilis** – this has three stages of growth, and it is during the first two that the disease is highly contagious. Symptoms appear early – from ten days to three months – but most women don't recognize them: small sores, rather like pimples, that appear on the vulva and edge of the vagina. They are painless and will disappear within a few weeks. The second stage develops within six months; the symptoms include fever, rashes, headaches, nausea, loss of appetite, red eyes and sometimes loss of hair. These can continue for months or years. The third stage of development may not appear for ten to twenty years, but can cause brain damage, blindness and heart disease. Syphilis can be cured with penicillin or tetracyclines at both the first and second stages.

**Genital Herpes** – this is a disease that has flared up to a serious degree over the past few years. The herpes group of viruses appears as fever blisters on or near the genitals. They can be extremely sore and irritating. It is type 2 which causes this particular infection, whereas type 1 is responsible for cold sores around the mouth. It is very much a disease of the young; it is extremely difficult to control or cure, and it usually recurs until a build-up of sufficient antibodies kills off the virus. There are promising treatments currently under experiment, and there's hope about coming to grips with it soon.

**Chlamydial** – not very well known, not even by doctors, but increasing breakouts are causing concern. There are no obvious early symptoms, though there may be a discharge, burning on urination, pain in the lower abdomen and abnormal menstrual bleeding. The trouble is that it can cause pelvic inflammatory disease, which is not easy to treat. Chlamydial can be cured with antibiotics over two or three weeks.

Genital warts can become a problem from the aesthetic point of view, though medically they don't cause concern unless profuse. They often occur between the vagina and rectum, beginning as little grains of tissue. They can be treated in a doctor's surgery by the application of a solution that causes them to fall off within two or three days. If they are allowed to develop, surgery is sometimes necessary.

## The Menstrual Cycle

Women past their teens come to terms with their own particular cycle, know what to expect and quickly recognize what is normal and what is not. Any change in timing, quantity of flow or continual bleeding should be checked at once with a doctor.

The average woman can expect to menstruate for thirty to thirty-five years of her life, and once the individual rhythm has been established, it usually continues smoothly until the approach of menopause. The complex sequence of events within the cycle is controlled by the ebb and flow of two hormones, oestrogen and progesterone. Women respond differently to the change in hormone levels. There is little difference from one woman to another as to the quantity release, but it is thought that it's a woman's individual sensitivity to the changes that determines pre-menstrual symptoms. It is now firmly established that the pre-menstrual syndrome (PMS) does exist; they are mostly behavioural and emotional effects rather than physical, and for this reason doctors have been predisposed to label a complaining patient as being neurotic or difficult. PMS can be effectively treated both through hormone and vitamin therapy, bringing symptoms to a much more tolerable level.

A woman knows very well what to expect in the way of problems, knows what she can cope with herself. There's no need to be a martyr today and suffer unduly. If there's a definite cyclical connection to symptoms, keep a diary, and consult your doctor. Don't be fobbed off with a pat on the back or tranquillizers. There is a way to balance hormones and supplement vitamin deficiencies – the level of Vitamin B-6, for instance, has been found to decrease in many instances prior to menstruation.

Most women have some physical sign that a period is coming. It's common to gain weight, feel bloated and lethargic, lose lust; concentration is poor, there may be aches in the lower abdomen and the breasts are usually sore and tender. Behavioural symptoms are not so widespread; it is estimated that they are suffered in moderate to severe degrees by between twenty and sixty per cent of all women. They include tension, anxiety, depression, mood swings, irritability, loneliness, crying spells, forgetfulness, clumsiness, difficulty in making decisions and inability to sleep properly. It's a long list, but of course, no-one is likely to suffer them all.

One of the biggest blows to a woman's feelings of confidence in her sexuality is the removal of a breast because of cancer. She feels disfigured and maimed for life, no longer a complete woman. There are now amazing results from reconstructive surgery (see page 211) and afflicted women have come forward to comfortingly explain that the aftermath is, in reality, not so desperate as imagined. The fear of being physically rejected is very real, but what often happens is that one's partner becomes more caring, affectionate and gentle, which can bring a new dimension to sex that wasn't there before. Because breasts have been branded as a prime sex symbol, it is no wonder that women equate losing one with losing sexuality completely. But our sexuality is made up of many parts, and it is the total image and sensual expression that counts.

## The Menopause

The menopause used to be thought of as the end of the line as far as sexuality was concerned. In the past, women have certainly suffered from the disadvantages of both their age and their sex. The menopause brings physical symptoms that result from hormone changes, but it also brings psychological problems as a result of society's attitude towards women. There are many myths that surround the menopause and today women are putting the record straight. Women are changing things because of the new way they feel about themselves and because they now know that severe symptoms can be treated.

The menopause is not the dividing line between youth and age. It is a metabolic change and readjustment in body chemistry. Some bodies need help to get the new balance right. The menopause is actually the term given to the time of the final menstrual period. The phase that builds up to it is known as the climacteric (an unfortunate term) and it is during this time that emotional and psychological problems crop up. Depression, irritability, anxiety and general tension are the most common effects, but how much is due to hormonal imbalance and how much to social pressures is hard to determine. Our attitude is still influenced by previous generations, who were expected to be difficult at this stage of life.

Menstrual periods usually stop between the ages of forty-five and fifty-three. After this, the ovaries cease to produce a monthly egg and the levels of the hormones, oestrogen and progesterone, fall. The build-up to this point is spaced over several years, and the first indication of the approach of the menopause is usually a change in the usual menstrual pattern. Sometimes the flow becomes less, the intervals between periods longer, while periods may be missed altogether. On the other hand, periods can also get much heavier, but any really abnormally heavy periods or floodings need to be medically checked – as should any bleeding between periods or after the menopause. There are no set guidelines as to the course the pre-menopausal phase will take; it is very individual and quite unpredictable. It has been known for periods to cease abruptly overnight, often causing concern about a possible pregnancy.

With the onset of the change of life, a woman's whole hormonal complex changes because of the decreasing function of the ovaries, the female sex glands. The control of ovarian function involves the hypothalamus (the body's regulating centre) and the pituitary gland. Together they instrument the release of hormones into the bloodstream and by means of these influence other endocrine glands such as the thyroid and adrenals. In fact, the output of hormones by the pituitary gland affects most metabolic functions, and because the endocrine system is an interrelated network of glands, if one is not functioning properly others can be affected.

The two hormones produced by the ovaries – oestrogen and progesterone – are a vital part of the hormone complex, as well as controlling the reproduction cycle of ovulation and the release of the uterus lining (menstruation) if fertilization doesn't take place. When a woman's allotted number of eggs are shed (about 400 in a lifetime, a figure established at birth) the most significant change is the less effective production of oestrogen. It doesn't stop being produced, but the level drops; it has actually slowly been decreasing since the middle-twenties, when a woman's body is at its most fertile. The oestrogen supply will eventually regulate itself and reach a plateau where it will remain. It's the adjustment period that causes problems. What happens is that the feedback system between ovaries, hypothalamus and pituitary gland is upset and the body has to find a way to rebalance the altered endocrine relationship.

Is the menopause obsolete? Biologically it exists, but a lot of information about the menopause is outdated. Earlier ideas were that a woman suffered emotionally because she was frustrated with marriage, not desired any more and not needed by her family. Social conditions have changed, and now it is understood that both physical and emotional upsets stem from changes in the hormonal balance and body chemistry.

## Know the symptoms and their relevance

The menopause is not purely a biological phase, but is accompanied by psychological aspects, which whatever their source – body chemistry or emotional turmoil – are nevertheless very real and at times more difficult to overcome than any physical change. Some women can manage to sail through these years without a hitch, though about three-quarters of women experience some symptoms while it's happening. For the majority (an estimated seventy per cent) the physical symptoms are not severe. If they are, it is usually due to a drastic reduction or cessation of oestrogen, which can be remedied with hormone replacement therapy. It is impossible to state exactly how long the body will take to go through the climacteric; it can be a few months or it can take years, stretching from well before the actual menopause date to years afterwards. If you are one of those unfortunate women who seem to be constantly plagued with symptoms, do not grin and bear it, nor accept the fact that it's normal for your time of life (many doctors will still say this), nor dose yourself with tranquillizers. You must seek specialized help where responsible and constructive treatment can be given. There are now several menopause clinics; also very supportive are the community groups of women who meet to give mutual support and exchange information. Check out the following guide to symptoms and see where you stand. Don't think for one minute you are likely to have them all! Some women experience only a few, but at least be aware of the possibilities.

**general symptoms** – overall tiredness and lassitude, nervousness caused by tension, heart palpitations, giddy attacks or dizziness, plus headaches particularly of the migraine type. Changes in blood pressure are a problem at this stage, while hormone imbalance can cause tingling and numbness in the hands and feet. Excessive sweating is usual which can affect sleep and general composure. Weight can increase, particularly a thickening around the waist (watch diet and exercise to keep in trim). Fluid retention can cause swelling of legs and feet. Hair may thin out, but there could be increased facial hair; skin often becomes drier. There can be joint changes and pain, and because of a loss of bone mass (osteoporosis) bones become thin and brittle and more prone to fractures.

**emotional aspects** – there are many contributory factors: problems from physical symptoms, social pressures, realization of change, biochemical imbalance. Tension and general irritability can lead to upsets at home and work. Mood changes occur – from apathy to aggressive behaviour, depression, crying fits, persecution complex, poor concentration and forgetfulness. Many women feel they should be able to control these moods and pull themselves together, but it's not so easy and constant nervous reactions can lead to longer-term depression and a breakdown.

**hot flushes** – the commonest symptom of the menopause and one that causes great distress. A flush can be just a warm feeling or a

The negative side of sex during and after the menopause is constantly featured in articles and books. This is because most of them are written by doctors, who naturally only hear the bad news. If a woman is having good sex and feels great, she is not likely to tell her doctor about it. If something is wrong, she does. So don't be discouraged by these unbalanced reports – sexuality can, and does, continue smoothly way into later years.

drenching sweat. They can be incapacitating and embarrassing. Many doctors think it's not serious enough to merit treatment, yet it can reach a point when it causes continual exhaustion and can trigger off psychological disturbances.

Flushing occurs when the nervous mechanism controlling the blood vessels is impaired. It usually begins with a feeling of physical and mental tension; it is first felt in the chest or abdomen, then there is a sensation of heat together with a blotchy reddening of the skin that spreads upwards over the chest, neck and face. It is followed by sweating, which cools down the skin's surface and relieves tension – quick cooling can cause shivering. A flush may last a few seconds or minutes, may occur several times in an hour or only occasionally within twenty-four. It can happen at any time during day and night and with no regularity of intervals. Night sweats can be particularly unpleasant, and many women find it necessary to repeatedly change clothes. The cause of flushes is metabolical, not emotional; the disturbance in glandular regulation of the body's processes causes circulation and capillary problems. Three out of four women suffer from hot flushes in varying degrees. They will stop spontaneously after a while, but if they continue and are really troublesome, seek treatment.

**genital changes** – physical alterations take place in the reproductive organs, but only one in ten women find them a serious problem. Most women are not aware of what is happening. The ovaries atrophy and shrink, reduced oestrogen causes dryness and shrinkage of the uterus and vagina; the outer genitalia can decrease in size, the folds of the vulva thin and the clitoris can become smaller. Breasts sometimes decrease in size and are less firm. Dryness can affect sexual and bladder function. The main trouble is the loss of glycogen which precipitates the decreased secretion of protective acid. This results in less lubrication, a thinned vaginal wall and less distensible vagina, plus soreness and itching. Non-prescription vaginal jelly or cream may help to relieve the symptoms, but permanent treatment is from local hormone treatment, oral oestrogen tables or oestrogen pessaries over a period of two weeks.

## Treatment: Hormone Replacement Therapy

Medical attitudes to women and the menopause have been changing for the better over recent years. It is not a disease, but a change, and a woman may need help in many directions to see her through it. A responsible doctor will take into account all aspects of your life and give general medical checks to establish if symptoms are menopause-related or not.

If the effects of the menopause are severe and constant, hormone replacement therapy is the answer. For over thirty years, gynaecologists have used oestrogen for chronic cases and it was only when the public became aware of oestrogen due to extensive publicity that it came under closer scrutiny and started a controversy. This was because of its indiscriminate use as a 'youth pill' (mostly in the

Several menopausal symptoms, particularly to do with a slowing down of both physical and mental capacity, might very well be due to a thyroid deficiency. Have it checked.

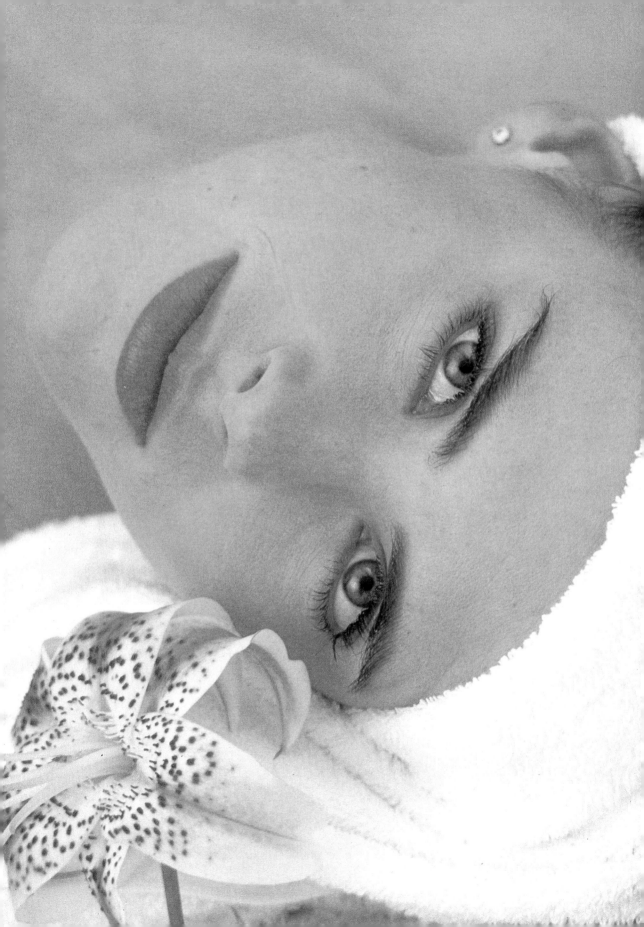

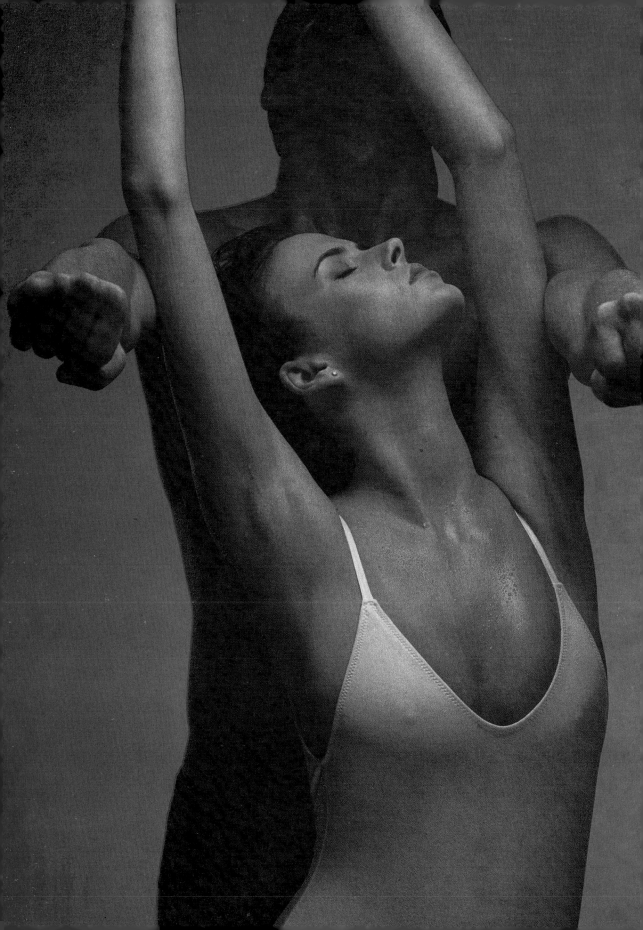

United States) and because there was a scare that it might cause uterine cancer.

Scientific evidence reveals that if hormone replacement therapy (HRT) is administered responsibly and under strict medical supervision, risks are reduced to the point of virtual elimination. As previously mentioned, most menopausal symptoms stem from an abrupt stoppage in the supply of oestrogen. Therapy involves adding oestrogen to the bloodstream in decreasing amounts over a period of time, which gives the body a chance to adapt to the final hormonal balance in a gradual way. It is effective for all menopausal symptoms, but particularly brings relief for hot flushes.

Treatment is usually in the form of tablets providing the smallest dosage of oestrogen. It is given in regular cycles, that is a few weeks of pills, a few weeks off. This can be continued for months or years if necessary, the amount of oestrogen decreasing all the time. Sometimes small doses of progesterone are added which stimulates regular bleeding. Some doctors believe that continued combined doses could counteract and even stall the effects of aging. At this point there is not enough evidence to back up the theory, but it may be the answer for the future. At the moment, it is known that HRT can help prevent decrease in bone mass and eliminate osteoparosis.

Side effects are proving to be minimal. The first few days may bring nausea, bleeding can occur if the dosage is too high. There is sometimes an increased tendency to blood clots if treatment goes on for a long time, but doctors are careful to monitor this with repeated checks and laboratory tests.

# STRESS
## Relax and make it work for you

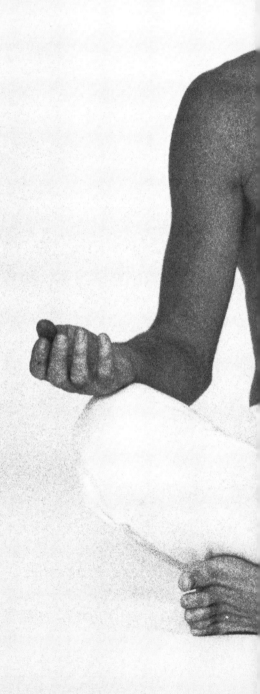

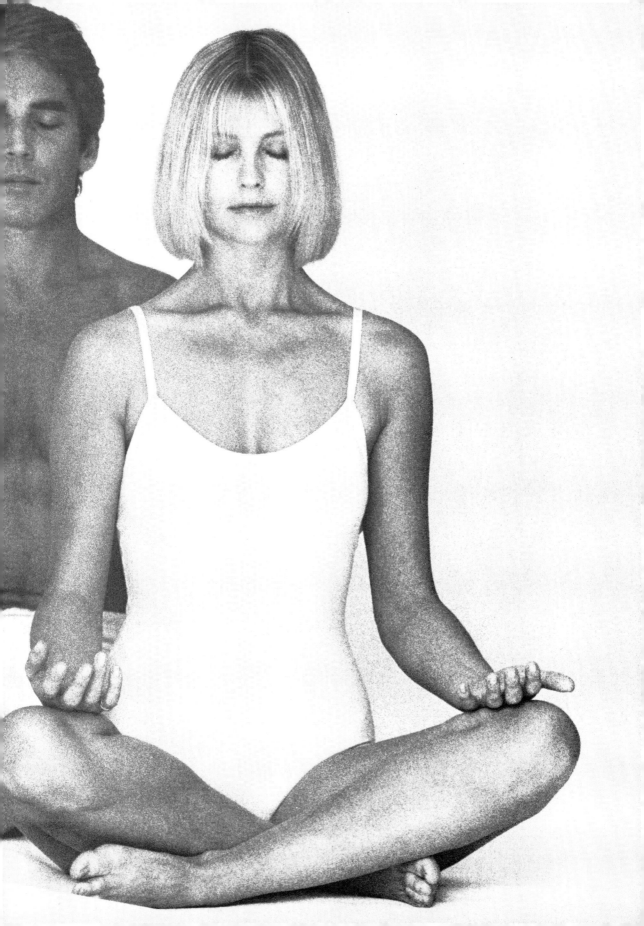

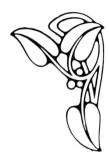

It is now considered a fact that mental and emotional stresses are the main causes of the degenerative diseases that lead to premature aging. Tension, anxiety, worry and depression will age you before your time, so will negative emotions such as hate, envy and jealousy as these can prey on your mind and obliterate any positive thoughts.

Life is filled with tension but a certain amount of stress is natural and cannot be avoided. It can even be beneficial as it can spur you on to achieve things you'd never think were possible, and you can make it work for you if it is counterbalanced by sufficient rest and relaxation. That is the important thing – being able to effectively put your body and mind at rest to recuperate both physical and mental forces. The problem is that very few people can do it, and this is what this chapter is all about. I'm not going to dwell on the woeful side of stress as we all know its negative results, but I'm putting forward various ways and means for self help.

Who suffers from stress? Anybody and everybody. We all have different levels of tolerance, but no matter to what degree, stress is present in all lives. Routine jobs can be as stressful as high powered ones, and the bored housewife is equally as susceptible as the business tycoon. It has a lot to do with our society being success orientated, and the constant reminders by the media about the achievement of others. It is often the exposure to the facts of what others are achieving that makes one feel inadequate. Before sophisticated communications revealed how the rest of the world lived, most people were reasonably contented in their slot. Now no more, the pressure is on.

Women are subject to more psychological strain than ever before. Ironically, fighting for equal rights has produced a whole new set of pressures, which many of us feel we would be better without. Women have got themselves in the position of trying to be all things to all people. We are in constant conflict between the old traditions and what is basically nature and the cultural preaching of ardent feminists. This in itself is a tremendous stress, and there is no way one can say what is right and what is wrong. It is entirely up to you to work out the balance, to decide where your personality and priorities stand. Personally, I feel it is terribly wrong for a woman who is perfectly happy being a wife and mother to be made to feel inadequate and unfulfilled by not accomplishing something on her own. In fact, it is nonsense that she should feel it necessary. Divided loyalties can cause incredible stress and result in divided families. Such a situation, however, does force you to look closely at your personality and desires, to make yourself aware of how you function as an individual and not in the shadow or context of others. What do you want out of life? What are you happiest doing? What are you doing for yourself? Then balance these with your obligations within relationships. The secret of alleviating stress is to balance your needs with those of others nearest and dearest to you, and to balance the liberated woman with the passive one.

Stress can be productive. A moderate amount of it can improve efficiency, urge you on to creation, force you into action. The plus things are that the mind becomes clear, reflexes are quicker, energy increases and speech can become more fluent. All these are assets, and some people need stress to function at all. Only you can establish your optimum stress level and you can only do this through experience. You can tell through observation what really gets you going and what makes you fall apart. Once beyond the peak, stress is destructive – you will feel agitated, tense, jumpy and be unable to think or act clearly. On the other hand, if stress falls below a certain level you will feel frustrated, bored, unfulfilled and void of energy. That is also a form of stress. The ideal is a level at which you feel your happiest, function to capacity and end the day feeling fulfilled at what you have achieved. Acquiring this level is not automatic, it demands realistic observation, assessment and readjustment. You've probably never looked at stress this way before, but if you do, you can use it to your advantage. Learn to distinguish between positive and negative stresses and work out the optimum balance for you.

What happens in your body during a stress situation? Practically every metabolic function is affected as the original animal fight-or-flight syndrome is instinctively put into action. It is our response to danger, though today's dangers stem more from mental and emotional sources than from actual physical threat. The response is totally automatic – the temperature drops and sweating increases, the heart beat rises by as much as one hundred per cent in order to increase blood supply to the muscles; the muscles tense and lactic acid is released into the blood stream which causes anxiety to increase; cholesterol is produced by the liver for fuel; the adrenal glands release hormones; breathing becomes faster and shallower, sugar is released from the liver into the bloodstream for energy, so is the subcutaneous fat; digestion closes down, the salivary glands stop and the mouth becomes dry. All this happens very quickly and studies show that these changes occur whenever the body is threatened regardless of the nature of the threat, be it physical or emotional. Danger is a primitive instinct and the body immediately becomes alert. If the body can physically let go at this point, it will quickly return to a calm relaxed normal state, but if not – which is usually the case with emotional stress – the body remains in a state of partial tension with all the consequential reactions and this is when the trouble starts. The tension that results from stress must subside, if not automatically, by training the body and mind to relax and let go. Otherwise, a continued state of arousal quickly leads to many disorders, initially manifested in headaches, digestive problems, general aches and pains.

tress can turn off sexual desire nd if you are ultra competitive ı your work, this can almost egate your female sexuality nd you'll find it difficult for oth mind and body to submit ɔ sexual responsiveness.

## COPING WITH STRESS

Stress has to be managed otherwise it will get the better of you. Th
most important thing is to acknowledge the value of rest an
relaxation. Life cannot be all go and the body has to calm down an
recuperate from time to time. Rest is as vital to health as th
right food and regular exercise. If you feel you are doing too muc
and getting het up about it, you need to stop for a minute and sor
out your mind, your attitude and your daily living pattern. How we
do you handle stress? Do you actually know how to or where t
begin? Here are some suggestions:

### Lifestyle Guides

It is often mismanagement of daily living that causes stress rathe
than some external trauma. Problems that should really be of littl
consequence can explode into high drama and seem insurmour
table. Putting everything into proper perspective has a lot to do wit
planning and expectation; it has a lot to do with pacing your day
with balancing work and pleasure, alternating activity and res
Conserve and recharge your batteries by occasional pauses c
simply doing nothing, or consciously relaxing (see how to on pag
168). The following are points to check:

**become more active** – physical activity of any kind counteract
stress. It will leave you feeling much more relaxed and if you follov
a regular exercise programme – even if it's only a long walk ever
day – you are less likely to get in a state of tension. Even doing
constructive household chore will relieve the pressure, and in an
case something positive will have been achieved – perhaps all th
ironing.

**manage time** – a great deal of stress is caused by falling behind i
work or household matters. It is at this point that you fee
everything is too much and you simply can't cope. However, this i
often more to do with how you manage time rather than the numbe
of tasks. A lot can be achieved in a day and if you work out
schedule and systematically allocate time, you'll be surprised hov
all the tasks can be fitted in. We all waste time – keep a record for
few days of what you do, and you'll be amazed how much time wa
spent fiddling around, doubling up on jobs and doing unnecessar
things. Careful daily planning can cut down on stress.

**establish priorities** – part of time management is to decide what ar
the most important things to get done. Make a list of jobs in order c
importance and methodically work through them. It is better to do
few things well than haphazardly tackle many. There's a terribl
feeling of frustration that comes from not doing anything properl
For example, if you are a working wife or mother, don't negle
yourself in desperation to keep the home straight. Make sure yo
look good every day as this will make you feel better about yourse
and spur you on to gradually get the house in order. So many wome

end up looking a mess and the home not that pulled together either. So there's frustration all round. There's little chance that everything can be perfect at one time.

**realize limitations** – today most women take on too much and the pressure is on for women to achieve something professionally and at the same time be marvellous wives and mothers. Not everyone can do everything, nor does everyone want to. It is very important to be realistic about your potential. By all means have ambition, but don't aim beyond the realm of possibilities. If you set yourself a goal and reach that, it can be very satisfying and will reduce the stress in your life; whereas if you are struggling to attain a dream, the strain on your mental and physical powers will be enormous. It is only a few women who are capable of becoming ministers, lawyers, doctors, writers, etc. – but bear in mind that applies equally to men.

**ration problems** – it is bad enough coping with one problem, but most of us have many churning around in the head, and the tendency is to jump from one to the other, grasping for momentary solutions. This causes more stress than the problems themselves, and it is also apt to exaggerate their number and seriousness. Try to disassociate yourself from these worries, putting them out of your head and holding them at bay for a while. Then pluck one back in for thorough inspection and analysis, and when you think you have solved that one, bring in the next. If you ration yourself to one worry at a time, it is so much simpler to solve them all. Start with the easiest, for example what to wear, when to shop, what to cook for dinner, etc. If ordinary everyday matters are solved, then the bigger ones to do with money, work, family and emotions can be approached with greater confidence. But remember – one at a time.

**limit changes** – it has always been said that a change is as good as a rest or a holiday, and so it is to a certain degree. However, too many changes can cause havoc. Frantic changes from house to house, job to job, man to man can seriously strain the nervous system. Scientific reports show that negative changes such as losing a job or a partner provide the highest degree of stress. Adjusting to any new environment requires great emotional effort – even a too hectic holiday can cause stress, just the matter of changing countries, language, customs or climate. There's a lot to be said for the comfort of routine; it only becomes monotonous and boring (therefore stressful) if no changes at all are made. So control changes if you can, remembering there are some over which we have absolutely no control – and to worry about those is a complete waste of time.

Don't take pills for stress, for anxiety, for depression, for insomnia. They may help you initially but in the long run can only make everything worse. Withdrawal symptoms from barbiturates and tranquillizers can be alarming. They can destroy the body's natural defensive mechanism. Have faith in the power of your body. If you treat it properly and have a persuasive mental approach, you can literally pull yourself together – as used to be said. Look into what you can do for yourself. Pills are a temporary crutch and then become a burden.

## Relaxation Techniques

Stress needs to be balanced with relaxation, yet the irony is that those who desperately need to relax find it the most difficult thing to do. Nervous tension has to be expended and if you can't do it through exercise or simply by putting your feet up to daydream or read, then you should systematically learn how to bring your mind and body to that necessary level of beneficial relaxation. It may seem paradoxical, but it is through discipline that you can finally let go. The way to do it is surprisingly simple and based on the proven patterns of Yoga. Serenity can be achieved by taking a little time, finding a quiet corner and following any or all of these routines.

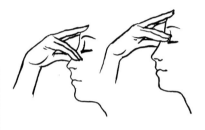

**breathing** – sit cross-legged or kneel on your heels, whichever is the more comfortable; place the first and second fingers of your right hand on your forehead, rest your thumb against the right nostril, hold your third and fourth fingers against the left nostril, closing it whilst you breathe in through the right nostril to the count of four. Now with the thumb close the right nostril, release pressure on the left and exhale through it to the count of four. Repeat five times. Reverse hands and breathe in through the left nostril, out through the right, follow the count of four rhythm and repeat five times.

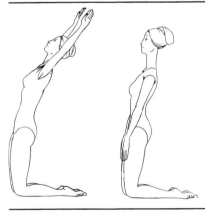

**rhythmic breathing** – kneel on the floor, curve the body over the thighs and relax with head on floor and arms back. Breathe in slowly, raising the body and bringing arms over the head; arch the body slightly, hold the breath for two or three seconds, then exhaling through the nose, slowly return to the original position, hold for a second, inhale and repeat the movement. Do six times. This is a good discipline to start the day.

**revitalizing slant** – a tried and true way to refresh the body and calm the mind, is a ten minute rest on a slanting board. Any board will do, raise one end twelve inches above the floor and cover with a towel. With head lower than feet, lie still, close your eyes and totally relax.

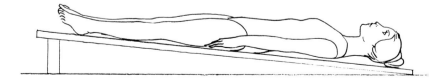

**pose of tranquillity** – as the name implies, this is a Yoga posture that helps the entire nervous system. It is recommended as a way to unwind at the end of the day or for relaxation before going to bed. Lie on the floor, arms stretched close to the head. Slowly raise the legs, bringing them over the head until they make an angle of forty-five degrees with the body. Then lift the arms, keeping them straight and place palms of the hands on the legs. Hold the pose as long as you can, keeping your eyes closed and mind free of hectic thought.

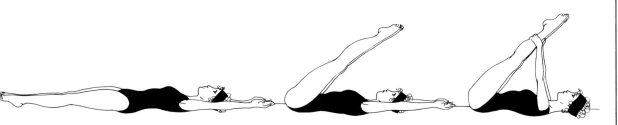

**letting go** – this is a way of getting the body in a completely relaxed state by mental concentration. Lie flat on your back, arms at sides. Take a few slow and deep breaths. Now try to visualize the patterns of your muscles. Get to know the sensation of movement and relaxation by flexing a toe, stretching a finger, moving the neck, holding in the abdomen. Now stretch your legs, brace the torso, stretch the arms, shoulders and neck. Mentally visualize the entire muscle build-up and hold in this stretched position for a few seconds. In slow motion, let go. Start at the top and work down, relax the head, the face, the jaws, the mouth, the neck and so on down through torso and limbs right to the toes. End up like a rag doll. Relax through will power.

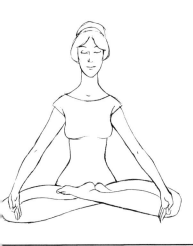

**meditation** – sit in the Yoga lotus position (see page 138) or cross-legged tailor-fashion. Close the eyes and try to concentrate on a single part of the body. The heart is a good choice. Think about what it looks like, its position, its beat; now turn from its physical aspects to the emotional ones and expand thoughts on the association of the heart with love, happiness or despair. Instead of looking inward, you can meditate on an external object – a candle, a light, a picture, a vase. Elements of nature are good subjects – flowers, trees, clouds, a river, the sea. Think deeply about the subject and develop thoughts and symbolic associations. It is often helpful to repeat a sound, or mantra. The most effective one for tranquillity is said to be that of O . . . M. Inhale and form the lips into an O, say the letter O until half the air has been expelled, then close the lips to say the letter M exhaling through the nose.

## Mind over Matter

If you accept the fact that stress can cause physical disorders and that it is negative thinking which triggers off adverse reactions, then it is only logical to reason that a positive mental attitude can improve health. It can – and it has been proved in laboratories around the world. This is, of course, the basis of many psycho therapies (see page 190) but it has also resulted in mental techniques that force the body into a relaxed state and actually bring about an improvement in many of the stress-related ailments. Two of the most significant are autogenic training and biofeedback. You may never have heard of either, but they are producing amazing results. This is how they work:

**autogenic training** – this involves learning a series of easy mental exercises, body awareness techniques and physical relaxation in order to turn off the fight-or-flight reaction to stress and turn on the relaxation and rest mechanism. The aim is to be able to do this at will, and balance all stress no matter what causes it.

It can be self-taught from a book, but it is much better to take a course, which involves an hour of instruction a week for eight weeks. (There's an autogenic training centre in London, see page 8 for reference.) Autogenics can be done anywhere, anytime and apart from mental control it involves doing basic exercises three times a day. Eventually you will learn to put yourself into a state of complete deep relaxation. Some people have very strong emotional reactions at first – tears, laughter, pain, for example – perhaps an indication they had been repressed for a long time. You can learn to generally balance stress, and finally master techniques for specific disorders. Its effectiveness is purely individual; some people have incredible success, others not so much. Only by training can you tell.

Stress-related disorders which benefit from autogenics include anxiety, circulatory problems, high blood pressure, digestive upsets, headaches, migraine, listlessness and insomnia. It has also helped those with dependency on alcohol or tobacco, and can slowly cut down addiction to tranquillizers, sleeping tablets and anti-depressants.

**biofeedback** – both mental and mechanical devices are used for this technique. Through instruments you have a continual report on your biological processes and as you learn to relax and calm down, your responses are immediately monitored for you to observe. Biofeedback is essentially a method of training the mind to control body functions which are usually involuntary. Normal relaxation response can be learned through biofeedback training.

It works this way: the recording equipment feeds back body reactions by way of sound, light or the movement of a needle on a chart. The louder the sound, the brighter the light or the higher the needle, the stronger the fight-or-flight reaction. The most basic response instrument is one that is attached to the palm or fingertips of the hands and measures the changes of polarization at the sweat

Learn to relax. But how! It's not easy, but it is essential if you want to keep up a younger vigour, a younger look. Make yourself rest, no-one can stand constant activity. Have an afternoon nap, just lie around and read a book, put on a record, simply do nothing. Don't feel guilty – the benefits are remarkable. One very well known beauty always took Thursday off, to lie in a darkened room all day, sipping lemon juice, having a massage, doing absolutely nothing. It clearly worked – she always looked marvellous.

gland membranes as this indicates the blood flow rate. There are also more sophisticated instruments which give a picture of what is going on in the mind. If you purposefully tense muscles, the sound or light becomes more forceful, and the needle swings high. If you consciously relax, all these indicators diminish in intensity. You can be taught thought processes that will finally stop all indicators completely. The ultimate aim is to find out what calms you down completely by observing the mechanical devices, and then being able to engineer the mental processes without the aid of a machine.

Biofeedback can help any illness where tension is the cause. It has been found to be extremely useful for headaches, migraines, irregular heartbeats, high blood pressure, strokes, gastric and duodenal ulcers and for a wide range of nervous disorders resulting from modern stress. It is a powerful preventive tool, as it can show you how the mind is able to control many workings of the body, and if you learn to use biofeedback for stress reduction and relaxation it could appreciably change your health level, but the skills learnt have to be incorporated into everyday life. Many hospitals now have biofeedback units, also private clinics and psychotherapy centres.

## SLEEP: the great revitalizer

To remain looking and feeling younger than your years, it is essential to get adequate restful sleep. The quality of sleep is actually more significant than the number of hours. It is not essential to have the traditional eight which is the average amount women require; each of us has our own individual biological clock. One woman may need ten hours sleep and another only four. There is no hard and fast rule. It is how you sleep that matters – four hours of peaceful rest is of much more benefit than eight hours of tossing and turning.

During sleep the body recuperates, not only physically but mentally; it needs this time to rebalance metabolism and regenerate energy. You only have to be without sleep for a while to realize how essential it is. Yet it is an extraordinarily natural thing – the body seems to know how much sleep it needs and unless influenced by outside distractions (a noise, an alarm) it will trigger wakefulness only when ready. Although there have been many scientific studies on sleep, how this mechanism works is still not quite clear. But what has been established is that the physiological processes involved in sleep include a span of biochemical changes and body movements which vary with age.

There are two phases to sleep. The first is a slow-wave sleep where muscles relax, breathing becomes regular, body temperature falls and the electrical brain wave patterns become slower and more even. The second phase is known as REM (standing for the rapid eye movements that go on under the lids) and though sleep is deep, body processes change considerably. Muscles relax more, but pulse rate and respiration become more rapid and irregular, while electrical brain wave patterns are similar to those when awake.

However, the most important aspect of REM sleep is dreaming, as it is now established that dreams restore the central nervous system, work out problems and reorder the psyche. Dreams can help in coming to terms with emotional problems.

Slow-wave sleep and REM sleep go in cycles during the night normally completing between four to six. Research has shown that if you are deprived of the slow-wave sleep it doesn't really matter, but if the REM cycles are limited, then tension and nervousness is increased. Dreams are good for mental health – whether you remember them or not.

Sleep is often disturbed by emotional problems, mainly anxiety and depression. In a depressed state you usually go to bed tired, drop off to sleep easily, but then wake up during the night – at any hour between two and five a.m. It is often very difficult to get to sleep again, because the mind is alert and intent on solving problems. Sleep usually eludes the depressed person in the early hours of the morning and although problems are sometimes solved, more often than not they become exaggerated.

Anxiety disturbs sleep even more. Sleep eludes the chronic worrier, even at the start of the night, and every fear is blown up out

*Lotte Berke* (aged 82 in 1983) 'My life philosophy – I refuse to be unhappy, to give in, to be ill. . . . I wake up every morning and say "Now what's happening today?" and I look for something that is good, that's going to make me feel happy. If I wake up feeling low I determine to find something, however small, that will turn the day into something better and make it all worthwhile.'

of all proportion. An anxious person may doze, but this is usually accompanied by alarming dreams. What can be done?

Getting to sleep and having the proper frame of mind for tranquil rest involves all the anti-stress and relaxation tactics. If you can manage to calm down at some point during the day, then there is a greater chance of your getting the essential nightly restorative rest. You may worry about not getting enough sleep and panic about your performance on the following day. But as I said before, not everyone needs a lot of sleep. Insomnia can result from this very concern, and many women seek treatment because they sleep only a few hours when it is only that amount they actually need. Complete insomnia is rare. People who say they can't sleep at all usually do so to some degree though they believe they lie awake night after night without closing their eyes.

Doctors usually describe a sleeping pill, barbiturate or tranquillizer – all these are disastrous as they add to the problem despite temporary relief. All can become addictive, whilst barbiturates immediately interfere with the essential REM sleep, which means that you often wake up more agitated than when you went to bed. It is better to leave them alone, and look at the many self-help and natural ways that will help you to get a good night's sleep with the maximum of benefit. Try any or all of the following:

- Are you getting enough daily exercise? If you are sedentary most of the day it's a good idea to take a brisk walk before going to bed, as this raises the pulse, increases respiration and makes you want to physically relax afterwards.

- Do you sleep in late? Force yourself to get up earlier, because if you do, you will want to get to bed at night and be anxious to fall asleep right away. It may be difficult for the first few days, but it is one get-to-sleep trick that works well.

- Only go to bed when you are really sleepy. Just because it is bedtime, there's no need to go. Do something calm and maybe creative until you are really tired. If you go to bed when your mind is still alert and reacting, you can delay sleep indefinitely.

- A warm bath is sleep inducive; a really luxurious soak in bubbles with music playing and maybe a book in hand. Not too long and not too hot, but just enough to relax; helpful aids are a few drops of the essential oils of lavender, orange blossom, rose or camomile.

- Before getting into bed establish a routine, a sort of security check on the household to set your mind at rest before going to sleep – are doors locked, windows closed, fire out, TV off, etc?

- Is your bed really perfect? You spend so much time in bed there's no point in skimping on it; invest in the best mattress, make an effort to have the prettiest surroundings.

- Check on pillows. Are they soft enough? You also shouldn't have too many nor should they be too high. The whole point of a pillow is to provide support for the curve of the spine in the neck area.

- Make sure you have not taken stimulants before going to bed, this includes alcohol, sugar, coffee and tea. Also the stomach should not be overloaded, though if you are out socializing, this is sometimes unavoidable.

- A milk drink is still a good idea before going to bed, it is calming and inducive to sleep – warm milk with honey or even a little whisky could send you out like a light.

- Stop worrying about sleep. The more you worry about falling to sleep and getting enough, the less likely you are going to drop off. Sleep should be a most natural thing – but if you think about it, it may elude you.

- Learn about natural tranquillizers and scrap the medical ones. A herbal tea of camomile or peppermint is soothing, so is an infusion of the simple lettuce (steep a few leaves in hot water for ten minutes), but possibly the best herb for insomnia and any nervous ailment is valerian. Infuse a teaspoon of the crushed root in a cup of boiling water; take in small doses, a mouthful at a time but no more than a cup a day. If you have a few doses during the course of the evening, by bedtime you should feel relaxed.

- Calming essential oils can be dropped into the pillow, the best are orange blossom, rose or sandalwood.

# HOW YOU CAN BENEFIT FROM THE PROFESSIONALS

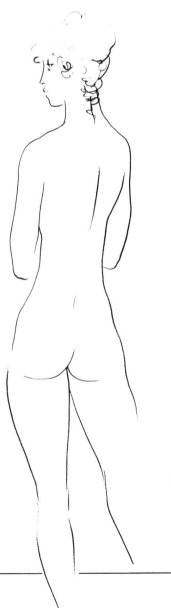

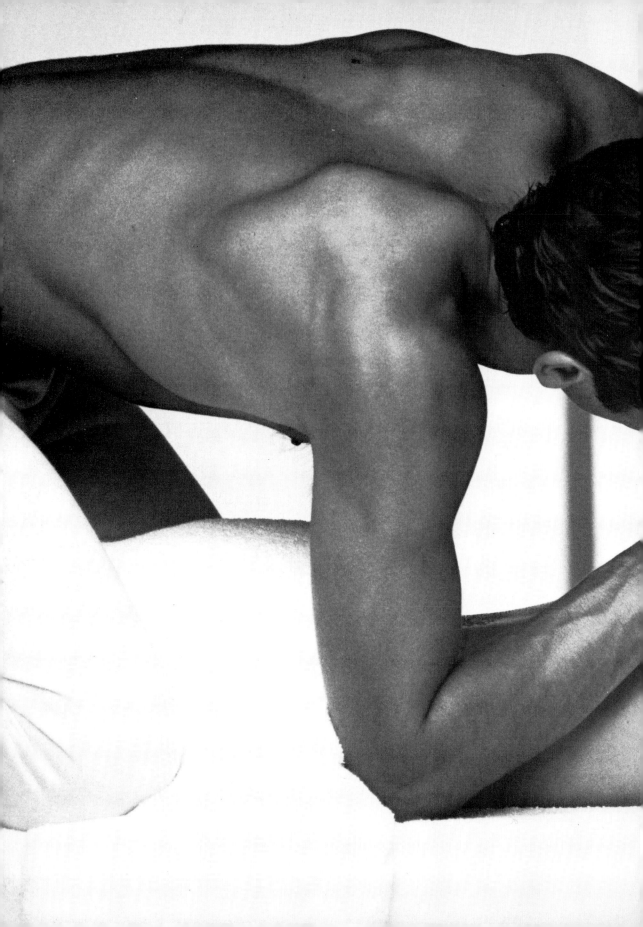

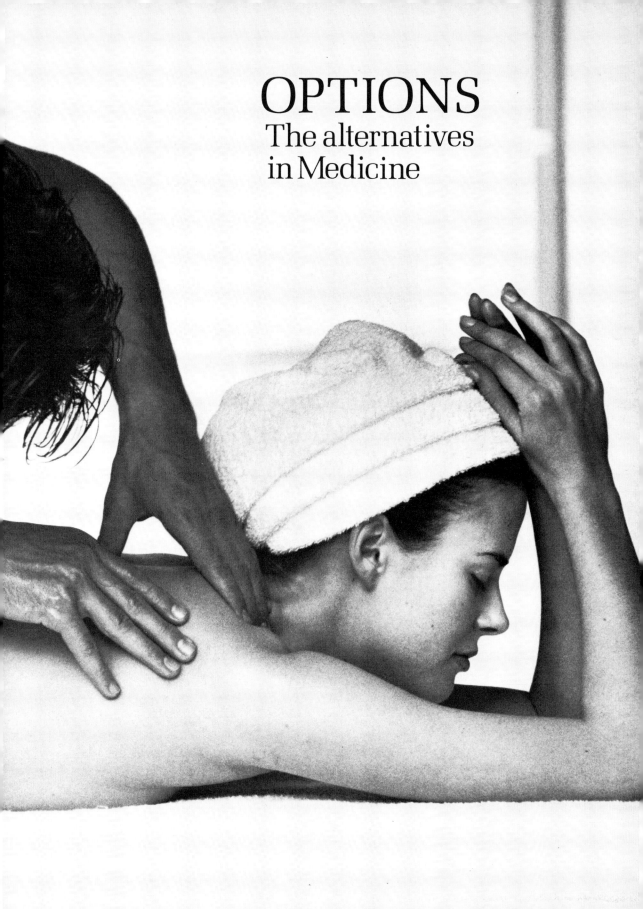

# OPTIONS
## The alternatives
## in Medicine

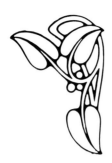

Over the past twenty years there has been considerably increased interest in other ways to treat disease apart from the usual allopathic one of relying on drugs and surgery. This interest, however, has been on the part of the patient and not the official medical establishment, who have been slow and reluctant to accept that the alternatives have anything valid to offer. We are on the brink of change, as orthodox medicine is going through a crisis of confidence particularly in the treatment of the degenerative diseases which have almost become an inevitable part of aging.

Improved hygiene standards have been responsible for the real leap ahead in healthier living and longer lives; inoculations and drugs now control viruses and epidemics; surgical skills become more impressive all the time. However, we seem to be stuck with heart diseases, circulation problems, digestive disorders, arthritis, rheumatism and, of course, cancer. Then there are the stress-related states that range from lethargy to depression, and the general feeling that you are simply not as well as you should be.

General medical practitioners have concentrated on treating physical symptoms with chemical remedies, prescribing pills, injections and tranquillizers – yet the side effects of drugs, some to the extent of actually causing another illness, are currently being questioned.

So what is the answer? The only sensible thing is to get to know what the options are. There are a surprising number of therapies, the majority of which could be termed 'natural' in as much as they rely for healing upon one force or another in nature's spectrum plus a belief in the human body's self-corrective mechanisms.

These are the auxiliaries to conventional medicine, not substitutes for it. Don't switch completely from one side of the medical fence to the other, but search and find out what is best for you from both. Any system that makes you feel better is good medicine. The most significant aspect of all natural therapies is that you are treated in a holistic way: that is, you are looked at as a whole person, not an isolated symptom. Body, mind, spirit and attitude are all considered to be of equal importance. A practitioner will ask not only questions about health, but about your lifestyle, your emotional and psychological states, your work, your domestic situation. The cause of the problem is thoroughly searched for, and it could come from any number of sources.

Although natural therapies work on a curative basis, they are especially valuable on the preventive level and therefore important for any stay younger programme. The capacity of the human body to improve and protect itself is far greater than you can imagine. You often need just a push in the right direction – a physical impetus, a mental suggestion. You can get to know your body much better and learn to recognize its warning signals through natural therapies, and start to take more personal responsibility for your health.

Here's a guide to the most important alternatives to orthodox medicine. Many of them go hand in hand and practitioners are often trained and experienced in more than one. If you go to a

Learning about natural medical therapies is an important step towards taking more responsibility for your own health. You'll discover fundamental facts about diet, body control, energy flow, early disease symptoms and how to cope with stressful situations.

naturopathic clinic or health farm, for example, you will find the nature cure attitude towards diet, hydrotherapy treatments, invariably a consultant at hand for chiropractic or osteopathy, often a homeopathic doctor, an aromatherapist, a Yoga teacher etc. All are members of the same family. Check the reference on page 8 for details of authorized practitioners. It is important to do this because alternative medicine doesn't come under the jurisdiction of official medical boards, so anyone can hang up a sign saying 'acupuncturist' for instance without fear of reprimand. The individual societies do have standards on training and qualifications and are only too happy to give out recommended lists as this is the only way to put out of business the charlatans that give fringe medicine an unnecessarily bad name.

## ACUPUNCTURE

Although practised in China for thousands of years, acupuncture only became generally known in the western world in the 1950s. It is completely different from any other medical therapy and one that at first may sound alarming. Fine needles are pricked into the skin at certain points in order to restore the flow of energy, called chi. Acupuncturists believe that health exists only when this energy flows freely and is in a state of perfect balance – and that depends on the two energies of yin and yan, the negative and positive forces of life.

The history of acupuncture goes back 5,000 years and is the very earliest form of Chinese medicine. It has continued to be used in the Orient, but only became known in the western world this century, due mostly to colonial Frenchmen who were impressed by its beneficial effects. Twenty-five years ago the Chinese invited a group of distinguished doctors to see for themselves how modern, sophisticated acupuncture successfully worked as an analgesic.

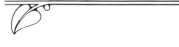

There are approximately 800 points for needle insertions over the body and they join vertically to form twelve main groups, called meridians, which are energy channels to the major organs. The needles are fine and can be of gold, silver or copper, and are used in numbers varying from two to three to a dozen or more. Often there is no feeling when needles are inserted, but some areas may be sensitive and there is a tingling sensation. The spot where they are inserted may be far removed from the complaint area – a needle in the foot for backache, for example – but it is the whole meridian that is being treated. Needles may be inserted vertically or at an angle. They usually just penetrate the skin, but sometimes can go in an inch. The needle is moved to stir up the energy – rotating it rather like a screw or moving it up and down. The time the needles are left in varies according to the disorder and the individual technique and instinct of the practitioner. Treatments can take from twenty minutes to an hour.

Diagnosis is interesting. Medical history is recorded, but you will also be observed very closely, particularly in connection with breathing, movement and gestures which are prime indicators of energy failings; a tongue inspection is also considered very important. A special point is the taking of the pulses – yes, plural – because there are twelve to check, one for each meridian and six on each wrist. This pulse diagnosis is fundamental in acupuncture as it gives the readings of the energy flow. Past and present illnesses can be revealed, but it is also possible to predict future problems before physical symptoms appear. This makes acupuncture a worthwhile preventive treatment. Actually in China, doctors were paid to keep patients well in this way. It's a check-up system that therapeutically treats at the same time. A course of treatments is usually required depending on the disorder – a minimum of six sessions is considered average because by that time you should be able to judge benefits. Reactions naturally vary, some patients claim to feel invigorated right from the start, while it may produce tiredness in some and actually initial aches or rashes – these are caused by the body's energy flow and will disappear within a few days.

Conditions which acupuncturists say they can treat with confidence include headaches, migraine, neuralgia, ulcers and digestive troubles, lumbago, arthritis, rheumatism, sciatica, dermatitis, eczema and other skin conditions, asthma, bronchitis and colds; it is also said to help anxiety and depression. It is commonly used for pain relief, indeed in China it is the method of anaesthesia for surgery. On the whole practitioners do not like to stress help for a specific illness, for they always treat the entire body, generally tuning up the entire system so that it is capable of healing itself.

## ALEXANDER TECHNIQUE

This is a method by which general health can be improved and certain disorders helped by making postural changes. It is not manipulation done by another, such as in osteopathy and chiropractic (detailed on pages 190 and 183), but under the guidance of an individual teacher you learn to correct your own body. Posture is fundamental to wellbeing because the spinal column is literally the backbone of health with its concentrated network of nerves and vessels.

We all misuse our bodies to some degree, causing physical and organic disturbances. Poor posture leads to faulty co-ordination and movement, to wrong use of muscles, to incorrect breathing, to nerve blockages and invariably to pain and tension. Its effect on general health can be far-reaching.

It was an Australian, Matthias Alexander, who brought the posture principle into medical focus around the end of the nineteenth century. He was an actor and suddenly began to lose his voice for no apparent reason. Finding no satisfactory medical answer, he diligently and systematically observed his own body and discovered the cause: he was moving his head oddly and misusing his spine. He corrected his faults, recovered his voice and developed a technique of showing people how to rethink posture to regain health.

The basic concept is that spinal energy should flow upwards without any blockage, that the head should be on an imaginary string pulling it straight and high, and that all movement should stem from it.

As with most natural therapies, it is practically impossible to assess the value of the Alexander Technique in standard clinical trials, as more is involved than just correction of posture and movement. However, some very famous people have stood up to vouch for it – thinking people, more interested in its effect on mind and energy; Bernard Shaw, Aldous Huxley and Sir Stafford Cripps all considered it played a leading part in their personal growth.

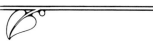

It is practically impossible to describe the Alexander Technique because although the principle remains the same, the method depends on individual problems. You take a course of lessons and you are shown how to correct your bad habits. But it is more than that – it's a reconditioning of body and mind, as through mental processes you change automatic body responses. It's a body training course of the highest order, and enthusiasts say it is one of the great experiences towards articulate body-consciousness.

There's practically no-one who could not benefit from an Alexander course because you just generally feel better. In fact a lot of patients are those people who don't know why they never feel completely well – always something like a headache, a backache, a pain here, breathlessness at times etc. Muscle, bone and nerve disorders are helped a lot, plus any movement difficulties. It is really a sophisticated form of rehabilitation and self-physiotherapy.

## AROMATHERAPY

As the name implies this treatment involves a sense of smell, but that is only part of it. Aromatic oils and essences are used to regenerate the nerve points, the skin and the mind. Aromatherapy was an important part of medicine in ancient China, Egypt and all old civilizations, but has only been revived in modern terms during this century. Scientific aromatherapists are analysing the chemical components of the essences and gradually discovering what it is that provides the special power.

Plant essences have been compared to blood as they contain all the healing elements and characteristics of the plants from which they come. The therapeutic agents act both externally and internally; the professional practitioner prescribes a combination of aromatics (there are around forty to choose from) in all applications – massage, inhalation and oral. The essential oils can be absorbed by the body through the skin and reach organs via the nervous system and sometimes the endocrine network. They stimulate internal metabolisms and muscles – not chemically, but by energy and radiation.

The aromatherapist is primarily interested in restoring the natural rhythm of the body; growing old, they say, is but a slowing down of body rhythm and to stimulate it is a preventive measure. The regeneration of tissue is seen in the fresher, livelier look of skin after even one treatment. It can help skin disorders including the effects of scars and burns. Bones and muscles benefit, so it is a boon for rheumatism and arthritis. Respiratory ailments respond well. Of great significance, however, is the effect of aromatics on the psychic and mental state, so any illness that is psychosomatic or stress-related can be helped. Certain scents can bring about complete relaxation and relieve tension; others can sharpen the mind and make perception and memory more acute.

As with other alternative medical therapies, it is usual to have a series of treatments. Diagnosis is detailed, personality and

Oils and essences were the backbone of Chinese and Egyptian medicine, in fact were in common use in all ancient civilizations and their healing power is even mentioned in the Bible. Incense and perfume have an effect on the mind as well as on the body, which is probably why they have always been used for religious and mystic ceremonies.

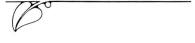

emotional patterns are as important as physical ones. Allied diagnostic aids may be used such as a check on foot reflex zones, blood crystal formations or energy messages from, for example, a strand of hair. Application and massage concentrate in the spinal area, from the base of the neck and around the shoulders, for maximum contact with the central nervous channels. Inhalation is also employed for respiratory problems, while digestive and urogenital disorders are treated orally.

The mixture of oils applied is individually prepared. It will contain essences of various densities and variable times of evaporation. Heavy resin-bearing scents and dense oils influence the quality of the tissues and the assimilation of food. Moderately fluid oils effect function and mobility, while the more volatile oils act on the mind.

Many beauty therapists claim to give an aromatherapy treatment, but this should really be called cosmetic, aromatic massage, because although it will benefit the skin and it does smell divine it should not be considered as a medically therapeutic treatment. You have to seek out a trained aromatherapist.

## BACH FLOWER REMEDIES

An original creation of Dr Edward Bach, a British physician who pioneered a new way of healing during the 1920s and 30s. There are thirty-eight remedies derived from flowers, but they are unusual in that they are prescribed not directly for a biological disorder, but according to a negative emotional or personality trait such as fear, worry, anger, depression. Dr Bach firmly believed that all illness stemmed from agitated mental states.

The idea that a flower can influence the mind so that it can cure the body sounds improbable, but there have been enough remarkable results to put the Bach remedies on a valuable therapeutic basis, despite scientific bafflement as to why they work.

The treatment is based on the principle of helping the body achieve its highest state of positive thinking in order to restore health or prevent disease. The remedies are benign and can be used in conjunction with any other form of treatment, orthodox or otherwise. It seems extraordinary that they can be harmless in themselves and yet capable of transmitting such forceful, positive energy. What is more anybody can follow Bach's instructions. You don't have to go to a special therapist, though many alternative medical practitioners use them in conjunction with their own particular speciality.

The remedies are available from health centres and homeopathic chemists together with the Handbook of Bach Flower Remedies – or you can directly contact the Bach Centre at Wallingford, near Oxford. Self-treatment requires sensitive and honest observation of your feelings, emotions and reactions when in a crisis, under stress or tired. Two or three drops of the concentrated remedy are diluted

Dr Edward Bach was originally in orthodox medicine as a pathologist and bacteriologist, but becoming dissatisfied he switched to homeopathy (see page 185 and that led to his belief that it was the emotional state that causes disease. He turned to flowers for the answer and roamed the countryside to find the right ones growing in the wild. He selected through intellect and instinct, and became so sensitive that he only had to hold his hand over a flower to detect its possible healing properties.

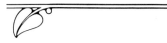

in pure water in a special treatment bottle; two or three drops of this highly potentized solution are taken in a glass of water whenever necessary. There is no chance of taking too much – in urgent cases every few minutes until there is improvement, in severe ones every half an hour, as a preventive once a day.

Remedies are divided into seven groups; fear, uncertainty, lack of interest in the present, despondency and despair, over-care for others, loneliness, over-sensitivity; and each group is subdivided so that the whole spectrum of emotions is taken care of, even those of jealousy, guilt, hatred, suspicion and resentment.

## BIO-RHYTHMS

This is not exactly a therapy, but it is a way of establishing your biological ups and downs which could be very important as you grow older in helping you to know when to conserve energy and when you can push yourself to the limits.

Variations in capability, performance and mood depend on energy. We have three cycles: the physical, the emotional and the intellectual. All cycles commence at birth, but each is of a different length. The physical cycle has a twenty-three-day span and controls strength, stamina, general health, protection and recovery from illness. The emotional cycle is twenty-eight days and affects moods, emotions and creativity. The intellectual cycle lasts thirty-three days and governs mental ability, concentration, memory and rationality. Each cycle has a positive stage when energy is flowing freely, a transition period when it ebbs and flows, and a negative stage when there is less energy. There are periods when all three cycles are simultaneously at the peak or at their low, which, if you hadn't thought of it before, accounts for feeling so on top of the world at some points in your life and so despondent at others.

It is possible to obtain monthly charts from agencies – calculations are now simple due to computers – or work them out for yourself from detailed books. They will reveal the pattern of energy variations, but how you react to them is up to your situation at that moment. Bio-rhythm knowledge is a useful tool, for it gives you the opportunity to take advantage of energy when it's there, and be cautious when it isn't. This means you can avoid frustration and reduce tension, thus preserving your body and mind for a longer, more rewarding life.

## CHIROPRACTIC

This is a manipulation therapy in relationship to the nervous system. Chiropractors believe that displacement of joints and muscles, particularly those of the spinal column, can cause illness because of nerve irritation. If any of the vertebrae of the spine are out of line, it is not just your back that will ache, but you may also suffer from headaches, indigestion, asthma and psoriasis. This therapy is

---

There is still no definite evidence that bio-rhythms exist, though research into illness zeniths and deaths reveal these occurred in more than fifty per cent of the cases on critical days. A German physician, Dr Wilhelm Fliess first developed the idea, but it was an Austrian, Professor Herman Swoboda, whose research gave it more credibility. Extended studies now also take into account circadian rhythms, which are daily cycles.

very close to – and is often confused with – osteopathy (see page 190). Both treat by manipulating the spine, but chiropractors use more direct and repeated thrusts; they also make use of X-rays to verify the extent of bone deviation or lesion.

Most people who go to a chiropractor suffer from back pain, sciatica, hip, leg and knee problems, shoulder and arm pains and headaches. These are all the disorders that orthodox doctors just don't seem to be able to cure, and merely prescribe pain-killing drugs. A turn to chiropractic is often the last resort; in fact, it should be the first.

Your initial consultation will involve a detailed case history, a thorough physical examination, an X-ray and possibly blood and urine analysis. You just don't go to have your back put into place, as is generally thought. The immediate task, however, is to adjust the spine; this may require several visits before it is correct on a permanent basis. You are guided in posture, movement and relaxation exercises. An interest in Yoga is encouraged, as are remedial massage and water therapy. Chiropractic is a notable preventive measure, since health depends very much on good transmission of nervous energy.

Chiropractic was founded by Daniel David Palmer in North America at the end of the last century. It was an accidental discovery. He heard someone explaining how he had lost his hearing many years previously after bending over and feeling something 'go' in his back. Palmer found a vertebra out of place, adjusted it and gradually hearing was restored.

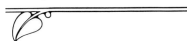

## HERBALISM

Remedies are either in the form of medicine to be taken orally or for use on the skin either as an ointment or a poultice, but all are prepared from the roots, leaves, stems and seeds of plants. The use of plants for healing was one of man's earliest instincts – and one that animals still have – though it went into decline when synthetic drugs came into being. Now herbs are back in favour because faith in manufactured pharmaceuticals has been shaken due to reports that they can in themselves create illness, cause allergies or breed resistant strains of bacteria. Herbal remedies are neither toxic nor habit-forming.

This renewed interest in the merits of herbalism has resulted in scientific research to find out exactly what the power parts are. Manufacturers, of course, have ideas to isolate the substances to finally market them. But an interesting fact has been revealed: it is the whole plant that provides the benefit and sometimes the key element doesn't work when isolated, or on its own may produce adverse side effects. It is thought that nature gives plants a balance, an interaction of active parts where one element backs up the work of another – or that passive elements may be there to act as a buffer, to help modify any harsh action. This is known as synergism, and such natural joint effort is absent in synthetic reproductions.

Another result of modern, analytical, techniques on plants is that they have shown these therapeutics do contain compounds familiar to medical chemists and do have the antibiotic and chemical properties claimed for them. A major complaint against herbs has always been that they are not standardized. This is true because

Herbalism originated about 5,000 years ago in the Far East. It was an essential part of Greek and Roman medicine and continued as an instinctive remedial source until the Middle Ages when it lost its original natural character by acquiring overtones of astrology and magic. The monks and nuns, however, continued to cultivate herbal gardens for the benefit of the sick. Herbs continued as the basis of country cures and remedies were handed down from generation to generation.

With regard to age prevention, one of the best elements in the herbalist's repertoire is an oil extracted from the seeds of the evening primrose plant. It has shown to have remarkable results with many of the ailments associated with middle years and onwards both physical and mental. The oil is a valuable source of an essential fatty acid known as gamma-linolenic acid, which the body can produce but finds it increasingly difficult to do so as it ages.

their quality and strength vary according to the soil, the climate, the time of year – and sometimes the time of day – when they are picked. But nature has a remarkable capacity for adjustment – and after all, human beings aren't standardized either.

Herbs, of course, are available to anyone – for the picking or over the counter of a specialist shop. There are a wealth of books giving advice, giving almost too long a list of herbal suggestions for everyday disorders. Deciding which to use is a matter of trial, error and your personal palate. For general health, drinking herbal teas instead of coffee and tea can be a start. Don't be too ambitious; begin by getting to know just twelve and end up by using the ones you personally find improve your health. A suggested list: basil, borage, burdock, camomile, comfrey, dandelion, mint, meadowsweet, parsley, sage, sorrel and wild oat.

Consulting a medical herbalist is another matter. Although they will prescribe remedies specially blended for each patient and each illness, today's herbalists like to take the holistic approach and think of the remedies as just part of treatment. Many herbalists are also naturopaths and your entire physical and mental pattern is discussed, plus details of your reaction to chemical drugs and inoculations.

Herbalists take the attitude that as well as counteracting the symptoms of a disease, they are more able to get to the source of trouble with a formulated plant remedy than with a standard chemical one. They also point out that it is specific patients rather than specific disorders that benefit. However, apart from this overall approach, herbal medicines have helped, and do help, the annoying everyday disorders such as colds, coughs, tonsilitis, headaches, rheumatism and arthritis, skin troubles, digestive problems, nausea, constipation and diarrhoea. They help keep the body in good working order and should be regarded as prime disease preventives. A trained herbalist will be able to tell you what individual concoctions you should take to maintain good health – and your prescriptions will be different to anyone else's. And ask about the herb home first-aid kit: treatments for burns, cuts, bites, bruises etc.; they really work.

## HOMEOPATHY

In practically every way, the homeopathic approach to disease is completely opposite to that of the orthodox medical practitioner. At the crux of it is the interpretation of symptoms. We have been brought up to believe that symptoms are the result of a germ, a virus, an internal toxin or foreign body, and that the essential thing is to get rid of the symptom with a counteracting remedy. The homeopathic belief is that symptoms are the tangible manifestations of what the body is using to resist and repel the disorder – and the body should be helped by giving it more of the same thing, as an extra boost to what it is doing itself. This is not easy to comprehend

Homeopathy was established almost 200 years ago by Samuel Hahnemann, from Saxony. He had trained as an orthodox doctor and had done considerable research in pharmacology. He turned away from the cruelty of medicine at that time and believed the patient's life force was sufficient to cope with illness if it was given the right push. He was exceedingly diligent in his initial provings of remedies, trying them first on himself, then others. Recently many of his early remedies have been 're-proved' and the original work scientifically endorsed.

for anyone ingrained with established medical explanations. But think of it this way: if you have a fever, you are normally given a drug to bring it down; however, a homeopath would give you a remedy to induce more fever.

That is not the only radically different approach, the other is in the strength of the remedy. We usually believe that the stronger the medical dose, the better; homeopaths say that the more diluted the dose, the more powerful it is. Little wonder that orthodox practitioners find it hard to accept homeopathy as valid treatment. Traditionally homeopaths have first completed a training in orthodox medicine, but now homeopathic remedies are frequently used by natural therapists.

What are the remedies? They are all from natural sources, mostly from the plant and animal worlds, but minerals are also used. They are selected for their ability to provoke a similar set of reactions to that of the illness if given to a healthy person. For example, if a fit person is given a dose of quinine, it produces a high fever of the type that comes from malaria; therefore quinine is given to cure someone who has malaria. And it does. There are about 2,000 such remedies in the homeopathic pharmacopoeia. They come as pills, tinctures, powders, granules and ointments. They are personally formulated and to a potency decided by the practitioner.

Clinical trials in conjunction with orthodox methods have shown the effectiveness of homeopathic drugs, but although cautious approval has been conceded by orthodox groups, it is by no means an overall concession. Homeopaths offer alternatives to all conventional medicine, plus freedom from side effects, but because homeopathic remedies work slowly allopathic antibiotics are advised when a virulent infection threatens life.

A consultation with a homeopath is more or less along the same lines as that with an establishment doctor except that diagnosis takes longer and goes much deeper. Emotional, psychological and sociological aspects are probed, plus personality. This is because for each symptom there are many remedies and the choice depends on the many possible variations. In this way, homeopathic therapy is extremely individual and finding a drug to match the temperament is as important as matching the drug to the symptoms.

Although science cannot fully explain why and how homeopathic therapy works, there is a relationship between it and the orthodox method of inoculation: a very small amount of the disease is injected into the body so it can reject, or better combat, that virus should the body ever be exposed to it. In this way epidemics of smallpox, cholera, diptheria etc. have been controlled.

## HYDROTHERAPY

Water has always been widely used as part of a general nature cure, but even the individual aspects are beneficial on their own. Hydrotherapy is often prescribed by a naturopath and is always available at health farms and spas. It has many facets: water as a cleansing agent, beverage, baths, steam treatments, hot and cold compresses, underwater massage and internal irrigation.

Therapeutic centres are usually concentrated in areas where special mineral waters are to be found. Many mineral waters are particularly beneficial for connective tissue. All water, however, can be health-giving providing it is fresh, clear and uncontaminated. Running water exposed to the sun is said to have special curative power as it absorbs solar energy and passes it on to the body.

Water can be used to relax or stimulate. The body responds to a cold stimulation by producing its own heat, which automatically increases the blood supply. Cold compresses applied locally cause perspiration and help eliminate toxic matter – the body is wrapped in blankets to exclude air. Sometimes the whole body is wrapped in a cold, wet sheet then covered with blankets. Cold showering from a forceful hose or jet is considered most invigorating. The stimulus of the cold bath varies according to the area immersed. A cold footbath draws blood away from the head and chest; a cold sitz bath – you sit in a bath so that water covers the area from upper thigh to the abdomen – stimulates elimination and reproductive organs. The combination of alternate cold and hot baths are often prescribed for internal problems.

Hot water treatments are in the form of moist (steam bath) or dry (sauna) heat. Both promote sweating and help eliminate toxic matter from the body. For a steam bath there are special cabinets where the body is shut in, but the head left exposed. A sauna is taken in a little wooden slatted cabin with a temperature anywhere from 100–200°F (38–93°C). It is usual to stay in for ten to fifteen minutes, then expose the body to cold air or water – a really cold plunge is the most beneficial – and return to the sauna for another ten minutes. Anyone with high blood pressure should not take a sauna.

Thalassotherapy is the name given to sea water treatments. The sea is extremely rich in minerals and sea air is high in fortified oxygen molecules that can revive and stimulate both the respiratory and circulatory systems. Some naturopaths recommend drinking 1oz (30g) daily to provide the essential minerals to the body; other treatments include baths, seaweed compresses, jet sluices and inhalation.

Hydrotherapy is a marvellous way to keep the body healthy and toned. You can often make an arrangement with a health farm for a day visit, while some beauty therapists have steam cabinets and health clubs usually have saunas. A final word: ask about underwater massage (see page 225 for details) as it trims and tones.

## MASSAGE

Massage may not appear to be a medical therapy, but there are varying degrees of it. In its most widely used form it promotes relaxation and eases tension by manipulating the soft tissues. When a special method, called rolfing, is employed it can reshape the body through muscle massage and is said to bring new awareness to the mind. The orientals go even further in their acupressure and shiatsu methods using pressure and touch to free the energy flow and therapeutically help all organs and disorders. Here's a summary of all types:

**General massage:** this is for relaxation and pleasure and once you start having a massage you could easily become addicted to it. Many women have a weekly massage, but it is an expensive luxury. A massage helps preserve muscle and skin tone; it also makes you very conscious of your body shape and encourages you to take maximum care of it – or improve it. The techniques of massage vary according to the therapist and some apply more pressure than others. Does it hurt? Generally no, but in areas of tenseness or where there's been muscle stress, there can be a momentary pain that quickly passes. Also your preference and reaction is important – some people like a gentle massage, others a more forceful one. Even if you've never had a massage before, you'll very quickly realize if you find it enjoyable or not.

It is usual to be massaged in the nude, but covered with a towel, on a massage table. Treatment almost always begins with stroking movements which is a gentle introduction to body contact and is also used to spread on oil or cream; then you can expect friction, vigorous rubbing and kneading. First you are on your back, the feet, legs, hands and arms are massaged, then the stomach. You turn over and first the legs and the buttocks are massaged, then the back and shoulders with emphasis on the spine and the nape of the neck to finally ease all tension.

**Rolfing:** a special form of massage that stretches and moves the connective tissue back into a symmetric state. The idea is to get the body free of knots and muscle misplacement so that energy is not lost on coping with a misaligned body. Rolfing is a way of rebalancing the body so that gravity works for and not against it. Fighting gravity causes stress. Rolfing claims not only to restore physical balance but to restore mental balance as well.

It is necessary to have a series of ten sessions, taking place once a week, each lasting about an hour. On the first visit, after your case history has been discussed, you will be photographed back and front. The therapist works with the connective tissue using fingertips, knuckles and sometimes elbows. The aim is to stretch and separate the connective tissue. Individual parts of the body are systematically rolfed in sequence. The sensation is a combination of pleasure and pain. After the session, another photograph is taken for comparison. During the final three sessions of the course, the whole body is taken into consideration, realigned and balanced properly in relation to the gravitational pull. Rolfing is not for any specific disorder, but because it relieves stress it also helps head-

Massage can be found in different forms all over the world, as body contact through touch is the most primitive form of soothing the body to feel better. Body touching has developed into sophisticated methods of tissue, muscle and bone manipulation to such a degree that disorders, seemingly far removed from the point of contact, are helped.

aches and backaches. It is a way to gain and keep the entire system in a healthy state, and therefore considered both a constructive and preventive therapy.

**Acupressure and shiatsu:** both are a form of finger, hand and sometimes foot pressure; they are very similar, the first is the Chinese version, the other how it is practised in Japan. Rather like acupuncture, the therapy involves the restoration of an even flow of energy along the meridians which are in contact with the body's vital organs. Pressure is put on the points that are known to ease pain and push the energy into a healing action. Both are thought of as first class preventive therapies and for early diagnosis of disease.

You wear easy, unrestricting clothes for acupressure and shiatsu. Case history is taken and the acupuncture pulse points (see page 179) are checked. Pressure is applied in many ways – light finger touches, the bulb of the thumb, the palms, the feet. Sometimes it is the strength of the arms that provide the force, but at times the body of the therapist is so angled that his entire weight is levered on your body through arms and palms. Pressure is applied for a few seconds and may be repeated several times on the same spot. You can experience some pain, but usually after two or three pressure applications it gets lighter and finally goes. Sessions last about an hour and it is up to the practitioner to work out the number you need and at what intervals. Both acupressure and shiatsu are recommended for headaches and backaches, for mental fatigue and depression, for insomnia, digestive and elimination problems.

## NATUROPATHY

This is precisely what the name implies; this therapy has everything to do with nature and natural functioning of the body and nothing to do with the intervention of chemical drugs. It is the oldest form of medicine and practically all the alternative therapies are offshoots from this base and are frequently integrated into it.

The principle is that if the body is treated correctly and fed the right things, it is capable of healing itself. Fundamental is food. A diet of fresh natural foods is the core of all naturopathy. On a curative basis, naturopaths believe in the power of a fast of just water or raw food to rid the body of all its poisonous, toxic matter and so restore health. It's not just a belief, it's a fact, and some of the most famous clinics in the world have case histories to prove it. Healthfarms and spas follow the naturopathic doctrine.

After food, the next most significant part of naturopathy is hydrotherapy (see page 186) and then the manipulative therapies such as chiropractic (see page 183) and osteopathy (see page 190). Very strict naturopaths don't use any remedies at all, but some integrate homeopathic elements into treatment. Great use is also made of pure fresh air and controlled sun in treatments.

Many people go to a naturopath when they are desperate about lack of improvement under orthodox medical care. It should be an

Naturopaths believe that to achieve and maintain optimum health it is necessary to live as close to nature as possible. This age-old philosophy states that it is the entry of unnatural elements that causes disease, and that once all toxins are eliminated, recovery is at hand. This means pure food, uncontaminated air, freedom of movement and spiritual tranquillity.

early consideration because just about everybody can benefit from eating the right food and allowing the body to perform in its most natural way. Food can be your best medicine and every disorder connected with body function has been improved, if not cured, in this way – from headaches, migraines, liver and kidney problems to cancer. A lot of people refuse to believe it, but the evidence is there if you choose to investigate in detail.

A consultation with a naturopathic doctor is similar to that with a general practitioner, but less emphasis is put on tests and more on the way you look, move, stand, breathe – plus, of course, a discourse on the type of food you eat and your style of life.

## OSTEOPATHY

A close cousin to chiropractic (see page 183) this manipulative therapy is centred on problems in the spinal area that cause disfunction of both the nerve and blood channels to the vital organs. The osteopath, however, is not just concerned with misalignment of the vertebrae, but looks for deviations in joints, muscles and tissues which are referred to as 'lesions'. They are caused by falls, sprains, strains, blows and bad posture and also, it is thought, by tension and the wrong diet.

The lesions are manipulated to coax the area back to normal. Many patients require gentle treatment, but others benefit from a sharp thrust which may be painful, but only for a moment. In fact, the latter method is often the quickest way to remove what was previously a nagging ache or pain. Osteopathy depends on extensive manipulation, whereas chiropractic is more direct and forceful.

The majority of people who seek advice from an osteopath are those with bad backs, and again because conventional medicine can offer little more than rest and painkillers. Perhaps a back has just been 'put out' by sudden movement or bending. However, osteopaths stress that many disorders are spinal related and prefer to take an overall view of health. On consultation, a general case history is asked for, but as with all body-connected therapies, emphasis is placed on observing stance, movement and gestures in relation to subjective information. You will be examined for areas of joint or muscle strain. The length and number of treatments is dependent on the problem.

## PSYCHOLOGICAL THERAPIES

The effect of mind over matter is a real and remarkable thing. There are two sides to it though – positive and negative. Your mind can work for or against your health, and it is now an accepted fact – in orthodox circles as well – that many illnesses are psychosomatic. However, the practice of psychotherapy embraces so many different theories and techniques that it is difficult to sort your way through them. Some are accepted by the establishment and others are

Osteopathy was founded in America towards the end of the last century by Andrew Taylor Still. He was a general practitioner but became disillusioned with orthodox medicine and from experience with patients became convinced that the spinal column was at the root of all trouble. Misuse and lack of spine stretching – instinctively done by animals after any rest period – were responsible for blockage in tissues and misalignment of the vertebrae.

considered too oblique. On the other hand many general practitioners tend to dismiss it completely and you will be told to pull yourself together and take some tranquillizers. That simply isn't good enough, and if you think you are ill simply because you can't pull yourself together, then you may very well benefit from some kind of psychotherapy.

Many women are very reluctant to seek psychological treatment because they think it is rather defeatist and at the end of the line. There is no need to feel embarrassed about it because the fact is that many women reach a point when they simply need some help in order to help themselves. All psychological therapies bring a degree of self-knowledge that sets you once again on the path to being self-reliant and self-assured. All therapies involve a certain amount of honest soul-searching, so it is not an easy road to take. You have to be prepared to face facts, to maybe change your attitude and possibly your lifestyle. But it can be very rewarding.

There are many approaches to psychological problems but all involve getting rid of negative thoughts and processes, and mobilizing mental energy for positive action. They range from meditation and relaxing sessions (see page 168) to group therapy and if really necessary to psychoanalysis. There are also the sensory therapies such as those of colour, music and art, while relevant facts can come from analysing dreams. The first step is to seek out a psychotherapist.

Psychotherapy is a means of finding out what is behind the mental triggering of an illness. In women it is usually a combination of daily stress and general anxiety. It could be frustration about age or position in life. It could be worry about the future, a total negative attitude as to what lies ahead. Whatever the cause, there are standard disorders for a psychosomatic condition: depression, anxiety, insomnia, overeating and obesity, sex difficulties, high blood pressure, breathing difficulties, asthma, constant lethargy. All stem from an inability to cope.

If you embark upon a course of psychotherapy you must have complete confidence in your therapist as you will have to reveal intimate details of your life. The idea is to understand, and ideally solve, problems by talking them over with a doctor. A common problem with women, particularly now that demands of achievement on all levels are high, is that they find it difficult to accept who they are and what they can do compared to what they imagine they should be doing. The aim of therapy is to change the patient's concept of herself, but it could also involve a personality change which puts great pressure on emotions. It may take time. Most therapists hold weekly sessions of about forty-five minutes, and these continue until you are no longer getting anything out of them, or are confident enough not to need them anymore.

Group therapy is a treatment that is becoming increasingly popular, particularly for women approaching or in the menopause. A group of six to ten women meet under the guidance of a therapist to discuss and share experiences. The aim is to define problems,

All psychotherapies derive from the preparatory work done by Sigmund Freud. At the turn of the century, he was initially involved in hypnosis using it to treat symptoms. While in a semi-conscious state, patients would often reveal past traumas which they had erased from conscious memory. Freud believed these were responsible for neurotic symptoms and many disorders. If hidden thoughts and experiences could be brought out into the open and finally acknowledged by the patient, a new mentally and physically healthy life could begin.

rationalize them and work out how to adjust or cope with them. It i often comforting to discover that you are not the only one with similar problems; you can identify with another member. Although members help each other, rely on each other for support, it is the therapist who is in control. The aim is to go from mutual acknowledgement of problems to group dependence to the confidence of facing anything on your own.

Psychoanalysis is the most intense form of psychotherapy. What distinguishes it from the freer forms is that the patient is unlikely to be aware of what is at the core of the problem. It is usually lengthy and expensive – and extremely demanding on the emotions of both the patient and the therapist. It is not uncommon to have daily sessions at first, eventually going down to two a week – but that could continue for a year or more. Every facet of the patient's life i probed into – personality, emotions, disturbances, professional and social ambitions – within the context of relationships and past experience. The first aim is to gain insight into self, then accept i and rebuild confidence from there.

Hypnosis is also a branch of psychotherapy where the power o suggestion, while the patient is in a temporary semiconscious state can be effective for disorders that have to do with stress or emotions It is a method of disciplining the mind to control the body. It can often help high blood pressure, insomnia, headaches, migraine and asthma. It has also proved valuable to counteract addiction to cigarettes, alcohol, drugs and sugar. Many people are nervous about its safety – will they come to, could the wrong things be suggested Actually, hypnosis is a temporary condition similar to sleep bu most of the faculties are functioning. You can come out of it at any moment, quite suddenly, in fact, particularly if something i suggested that goes completely against the sub-conscious will. You undertake hypnosis because you want help for a certain disorder so your mind is already in that direction and just a further push i needed to strengthen the will.

## REFLEXOLOGY

This is another therapy based on the belief that the most important way to good health is a clear energy flow, but unlike acupuncture the reflexologist asserts that the significant points of contact and pressure are in the foot and from there stem ten channels to all the vital organs. The soles and parts of the upper foot are said to make up a complete chart of the parts and functions of the body – rather like a contour map. Reflexology is considered both a diagnostic and therapeutic method.

Diagnostically, all parts of the body have a reflex point on the fee – and the organ affected is sometimes different according to the foot Most therapists prefer not to know before hand what you think is wrong, because by applying pressure at certain points and measuring your pain reaction, they are better able to detect for themselves

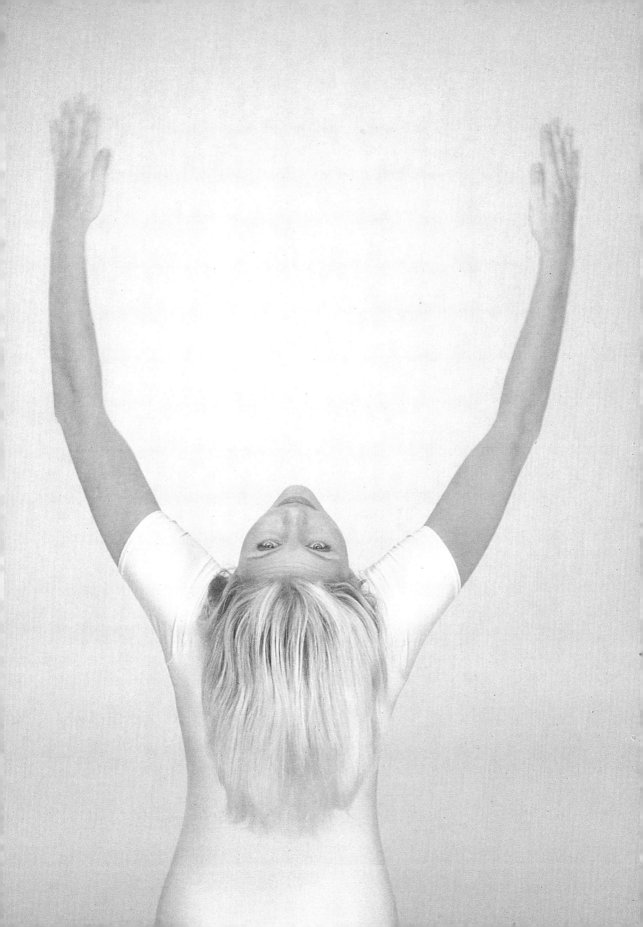

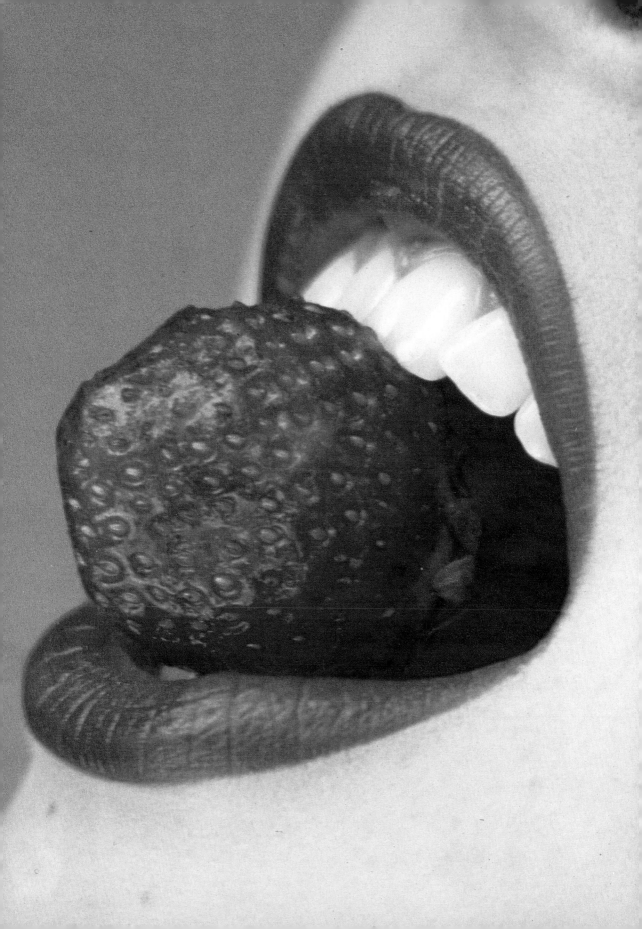

t is believed that a type of
reflexology was used in China in
the earliest days, and there is
pictorial evidence that it was
also performed in Egypt about
5,000 BC. Its introduction to the
western world was only around
the turn of this century, by an
American doctor, William H.
FitzGerald. It was finally
popularized in the 1930s by a
masseuse, Eunice Ingham,
whose methods and charts are
still used today.

what the disorder is. And it might very well be one you were not
aware of.

You will either be sitting or lying down for treatment, according
to the therapist's preferences. Initially the foot will be gently
explored with the fingers moving more in a massage way with
considerable stroking, plus manipulation of the toes. Then pressure
will be applied at the reflex points, rotating movements are often
employed, and you may feel pain either in the foot or in the organ to
which the energy channel is relating.

The aim is to unblock the energy channel, and an experienced
reflexologist does this by detecting a crystal-like deposit or a
shallow depression on the foot. Under pressure these are broken up,
absorbed by the body and finally expelled – and thus the channel is
clear. Treatment lasts about twenty minutes; a second session is
recommended after a few days and therapy could be continued on a
weekly basis if necessary. Reflexology often detects problems early
on so it should be considered as a preventive therapy as well. It
particularly helps conditions of congestion – migraine, sinus
problems, stimulation of pancreas and liver, kidney disorders and
constipation. It has had success with arthritis and circulatory
diseases, also in the relief of pain in the back.

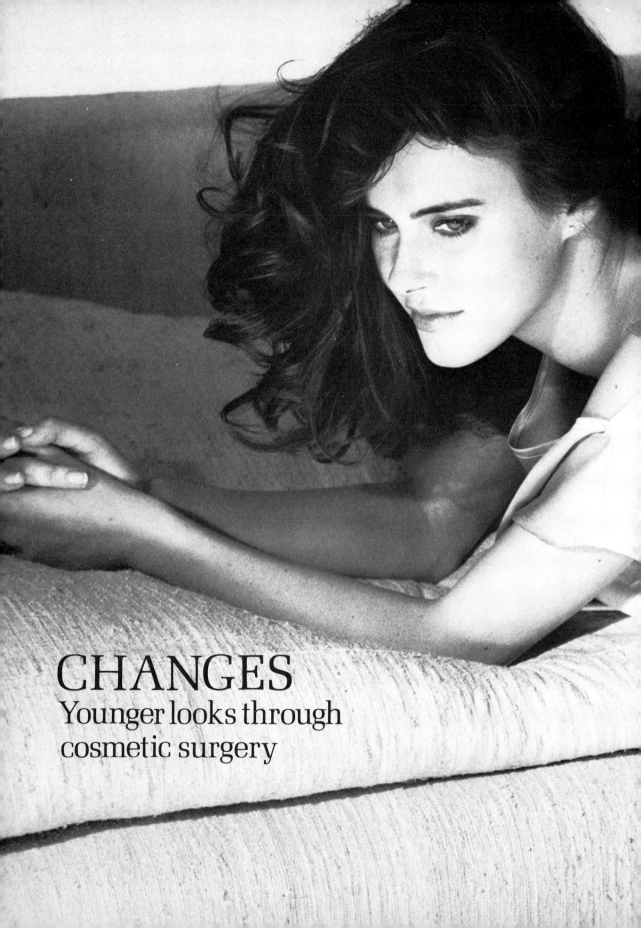

# CHANGES
Younger looks through
cosmetic surgery

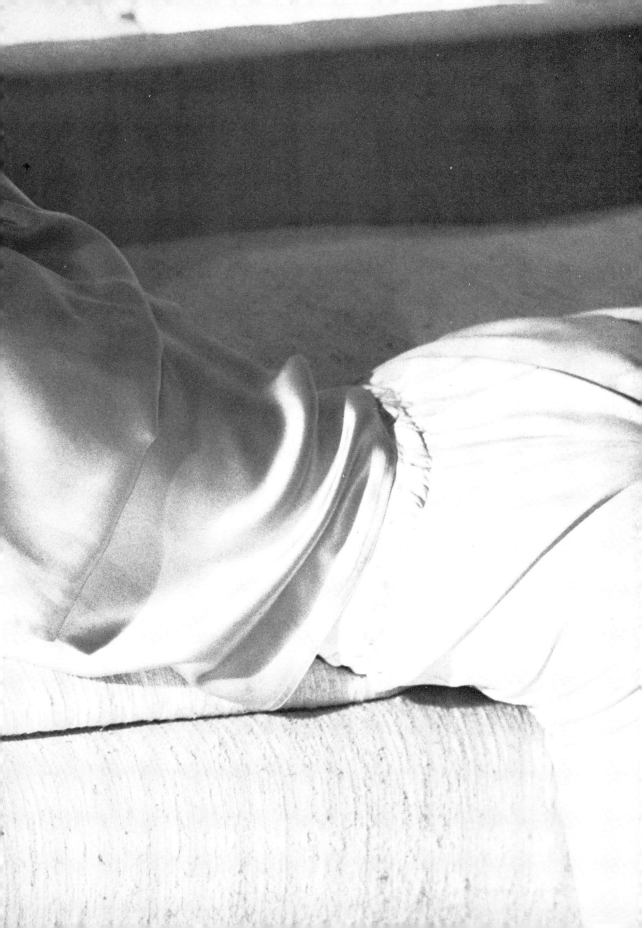

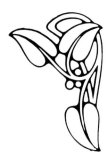

How far do you want to go on the stay younger path? Do you draw the line at cosmetic surgery? Many women do, not only because of cost and fear of the operation, but because there still lingers the Puritan ethic that it's too self-absorbing and too vain. And what would other people think? Would you even tell them? Is it wise to meddle with nature?

Cosmetic surgery is not such a secret issue as it once was, but many women are still reluctant to let the world know they have undertaken it. Yet if one looks at it sensibly, to erase some of the signs of aging of the skin should be equally acceptable as colouring the hair. Is it neurotic or psychologically healthy to want to look better and stay younger? Only you can answer that, but there are a great number of well-balanced women who say that cosmetic surgery gave them that extra degree of self-confidence to adjust to growing older and in many cases to go out and start a new career or change a lifestyle.

Cosmetic surgery is the art of the possible, and if you look at it in anti-aging terms instead of a way to perfection, it takes on a different aspect. The problem with cosmetic surgery at any age has always been the unrealistic attitude on the part of many women as to what it can achieve. You are not going to become a great beauty or a sensation overnight. You are not going to wipe away every line and wrinkle – nor should you, as faces need lines of expression. You are going to be the same, only looking better and looking younger. You will boost your morale and get a new lease on life.

The face lift is not the only way to help smooth out lines and wrinkles, the skin can also be chemically peeled or mechanically abraded. Maybe just an eyelid correction will take years off your face. More drastic is body surgery, which can help sagging breasts and thighs, though not all surgeons will perform the latter. Teeth too can be cosmetically changed with caps and other devices. All these changes should be considered with a view to how they could provide a more pleasing self-image. You should evaluate them according to your own reaction, not for their effect on others.

The best attitude is to be realistic and optimistic. You must also have it clear in your mind that although some procedures sound simple, it is after all surgery and involves an operation under local or general anaesthetic. There are stitches, there is going to be scarring – most of which will fade with time – there is some discomfort, bleeding and swelling, and there are risks, though slight. However, today's anaesthetics and proven surgical techniques make it possible for the well-trained plastic surgeon to perform complex and delicate operations safely.

To get a consultation with a plastic surgeon, you need a referral from your general practitioner. He may prove uncooperative, in which case go to another. You may have heard of the reputation of a particular surgeon, but you still require your doctor's referral. It is essential to establish a good rapport with the surgeon. The first consultation is usually up to an hour and is a time for mutual appraisal. You will need to be explicit about what you require and why; the surgeon will explain what he thinks can be done and exactly what he will do. Don't be shy about asking questions, however trivial they may sound. You need to know what degree of improvement can be expected, the length of operation, the type of anaesthetic, where the incisions will be and what form of stitching. Then there's the matter of length of stay in hospital, what degree of post-operative discomfort to expect, how long for recuperation and what precautions to take both before and after the operation. At some point before surgery, photographs will be taken not only for later comparison but also for use as a guide for the surgeon.

## THE FACE

No matter how well you have taken care of your skin (see page 48) through diligent daily attention, a face will inevitably start to show its age in one form or another. The process of aging begins gradually, so much so that you'll not notice it. It starts at about twenty-five to thirty but because you are living with your face you are not conscious of lines and sagging until they are clearly obvious. Time robs the skin of its elasticity as the underlying layers of fat and muscle begin to shrink – though facial exercises will help prevent this (see page 47).

Fine, fair skins show signs of age earlier than olive and dark complexions, though the good news is that these usually respond better to surgical and mechanical treatments than the duskier types. In the interests of looking younger the face is of prime importance; it's the main expression of your time clock. As it ages, should you philosophically just accept it, or do something definite about it? Women have been asking themselves this question for years, and there's still no cut and dried answer. It is purely a personal decision. Motivation should go beyond vanity; it should be a matter of a desire to look fitter, healthier, a little younger, more lively – not decades younger, nor more beautiful. In these terms, doing something to save your face cannot be considered frivolous or narcissistic, but a sensible decision on the part of a modern woman in a modern world.

Most women think the only solution is a face lift. Actually, this is but one, and the most extreme, of many possibilities. If your skin is lined and a little wrinkled, it may respond well to a skin peeling or planing (see page 203). Maybe it is your eyes that look tired and haggard, bags and lines underneath, droops of the lid above. You may very well only need an 'eye job' which is one of the simplest and most successful of cosmetic procedures. It can make a world of difference to a face, taking years off it. Only when the skin is sagging and no longer seems to fit your face, is a full face lift called for. It is a superb repair job, where the lifting and tightening of the skin of the face and neck creates a more youthful appearance. It can bring a feeling of self-confidence and provide a psychological lift. And there's nothing wrong with that.

A face lift does not bring you a new face, but can restore some of its earlier symmetry and contours. Also it cannot stop the biological

*Brigitte Bardot*
'Now I am 48 I view old age without fear or qualm. I just view it, that's all. I shan't have any face lifts when I am old. I want my face to be as old as I am.'

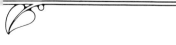

clock; after a successful lift you could look thirty-five at forty, but you won't stay that way as the aging process carries on as before. Nevertheless, you will probably always look younger and better than your age. And you can always have another lift. Age offers no restrictions for people considering face lifts if they are in good physical and mental health. The ideal is to have a lift before lines and sagging become really obvious. Surgeons say the very best results are from women in their late forties or early fifties with a minimum of wrinkles, with skin that still retains a degree of elasticity and has little underlying fat. Of course, most women don't think or plan ahead in this way, but there's a lot to be said for the early lift – a stitch in time, saves nine. But don't be talked into the so-called 'mini lift' – it is ineffectual; you may as well go for the full lift or none at all. The face lift is not a cure-all; it does tighten and smooth out the skin, but it cannot:

- remove bags and crepy skin around the eyes; this requires an eye job.
- get rid of a double chin; a separate procedure is needed to remove the fat pad.
- delete fine bleeding lines from the upper lip; dermabrasion or chemical peeling helps this.
- erase a network of fine wrinkles; better results are from dermabrasion or chemical peeling.
- eliminate furrows on the forehead; sometimes chemical peeling helps.
- treat lines radiating from the bridge of the nose; only silicone injections help, but not all surgeons will do them.

### The Face Lift

This is known by a number of technical names – rhytidoplasty, rhytidectomy and meloplasty – none of which are as memorable nor as descriptive as 'face lift'. It is not minor surgery, for it involves major dissection of the skin and is a complex and painstaking procedure. To put it simply; the surgeon incises and detaches the skin from the face and neck, tightens and rearranges the tissues and muscles underneath it, then lifts and redrapes the released skin; excess is cut off and the face is unobtrusively stitched up. It is a great challenge to the surgeon and its success lies equally in artistry and skill. Too drastic a lift can be more of a disaster than not enough – and there's a very fine dividing line.

What about scars? Concealment of scars is considered as important as the surgery itself. The incisions are made in areas covered by hair, behind the ear where it cannot be seen, and in front of the ear in the natural fold of the skin, which becomes almost invisible after a few months. If you have more than one face lift, the new incisions are made so that scar tissues from previous lifts will be taken away, thus leaving only one stitch line.

How long does a face lift last? It depends on your age and type of skin, but generally it is from five to ten years or even longer. If you are in your forties, the lift will last longer than if you have it done in your fifties or sixties because the younger the skin, the more elastic and resilient it is. Can a lifted face suddenly drop? There's no chance of this, though it's widely believed possible. The youth-giving effects of the face-lift will gradually diminish over the years.

Patients are hospitalized the day before surgery, given routine tests and started on sedation; hair and face are washed with special soaps. The operation is done under local or general anaesthetic depending on the surgeon, though most prefer local as the patient's reactions can more easily be monitored. You will be drowsy from sedatives by the time you are wheeled into the operating theatre, and you will feel no pain or discomfort during the operation.

The face lift operation takes from two-and-a-half hours to four hours depending on what has to be done. All surgeons have their individual techniques and procedure, but generally the first incision is in the temple region just inside the hairline – the hair is first parted to indicate the exact line. The incision continues down to the ear (see sketch) then follows the natural crease in front of it, goes around the base of the lobe, then up along the back of the ear and finally sloping diagonally downwards into the scalp.

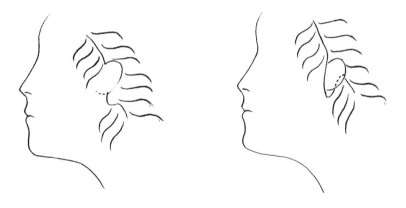

The surgeon then separates the skin from the underlying fat and muscle, starting at the back of the ear and working towards the jawline. This is called undermining and the extent of it depends on the amount of sagging and the location. Great care is taken of facial nerves, blood vessels and muscles. Sometimes nerve endings are broken which will cause numbness after the lift, but within a few months they heal naturally and normal sensation returns. The next step is to 'rotate' the skin, manoeuvre and drape it so that it fits the bone structure in the best way possible. This is the moment that requires judgement of the eye as well as technical skill. The two sides of the face are done in sequence. Excess skin is cut away and the incisions are sutured. Quite often small soft tubes are left in the incisions to allow drainage of blood (and other secretions) which helps prevent excessive bruising. The patient's head is then wrapped in a large cocoon-like bandage, which will stay on for one or two days.

It is better to remain in bed until the bandage is removed, and for this reason the hospital stay for a face lift is three or four days. You will have swelling and bruising, but exactly how much is difficult to estimate – again it depends on the extent of the operation, the type of skin and the speed of healing. The stitches are removed in stages but all are usually out by the tenth or twelfth day. You will probably be presentable in two weeks, but surgeons recommend three weeks for convalescence. Hair can be combed gently after four or five days; make-up can be applied after a week. There are weekly check-ups with the surgeon for the first month, afterwards less often.

Can anything go wrong? Complications can occur in all types of surgery. In face lifts they are rare, but there are effective counter treatments. As mentioned, nerve injury is possible, but this clears up. Infection is rare because of the excellent blood vessel system in the face. Hematomas (swellings filled with blood) are the most common problem and they occur within the first forty-eight hours after surgery. The small ones are absorbed within a few weeks; the large ones have to be promptly treated, but they respond well.

### Double Chin Refinement

A face lift can correct a sagging neckline but it cannot do anything about a double chin, which is a large deposit of fat under the chin line. A special procedure is used – either on its own or in conjunction with the standard face lift. An incision is made under the chin (see sketch) and the fat removed; excess skin is cut away and the incision sutured. The scar is a fine, hardly discernible line lying in the natural fold between chin and neck, an area rarely in direct vision.

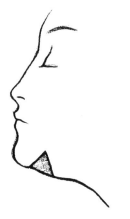 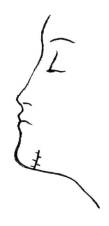

## Eyelid Correction

Medically referred to as a blepharoplasty and by almost everyone else as an eye job, it is the most frequently performed of all cosmetic surgery procedures. Plastic surgeons are unanimous in their opinion that of all the anti-aging possibilities, this is the one that can have the most dramatic results. The eyes are not only the most expressive feature of the face, but they are the first to mirror emotion, to show tiredness or stress – and they are the main focus of attention. But it is not just the eyes themselves, but the surrounding tissues that also play a great part in the look and expression of the eye.

There are two main aging problems with eyes: because the skin of the upper lid is extremely thin, it is subject to early wrinkling which gives it that droopy crepy look; underneath the eye are three fat pockets, and these can sometimes bulge against the muscle and skin causing bags and pouches, and the area here can get wrinkled and saggy very early on in years.

However, it should be reassuring to hear that the eye correction is not only one of the most satisfactory operations, but it is the shortest and the results last longest. Once bags are removed they rarely re-occur, and the skin on the upper lid will remain tighter and smoother for life. The gradual process of aging continues as usual, of course, but the endurance of an eye job is longer than that of a face lift – usually ten to fifteen years. It is certainly the first plastic surgery I would consider personally.

Drooping lids and under-eye pouches can be hereditary and actually can appear early in life, but after forty-five they are a common condition and have everything to do with aging. It is mainly because the skin becomes thinner and diminishes in elasticity; also subcutaneous fat and muscle tone decrease so the skin is no longer supported for smoothness. At this point no creams or exercises will help – though on a preventive level they are of considerable value (see page 76) – the only solution is surgery, but it cannot accomplish miracles. It improves only the eye area, it takes away bags and droopiness of the lid, it 'opens up' the eyes considerably which in itself is more youthful; it cannot eliminate all wrinkles; though most are smoothed-out the horizontal expression lines that radiate from the outer corner of the eye remain almost the same. This is really a good thing, as blank expressionless eyes are awful and instead of making you look younger would only make you look foolish and clearly a product of over-done eye surgery.

It is usual to go into hospital the day before surgery, and although there is a recent trend to do the operation in the doctor's private surgery, most responsible surgeons still prefer the facilities of a hospital. As in a face lift, the skin and hair are thoroughly washed with special soaps.

The operation is performed under general or local anaesthetic; the choice depends on the surgeon but most prefer local. Because of sedation patients are in a haze during the operation and feel no pain

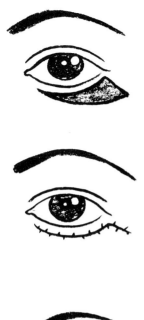

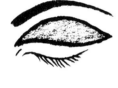

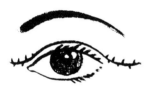

but have some sensations. The operation lasts between one-and-a half and two hours. First the surgeon marks, with a special coloured pen, the areas of skin to be removed; these are strategically placed so that the final scar will be hidden in the normal skin crease of the open eye. It is the lower line that is the one for final stitching (see sketch). After incisions, the excess skin is removed, then the troublesome fat lying under the muscle layer is taken away. Muscle fibres are joined and the eyelid stitched. The lower lid is trickier to do than the top. The most crucial decision is how much skin to remove. If too much is taken away it results in a drawn, pinched look, or too much exposure of the whites of the eye, or a pull downwards at the outer corner. The first incision parallels the lower rim of the eye from the inner corner to the outer point; the other incision forms a crescent-shaped segment of skin that is taken away. The final stitching line will be under the eye and concealed by the lower lashes. The area exposed is undermined; the muscle fibres are separated to reveal the fat deposits, which are diminished to a degree where just enough is left to support the skin. If too much is taken away there will be a hollow under the eye, which is almost as bad as a pouch. The surgeon's judgement is the key to success.

There's another aspect to an eye job that few women consider: the eyebrows. If you have droopy lids, chances are your eyebrows will have dropped too over the years. These can be lifted by cutting away a small crescent of skin above the outer area of the brow (see sketch). It is, however, difficult to end up with an invisible scar here, but eyebrow pencil will deftly conceal it.

After an eye operation, eyes may be bandaged, but not always. A lubricant is usually applied and sometimes ice packs to help swelling and bruising. There is rarely pain after the operation, but there is a pulling sensation which can continue for several months until the skin readjusts itself. There is swelling after surgery, also discolouration and the eyes may water. Stitches are removed after only two or three days. You can sometimes return home on the day after surgery, but definitely the following day. Make-up can be worn after about a week – but ask your surgeon's advice on this. After two or three weeks your eyes will be absolutely presentable without dark glasses. As previously mentioned, it takes a few months for the tight feeling to ease, but that is only a subjective reaction – you don't look tight or drawn. Follow-up visits are necessary to the surgeon's office.

There can be complications, but these are temporary. Infections are rare, but there is always the chance of hematomas (swellings of blood) as in a face-lift which can be efficiently dealt with. It is common for the eyes to water for the first two days. You may have double vision for a few hours after surgery. It is also quite usual to have problems completely closing the lids for a while, but as the skin stretches, this corrects itself in time.

## SKIN IMPROVEMENT

Once past the twenties, no-one can help but notice the signs of aging on the surface of the skin. First there are faint lines that etch the face and these finally deepen into wrinkles. No matter how well you have taken care of your skin, it will eventually lose some of its elasticity, become less smooth, it may get patches of pigmentation – and it will wrinkle and sag. The time and the degree of degeneration depends on genetic factors and preventive care (see page 48).

Apart from the face lift (see page 198) there are other ways of dealing with the skin; these will not help sags and pouches, but they can help erase wrinkles and blemishes. The first is a chemical peeling, which involves the use of a compound that burns away the top layers of the skin. Then there is dermabrasion, a method of planing the surface of the skin, which has proved effective for both wrinkles and scars. A third method is the use of a cold laser beam to give the skin an overall more youthful appearance. A fourth, though controversial treatment, involves injections of liquid silicone, which plump out the wrinkles and smooth the skin's surface. All procedures are complicated and absolutely must be done by physicians trained in the specialized techniques – cosmetic surgeons or dermatologists. Some beauty salons offer such services, but it is wise to check first who will be performing the operation because, in the hands of a lay person, permanent damage and scarring could result.

### Chemical Face Peel

This is also known as chemosurgery and chemabrasion. It is the ultimate in exfoliation and surprisingly enough was perfected a century ago – by the German dermatologist Unna. The peel is, in fact, a second degree burn; after the application of the chemicals, the treated surface tissue remains in place, while the new skin is formed underneath. There is no destruction of the cells involved – the outer layer (epidermis) and the upper layers of fibrous, connective tissue (dermis) that are just below it, become detached from the skin, remain intact and finally are taken away. There are only a few chemicals that have the property of detaching the horny layer of the skin (the wrinkled or scarred surface) without destroying it. One is phenol (carbolic acid) and a derivative called resorcin. These two are the most frequently used basic agents for the chemical peel. The phenol is partly absorbed through the skin and into the blood stream and it could be harmful to the kidneys. Therefore, anyone with any malfunction of the kidneys is advised not to have a chemical peel. When properly used, the toxic qualities of phenol are negligible, though many lay people who use peels do not realize that the more diluted the substance, the greater the chance of it going into the bloodstream. This is because in its strongest form, the phenol immediately forms a mechanical barrier and prevents seepage.

The chemical peel is regarded as valuable in improving forehead wrinkles, creases, cheek lines and the fine network of lines around the eyes and lips; it can often eradicate facial pigmentation. The skin will finally appear firmer and smoother. It is very effective when used in conjunction with a face lift – areas around the lips and lines on the forehead are not always smoothed out with a lift.

Who can benefit from a chemical peel? There are better results with fair skins than with darker complexions. Olive skins frequently show too noticeable a contrast between the treated and untreated areas and when the skin finally settles down it could be blotchy. Black skins do not respond well, not only because of the colour and pigmentation problems, but also because black skin tends to form keloids on healing. If the surgeon has any doubts as to the reaction, it is usual to do a patch test in front of or behind the ear. reaction is checked over a period of four weeks before the final decision is made.

Be prepared for an uncomfortable experience, not so much the operation itself, but the aftermath when the healing crusts on the face can be physically and psychologically disturbing. It may be necessary to be housebound for a minimum of ten days. If only a segment of the face is being treated, say mouth or forehead lines, it can be done in an office, but most surgeons insist on a hospital stay of three days for a full face. No anaesthetic is used during the operation, but the patient is premedicated for ultimate sedation.

The peeling agent used depends on the practitioner, but the compound has a phenol base combined with catalytic and buffer ingredients. It is applied with a brush or a cotton-tip applicator. During application the skin is stretched to make sure the solution gets into the grooves of all lines and wrinkles. There is a sharp momentary burn and then the area is anaesthetized. The skin will first turn white for two or three minutes, then it swells and becomes red.

The face is treated in sections, slowly and methodically, starting at the forehead and working down. To avoid any possible demarcation lines, the application is taken into the hairline and under the jaw. Sometimes strips of adhesive tape are layered on to the treated skin, leaving eyes, nostrils and lips free.

Immediately after the operation, the skin starts to swell and within a few hours will turn brown and give off a clear fluid. You will not be aware of this – and it is not advisable to look at yourself in a mirror at this point – but you will feel uncomfortable and may need medication for relief. Swelling of the face continues for three to four days; the eyelids may swell to the point of shutting. Bed rest is recommended for the first forty-eight hours, and if lip lines were treated and the area is swollen, a liquid diet is sipped through a straw.

The next step – around the third day – a crust starts to form and the swelling goes down. Because of the crust, which is after all a huge scab, the face can begin to itch; it is imperative to resist all inclination to scratch it. It will begin to crack and loosen, oozing sepsis here and there. On about the fifth day, cream or a specially formulated ointment is applied to facilitate the separation of the crust from the new skin layer. Now the crust starts to break away, but it is only after ten to fourteen days that it will have completely sloughed off, leaving a clear, firm skin underneath. However, the colour may be unnerving as this can be any degree of pink from almost crimson to a deep blush tone.

If the face is taped, these are removed forty-eight hours after the operation and because it can be extremely painful, the patient is sedated first.

The first look at your new skin – colour aside – will be one of joy at its smooth and soft appearance. However, the skin is still swollen – indeed it will still feel tight – which in itself eradicates lines. Some fine lines will reappear; you can't expect every wrinkle or undulation to be magically carried away. At this point, the skin should be washed with mild soap and water, moisturized and possibly treated with a gentle conditioning cream. No make-up should be used for two or three weeks.

The colour will slowly fade; if it's crimson that should go in a few days, but all skins remain very pink for six to eight weeks, sometimes longer. Care of the new skin involves simple cleansing and moisturizing routines, and the cardinal rule is to stay out of the sunlight at all costs for six months. Even a minute in direct sun can cause blotchy pigmentation which is almost impossible to get rid of. You can preserve your new skin surface with diligent care, but don't overlook the fact that it will gradually age and at the same rate as before. Chemical peels can be repeated, at what intervals and how often depends on your reaction.

## Dermabrasion

This is a mechanical method, developed in America, for the removal of the outer layers of the skin to even out the surface. It is usually recommended for scars such as those from acne, but in the context of aging skin it is useful in treating fine lines and wrinkles and removing pigmentations caused by overexposure to the sun. This is done by virtually sand-papering the skin with a rapidly rotating wire brush or burr. Instruments today are finely attuned and adjusted to merely scrape the surface at a speed of about 24,000 revolutions per minute, controlled rather like a dentist's drill from a foot pedal.

Again it is people with light skins who get the best results, except that large-pored skins cannot be treated as the pores are often too indented for contact with the brush and any deeper planing would damage the underlying tissues. Dark skins are a problem because of marked change in pigmentation and possible keloid formation.

Dermabrasion can be undertaken in a medical surgery using a local anaesthetic, otherwise it involves an overnight stay in hospital. The local anaesthetic could be an injection or a freezing spray, if the latter is used the face is anaesthetized and planed in small sections. As with the chemical peel, dermabrasion continues into the hairline and under the jaw so there is no obvious skin contrast. It usually takes from thirty to forty minutes to do the full face.

The freezing process before the abrading can be painful, but you feel nothing during the actual process. After the operation, an anaesthetic is applied to reduce the burning and general discomfort. Gauze dressings are gently pressed on the surface and continually changed until the bleeding ceases; an antibiotic ointment is applied. Some physicians bandage the face at this point, but not all. In the hospital a general anaesthetic is used, so there is no need for an injection or spray.

The skin starts by being moist and may ooze a yellowish liquid. A crust soon begins to form and after twenty-four to thirty-six hours it should be reasonably firm. The face also swells in all areas that have been treated. The eyes can close and you may only be able to open your mouth to a mere slit, so food is taken in liquid form. On the third day, the swelling usually begins to subside, but it is important all the time to apply a prescribed cream or oil – or warm water compresses – to keep the crust soft.

After a week to ten days, the crust begins to separate from the renewed layer underneath and it will gradually crumble off. The new skin surface will be very pink but look incredibly smooth. There is still a certain degree of swelling at this point which plumps up any remaining fine lines. As the skin shrinks to its normal coverage – from three to four weeks after the operation – small lines are likely to appear. This should not give rise to disappointment, as it is impossible to completely smooth out the skin; what's more the presence of a few tracings give a much more natural appearance. The pinkness will take a couple of months to fade, and during that time great care must be taken to stay out of the sun and to treat the skin with mild washings, moisturizers and conditioners.

## Cosmetic Laser

This is a concentrated light beam that stimulates cellular activity and in doing so gives a plumpness and freshness to the skin, helps to alleviate lines and wrinkles and generally makes the face more youthful. It is heralded as a face lift without scars, though in actual fact because it cannot do any lifting, nor get rid of sags and pouches that really is a misnomer. There are also many surgeons who claim there is no improvement, but that may be jealousy. Nearly all the women I have talked to are very pleased with the results of a series of treatments, and they are fully aware of its limitations. It may very well be the preventive tool of the future, but these are really early days to estimate the extent of its use and benefits properly. One should look at it with more hope than scepticism.

The laser is one of the twentieth century's newer technological offerings, though it was actually predicted by Einstein back in the twenties. The word laser comes from the initial abbreviation of its function: Light Amplification by Stimulated Emission of Radiation. If I've lost you here, in simple terms it is the directing and focusing of a single part of an ordinary ray of light. Light is composed of many wave lengths going at various speeds and in different directions. If one frequency is isolated and channelled it can result in a beam of incredible power. Lasers are used in such diverse worlds as heavy industry and precise medical surgery. This is because they have the ability to cut faster and finer than a knife; they also have the capacity to burn and heal. Power depends on brightness and there are millions of degrees of that. The palest and gentlest is called the cold laser and this is the one that has proved extremely beneficial on a cosmetic level.

There appear to be two reasons why the laser works for the good of the skin. Research has shown that it has collagen-synthesizing properties, and it is the degenerative changes in collagen and elastin fibres that cause the skin to deteriorate and wrinkle, and the underlying musculature to collapse. The laser also has the ability to stimulate the acupuncture points (see page 179) of the face which means that there is a freer flow of energy to give a push to cellular activity and improve circulation. It works best when the skin still has some elasticity, so is ideal for women between thirty-five and fifty-five.

The treatment takes a maximum of fifteen minutes, but it is recommended to have between ten and fifteen sessions at intervals of a few days to get the best results. The face is first cleansed, then wiped with witch hazel to take away every last bit of oil or grease. The beam is focused on the skin through an instrument that looks rather like a large ball-point pen. First the beam zones in on the acupuncture points; a digital reading indicates skin reaction and areas in need of special treatment. This lasts for about five minutes. Then the beam traces facial lines – on the forehead, around the eyes, on the cheeks, and especially around the mouth. Finally the whole face is painted with the beam.

Judgement is purely on a personal level. Some women say they feel as though they've been out in the sun; others report a distinct tightening of the skin and underlying muscles. If you see improvement after the first session you are probably imagining it, or are exceptionally receptive, but after a few treatments there are obvious improvements. However, remember that everyone reacts differently, particularly when the treatments are non-invasive and come under the category of natural therapy, which indeed the laser does. Another point to bear in mind: cosmetic laser beams help to restore what is there – the tissues, the muscles, the cellular activity, the circulation – they cannot reshape or readjust a face.

## Liquid-Silicone Injections

Of all the treatments for younger-looking skin and therefore rejuvenated faces, this is the most controversial. In theory it should be the most perfect answer, silicone fluid can fill out wrinkles and lines, thereby smoothing the face to youthful contours. Silicone is an inert plastic and on the medical level there have developed formulations which have proved valid in many ways. No-one questions its value as an implant, but the liquid form has given some problems. When liquid silicone is injected in too large an amount, it often drifts around the body and ends up in a most undesirable location, posing as cysts and tumours. Once in the body, it is very difficult to remove, and can often clog up normal body mechanisms.

There are many physicians, however, who say that if liquid silicone is correctly injected, there is no cause for alarm. The problem in the past is that these treatments have been in the hands of those not specifically qualified. Indeed, the crux of the matter and the effectiveness and safeness of liquid silicone lies in proper administration. It must be injected a minute drop at a time and into the deepest stratum of the skin. Application has to spread over many sessions at well-spaced intervals, so it may take a month or more to fill out one small wrinkle.

For the injections, the patient lies down; the skin is cleansed but rarely is a local anaesthetic given. Injections are dotted along the wrinkle, and after each shot the area is massaged to evenly distribute the silicone. The body's reaction to the droplet is to surround it with protective fibrous tissue and in this way the silicone is locked in position. There is usually no pain after injections but there could be some swelling and discolouration. One of the most successful areas for silicone treatment is the bridge of the nose, where vertical lines are difficult to remove in a face lift.

## THE TEETH

It's for justifiable reasons that people getting on in years are described as 'long in the tooth'. This is due to receding gums caused by periodontal disease, which can be prevented and successfully treated if caught in time (see page 78). However, on the cosmetic side, the appearance of the teeth plays an important role in looking younger. Stained, badly shaped teeth, missing and overfilled teeth, plus ill-fitting false teeth, are all very aging. Cosmetic dentistry can work wonders today, not only for looks but much of the work is also protective and can help you keep your teeth longer – and may very well mean you can escape having false teeth altogether, or at worst have them very late in life.

Crowns, bridges, veneers and partial plates can be used with skill so that only your dentist and you know they are not as nature intended. Cosmetic dentistry is always expensive and it has to be carried out by a dentist experienced in restorative work. If the work is done well at the beginning, it could last a lifetime, whereas mistakes are costly and extremely difficult to put right. It is almost impossible to get such work done under socialized dental schemes, as it is considered 'non essential'. How very wrong!

The best procedure is to have a consultation with the dentist and discuss possibilities for the whole mouth. To establish an ultimate plan is much better than having a tooth capped here and there, because the mouth can then be approached from an optimal function and preservation point of view. Work can be done over a period of time according to exigency and money. Note the possibilities:

**crowns** – these are permanent and age well unless badly fitted in the first place. The cosmetic result is excellent if the texture and colour have been carefully matched to the surrounding teeth. Although synthetic, the caps discolour and stain more or less the same as natural teeth, so it is rarely obvious that a particular tooth is a capped one. The material used depends on the position in the mouth. Porcelain is the most natural looking but because it is rather delicate, it is usually only employed for front teeth and even then it is fused on to a gold or alloy underlay. Towards the back of the mouth, where more pressure is applied and therefore more resilient material is needed, caps are a combination of plastic substances, gold and alloys. Gold is still the most sturdy component and may be used to back the crowns or form a centre-piece on the molars. Don't stint on the gold, it is false economy in the long run.

Preparing a tooth for capping is an exact and lengthy procedure. The tooth is filed down to a point and about half of its original diameter. Many impressions are taken in order to work out the ideal size, shape and undulation. A temporary cap of dental cement covers the 'fang' until the permanent cap can be put in place – usually a week later. There is considerable drilling and shaving of the tooth, possibly the removal of the nerve and treatment of the root canal. This may sound awful, but it is now painless due to premedication, local anaesthetics and high-speed equipment. One tooth may take an hour or more to prepare.

It is extremely important to keep the area around the cap scrupulously clean, as any build-up of plaque could infect the gum and cause infection in the space between the crown and the tooth. The dentist will show you the hygiene necessary which will include the use of special brushes and dental floss.

**bridges** – one, two, three and sometimes four dummy teeth can be attached to neighbouring teeth, which have been crowned in order to carry the false bridge. Bridges are usually made from gold or a gold and metal alloy and covered with porcelain for naturalness. They are joined at the back, but so well that no-one can discern it. Bridges are the perfect solution for missing front and side teeth as they eliminate the need for dentures. The dental technician is of particular significance for bridges, as he determines the natural look through colour and texture, but most of all through the shaping of the tooth at the gum line. It must look as though teeth are coming out of the gums, not just sitting on the top of them.

**veneers** – these are synthetic coverings that look like artificial fingernails. They are bonded on to the tooth, then cut and drilled into shape. A veneer can also be a cement-like substance that is painted on to the tooth in layers, finally hardening. Veneers are used to disguise a stained and sometimes a chipped tooth; they are not expensive. The main snag is that as they are plastic they are absorbent and can discolour easily – tea, coffee, red wine and smoking are leading stain culprits.

**implants** – these are metal stumps that are fixed into the jaw bone and act as roots for visible crowns. In theory it sounds ideal, as surely the whole mouth could be treated in this way, thus avoiding false teeth and achieving a very natural look. In practice it is another matter, as very few people can tolerate the implants and within a few years they are rejected. At the same time they can infect both the bone and gum tissue, eating away at this essential foundation and even hindering the final easy fitting of false teeth.

**false teeth** – these are not so much cosmetic as essential, both for chewing and eating as well as maintaining the shape of the jaw and position of the mouth. False teeth are made out of plastics. A full set is held in the mouth by close fitting to the gum. Partial false teeth often have some metal attachment to hold them in place instead of having a plastic plate across the roof of the mouth, or plastic gums to secure any bottom teeth. Clearly false teeth are better than none at all, but at first it is difficult to adjust to having something extra in the mouth; speech can become slurred and there is lack of sensation when biting or chewing. There is no reason why false teeth cannot be made to fit perfectly – teeth that rattle are the result of bad dentistry, and not due to the odd shape of your mouth or inability to adjust to them.

## THE BODY

As the body ages, and if you have done little or no exercise to keep muscles toned, the tissues and skin will begin to sag. It is a combination of the skin losing its resilience and the relentless pull of gravity. Breasts will sag at any age; the insides of the thighs and buttocks may drop due to sudden weight loss or age; the stomach can acquire a fold, the upper arms become flabby. Can anything be done? It's a bit late to preach, I know, but this is one instance when 'prevention is the best if only way' should be printed in banner headlines. Such sagging need not come with age if you have watched your diet and your fitness consistently over the years. The substructure of muscles contributes greatly to a firm skin, and so does a limited amount of fatty tissue. A big problem is when you decide it's about time to lose weight when middle-aged. It's a very worthy decision, yes – but if you lose a lot too quickly, your skin can't adjust fast enough and if it ends up being considerably larger than the body it has to cover, it will naturally sag. Disciplined dieting and exercise might help, but not necessarily.

All these figure problems not only affect a woman's silhouette, but frequently her self-image and confidence. There are cosmetic procedures to help recontour specific areas of the body, but many surgeons are reluctant to do them. Breast surgery is the exception, and is widely accepted and performed, but other areas of the body are treated with trepidation. Body contouring does leave scars; to what extent depends on the operation and the patient's reaction, but they never disappear and some don't even become faint. You are really trading a silhouette for a scar, so body contouring is for women who want to look good in clothes but are not concerned how they look without them. Body contouring is major surgery. It is painful and convalescence can be considerable, and apart from breast surgery you will need to do some detective work to find a cooperative surgeon.

### Breast lifting

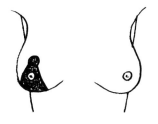

Even the smallest breasts can droop over the years – there is too much skin for the underlying tissue and the nipples instead of being pertly centred are hanging somewhere on the lower curve. The procedure is on the same principle as the face lift – cutting away excess skin, lifting what is left and stitching.

It is called a skin mastopexy and is very similar to breast reduction but in this case little of the breast tissue is disturbed, though areola and nipple must be resituated. If breasts are very large, then the surgeon will probably consider having a breast reduction instead, which is a more complex operation. Scars do remain after the operation, but in women who heal well there's a chance they will not be very noticeable.

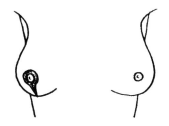

Hospitalization is required the night before surgery – and the stay is from three to five days. General anaesthetic is used, but before this is given, the surgeon sketches on the skin the area of skin to be excised and the new placement of the nipple. The segment to be taken away is a curve-base triangle stemming from a point above the nipple (see sketch). The final suture lines go around the nipple, a vertical one from there, then a curve that is hidden under the natural fold of the breast. Very important is the lifting and transposition of the nipple. In breast lifting, only a little undermining of the skin is done. Stitches are taken out gradually, the first around the fourth or fifth day and the last may be not until three weeks later. It is advisable to wear a bra continuously for several months. Complications are rare because it is the skin only that is being removed, not segments of tissue. Nipple sensation can be temporarily lost or lessened, but it does return.

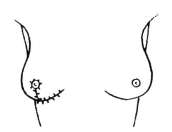

### Breast Reconstruction

Removal of a breast because of cancer (a mastectomy) can result in ambivalent feelings: it is a relief to have got rid of cancer, but not so great to have lost a breast. Some women can cope and manage perfectly well with special bras. To others it is a disfigurement which gets worse and becomes a real trauma. The general surgeon may not be sympathetic, but it is possible to have reconstruction plastic surgery – a procedure that has improved incredibly both in technical and aesthetic terms over the last ten years. It can be performed from six to eight months after the mastectomy. Not everyone is suitable, it depends on the extent of the operation, the scar tissue and the effect of any radiation treatment afterwards. Anyway, it is worthwhile to investigate.

It is contour that the surgeon considers his prime task, so that when a bra is worn the line looks natural and there is a definite cleavage between the breasts. The breast may look almost normal, but one should not be too optimistic. The operation is done under general anaesthetic. The position of the new breast is marked, the incisions are made and a 'pouch' inserted that will hold the implant. Sometimes a nipple is reconstructed at the same time, but many surgeons prefer to wait to see the result of the first procedure. The original nipple is sometimes preserved from the mastectomy, tissue is sometimes grafted from the other nipple, or a realistic one can be tattooed on to the skin. The operation for breast reconstruction takes about an hour; the hospital stay is from two to four days and not much post-operational care is required.

### Stomach lift

This is called an abdominoplasty and it can trim the contours, flatten and firm a sagging stomach. It is not surgery to remove fat, though a little is taken away; it is surgery to take away the loose folds of skin that result from age or from too quick a loss of weight. This operation is not as disfiguring as some of the other body procedures, because a considerable amount of the scarring is hidden by pubic hair, and the rest is more or less concealed in the natural crease between the thighs and torso.

General anaesthetic is used and the area to be cut away is marked. The aim is to try and remove most of the area below the navel, which is transposed to a higher point. The incision is triangular (see sketch) with a small indent at the base over the edge of the pubic hair. The final stitching line is the lower one. After the incision, the skin is lifted from the underlying tissue up to the ribcage, muscles are tightened and some fat is removed. The skin is

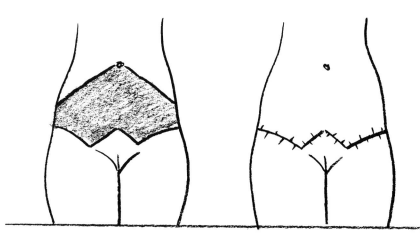

pulled downwards and inwards, but another incision is made around the navel, leaving it attached to the blood vessels. When the final position of the skin is attained, a new hole is made for the navel and it is stitched in place. The operation can take anything from three to five hours.

Afterwards there is some swelling and bruising of the stomach. Suction drains are placed under the skin and the patient must lie on her back. Hospital stay is five days, and after the second day it is advisable to start to walk a little, but this can only be done in a bent-over position. Some stitches come out after a week, others after three or four weeks. You are not allowed to stand up straight or sit down for a minimum of two weeks to avoid pain and pressure on the scars. It can be many weeks before the swelling goes down and you feel normal. You have to check with your surgeon many times during the first month.

## Buttock and Thigh lift

Inner thighs and buttocks start sagging from age, but redemption through surgery is neither quick nor lasting. Aging and pull of gravity can cause them to drop again, so they are very rarely operated on unless in conjunction with the removal of those thigh bulges of cellulite known as 'riding breeches'. The operation is lengthy, recuperation not easy and the scars can be very visible. It is not recommended.

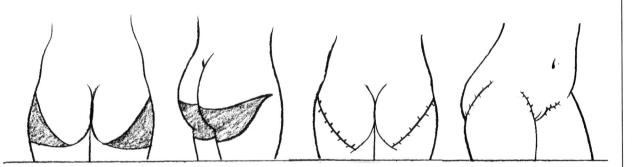

## Upper arms

So many women develop loose skin that sways from the armpit and can go down to the elbow area. Unfortunately nothing satisfactory can be achieved as the scarring in this area is very disfiguring.

## Hands

Again it's a matter of bad scars, though in theory wrinkles and sagging skin could be tightened. Dermabrasion cannot be used either because the skin is so thin. Some surgeons will inject liquid silicone, but it has to be so very carefully administered to prevent it travelling around the body and settling in an undesirable spot.

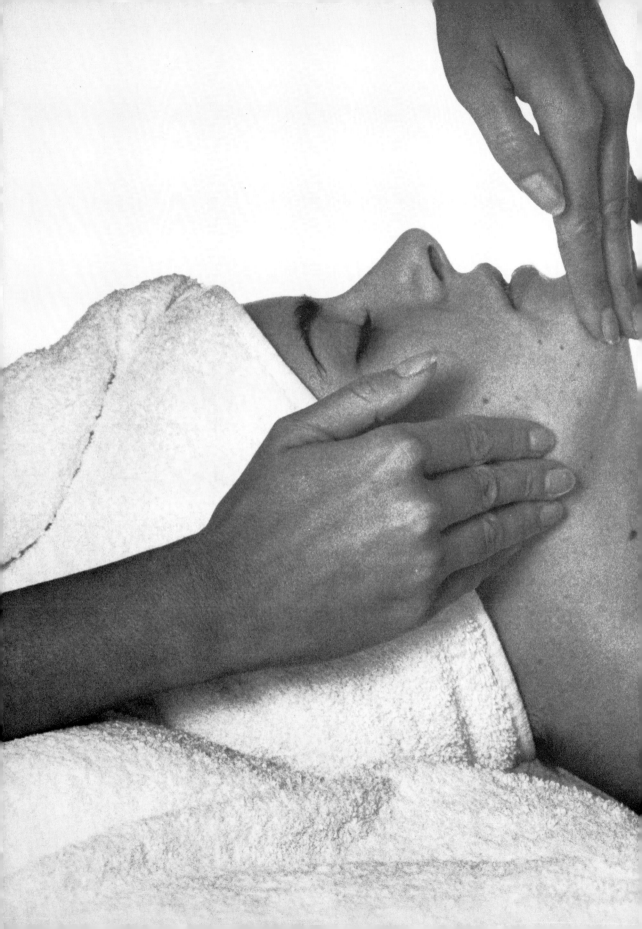

# TREATMENTS
Let yourself be pampered
now and then

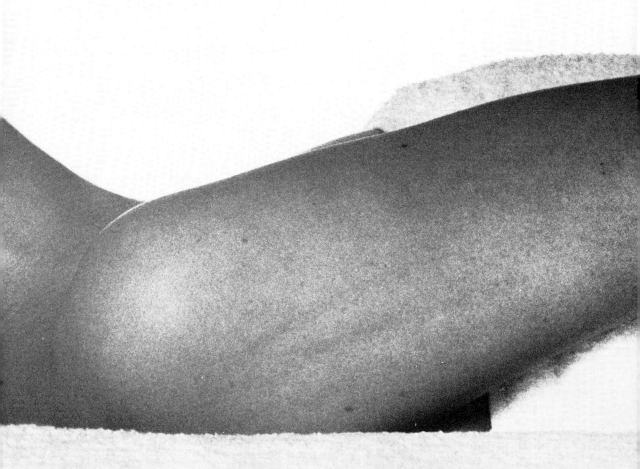

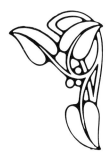

To many women the world of the beauty therapist is an unknown one and the goings-on behind those closed salon doors are mysteries full of promise. Actually a beauty therapist is simply someone who has been trained to perform more skilfully most of the things you could do yourself. There are, however, some skin specialists who have studied in depth the working of the skin, who have apprenticed in individual techniques (mostly in Europe) or who from sheer years of experience have the eye of an expert and the touch of a true therapist and have developed products and procedures of their own. This calibre of therapist is rare and precious, and when you find one you'll immediately know it. In general, beauty therapists do basic treatments and techniques that can be learnt by anyone, but as with many other things (hair, for example) beauty routines done by others invariably turn out being more successful than when you attempt them yourself. In any case – what bliss having it all done for you.

Does this justify the expense? Beauty treatments are not cheap, but they are luxuries that should be allowed every now and then because they are rewarding in many ways. First and foremost is the psychological benefit together with enforced relaxation. There's something marvellous about lying there, doing nothing and putting yourself in the hands of others. You just know you are going to come out looking and feeling better, and this optimistic, positive thought works for you. The mere fact that you are completely relaxed for any time up to an hour is benefit in itself. The therapist will take time with the treatment, doing it methodically and thoroughly, whereas at home you might be inclined to rush, cut corners and end up with a superficial job.

Needless to say, beauty therapists do not get much support from the medical profession and dermatologists are particularly down on them, saying that when it comes to skin treatments there is no lasting benefit. This is true to a degree, but it is unfair, because even a temporary improvement is worthwhile – and clearly visible – and the skin does get a thorough cleansing and conditioning which it may not get under self care. Of course, serious and persistent skin problems need to have medical attention, but because dermatologists generally can't be bothered with minor blemishes, the beauty therapist nicely fills in the gap between home and medical care. Although a beauty therapist can take care of such things as whiteheads, blackheads, general skin condition, superfluous hair and visual effects, don't let her interfere with warts, moles, red veins, bleach patches of dark skin or attempt skin peeling.

The best way to select a therapist is by personal recommendation and, frankly, by trial and error. It is only when you have been under the hands, so to speak, of several that you can properly judge who is good and who isn't. It has a lot to do with touch as well as method; you can feel confidence in some hands and not in others. Also, the training of beauty therapists is not always thorough or to a set standard, as there are a number of associations and institutes providing certificates after training (most of it practical) that could range from a few months to a few years. You can't always judge by the diploma, though some schools are run to standards set by a world wide beauty organisation – Comité International d'Esthétique et de Cosmétologie (CIDESCO) and this is usually a reliable sign.

The following is a guide to the most common facial and body treatments provided by beauty therapists; not all salons provide the full range of services; the electrical and mechanical equipment used is standardized and therapists are usually trained by the manufacturers as to use.

## FACIAL TREATMENTS

### Aromatherapy

This is where aromatic essential oils are used to condition and stimulate the skin, and at the same time provide mental relaxation through the calming effects of certain perfumes on the mind. In the beauty salon, it really should be called cosmetic aromatherapy, because it is but a transitory and superficial use of the technique, which in its therapeutic form and when practised by qualified professionals can be a curative therapy (see page 181). The therapist selects from a range of essences and gently massages one or a combination of scents into the skin. The more ambitious will also provide a body massage, but again bear in mind that this is not the true aromatherapy treatment, but a most pleasant and relaxing way of conditioning the skin. It is particularly valuable as you get older, because the skin becomes dryer and oil is one of the best ways to counteract it.

### Diathermy

A method for the permanent removal of superfluous hair on the face. A fine wire with a metal point is in contact with the hair root, and when an electrical current is passed through it, the root is killed. The sensation is that of a sharp touch with a needle.

### Ear Piercing

Done correctly, it is a painless and harmless process. The most common method is by a special gun which pierces the ears and inserts a sterilized stud at the same time. The studs are hypoallergenic and generally remain in the ears for about six weeks until the healing process is complete. Some therapists puncture the ear lobe by diathermy, insert a silk thread as a dressing and replace it after a few days with a gold ring or stud – these remain in place for a couple of months.

### Electrolysis

This can permanently remove small numbers of facial hairs – and also those around the nipple. It is a skilled procedure and if done properly is painless, but be sure to check your therapist is experienced in electrolysis otherwise there could be some scarring. A very fine needle, which has an electric current running through it, is applied to the hair root to destroy it for life. Only twelve to fifteen hairs can be treated at one time, so it is usual to have a series of treatments. There should be no inflammation, swelling or infection – if there are any signs, immediately consult the therapist and if the problem persists or worsens, see a dermatologist.

### Eyebrow Shaping

Certainly something you could do on your own, but there are women who simply can't bear using tweezers and pulling out hairs. A therapist does it with speed, so even if you have sensitive eyes they rarely water; also she is often better able to judge shape and thickness, can more easily make brows even and because tweezing is done under a bright, direct light, every little stray hair is removed.

### Facials

A facial is an extension of your own basic routine (see page 48) plus the addition of a treatment mask and massage – plus the advantage of lying down for any period up to an hour. A good facial has three important benefits: it leaves your face beautifully clean and glowing, it makes you relax and it provides a psychological beauty boost. I don't care what any sceptic says about the results only being temporary, because the positive effects are there to be seen immediately: you look better, you feel better and clean skin, after all, is better than the earlier sludged one. What's more, it is just about the best inducement to encourage you to carry on the good work at home. Once you've spent time and money in a salon, you'll be more determined to try and get the same results on your own. All these are valid points in the interests of youth and beauty.

There are many types of facials, but the basic routine is the same. You lie on a raised treatment table with shoulder and neck bare. The therapist works from behind. The room is usually dim with a bright light concentrated on your face when necessary. Hair is pulled back and the hairline protected with a cotton or tissue band.

The face is first cleansed with a lotion or cream, afterwards a toner is applied to get rid of any excess cleanser. Your face is then inspected to assess type, overall condition and any special problems. A good therapist will tell you what is good and bad, what you can do for yourself and what she considers she can improve. She will also clear your skin of whiteheads and blackheads. A cream or oil is then applied for massage, which apart from being very soothing, helps to exercise muscles and stimulates circulation. Movement is upward and outward, with gentle circular pressure around the eyes and the mouth. Whether the nutrient is an oil or a cream, it can only be of the best benefit to aging skin, which needs a lot of lubrication in its fight against dryness. Massage usually lasts about ten minutes, then the emollient is cleansed away and a face mask is applied. What type depends on your skin, the preference of the therapist and the type of products she uses. Masks are applied over the neck and face area, leaving the eyes free to be covered with a cooling cottonwool pad (dampened with water, a tonic, a lotion).

*Paloma Picasso*
'After a lot of experimenting I have settled for a look which I think best suits me. Sleeked-back Spanish hair, scarlet lips and squared and polished nails. I have to talk myself into taking trouble with my appearance. Cleansing is vital and I smother my face with a steaming warm flannel after using cleansing cream, and then I use a seaweed mask.'

The mask dries and tightens on the face, drawing out impurities, and you are left relaxing under a warm blanket for ten to fifteen minutes in a darkened room. If you have succumbed to the lulling effects of the facial, you may very well fall to sleep at this point – and so much the better. The mask is removed with warm water cottonwool pads, the face cleansed and a moisturizer applied. Most therapists prefer you to leave the skin this way for a few hours before applying make-up – and quite rightly so. Some skins can have an initial irritant reaction to facial treatment, but this is invariably due to the elimination of toxic matter, and the resulting redness or blotchiness will disappear within a few hours. It can be a sign that your face really needed attention.

There are no permanent benefits from facials, but the positive things they do are: get rid of surface dead cells, open the pores to allow impurities to get out, clear up whiteheads and blackheads, completely cleanse the skin, nourish dry skin, stimulate circulation through massage, temporarily shrink pores and give a more taut look to the skin. The ways and means to all of this involve many alternatives, the most used are:

**masks** – it is the commercial products that are mostly used, some of which are only available to beauticians and cannot be bought by the public. However, most are based on the drying power of clays. Some therapists will use natural products such as honey, egg yolk, avocado or glycerine.

**facial sauna** – this is steaming of the face, using herbal extracts in the water. The theory is that the steam makes the face sweat, opens the pores and helps cleanse the skin. It is refreshing and a useful treatment (though it can easily be done at home, see page 48) and is taken after cleansing before skin inspection and a mask.

**water-spray** – a fine spray of water under pressure (aerosol) is forced on to the face either to help cleansing or to remove masks. It gives a wonderful feeling and although there are those who say to splash on water is the same, somehow it is not – and those who use pressured sprays say that it is the tiny droplets that benefit the skin and that moisturizing treatments afterwards seem to work better.

**cathiodermie** – a special facial procedure that involves the extracts of sea plants, herbs, flowers and fruits together with electrical impulses that are brought to the face on miniature smoothing rollers. It claims to bring waste matter quickly to the surface, to cleanse deeply and provide an energizing element to the skin. It is a useful aid for oily and problem skins. It is one of several so-called galvanic skin treatments, where electrical vibration is used to help remove surface oils and introduce water soluble substances through the skin.

**faradism** – a type of electrical current which induces muscle contraction and thereby provides a type of passive exercise. It is used to stimulate facial muscles, which through movement improve local circulation.

*Barbara Parkins*
'I dance three times a week wherever I am. Once I dieted to an extreme so now I have found a more healthy method which consists of exercise and eating minimal amounts of nutritious food, especially fruit and vegetables. I believe that cleaning and moisturizing the skin should be a ritual and once a week I have a Cathiodermic treatment.'

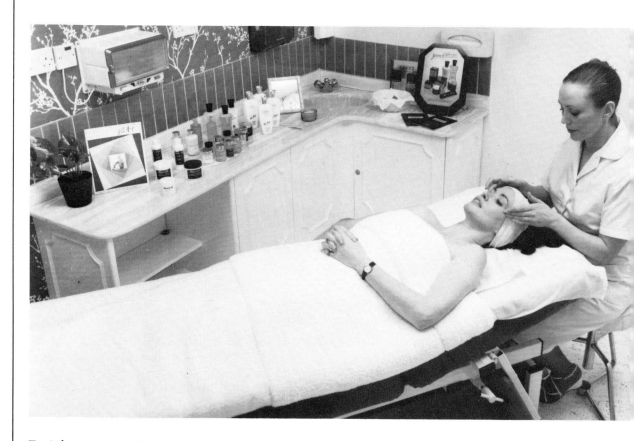

Facial treatment at
Champneys at Tring Health
Resort

**vacuum treatment** – a suction-like device, electrically controlled
that helps to remove blackheads and oily secretion; it also improves
circulation and generally cleanses the skin.

### Lash and Brow Tinting

If you want to darken these hairs it is advisable to let an
experienced therapist do it rather than attempt it on your own
because of the definite danger of getting dye in your eye – it is, of
course, practically impossible to do lashes with your eyes open.
Darkening lashes is useful in the summer when you are in and out of
water, as most mascaras run and smudge.

### Make-up

If you don't seem to get your face right, it's an idea to go and have a
professional make-up done and possibly a lesson at the same time.
However, don't go with the idea that you are going to emerge a
raving new beauty – you are more likely to come out over made-up
and not liking yourself at all. Not all beauty therapists are good
make-up artists – they may know how to use the products but don't
have that innate knack for knowing immediately what can be done
with a face. However, it is beneficial to have someone else's view of
your face and often you can learn a few tricks. What you can
definitely learn is technique, so watch what is being done in the

mirror – don't let the therapist lie you down – watch where the shading goes, how it is blended, when a brush is used, when a crayon. There are many salons that give lessons – you do everything yourself under instruction, and the big benefit is that there is a vast selection of products and colours to choose from. Your facial experiments can be done right there without the expense of buying preparations yourself for trial-and-error purposes at home.

### Ozone Steaming

This is an extra to some facials – a machine produces warm ozone vapour which is directed on your face, making it sweat profusely, opening the pores, increasing circulation and supplying the tissues with extra oxygen.

## BODY TREATMENTS

All beauty aids for the body have to do with skin and shape. As you grow older the skin of the body needs as much attention as that of the face, but rarely gets it. It does help to keep it smooth, keep it lubricated and maintain good circulation. Professional body treatments do this well. Many salons promote 'slimming regimens' where electrically controlled machines and devices are used. How effective are they? In themselves, not particularly, as when it comes to losing weight and toning up muscles for a better figure, it is really up to you (see pages 128–135). What you can get out of such courses is an extra boost, not a miracle cure with little effort on your part. Despite medical dismissal of these body treatments, many are beneficial and not just from a psychological point of view. Massage and water treatments help shape, circulation and skin. And, as I have said before, if you go to the trouble and expense of having special treatments for your body, you start to really care about it, become more aware of its shape and condition, more conscious of what needs to be done, what can be done. If staying younger is your goal, then the look of your body is of paramount importance. Check out the treatments below, try them and then decide which ones give you special benefit, and if you can afford it, start having them on a regular basis because that is where the beauty advantage lies; a once-in-lifetime massage, for example, is worthless, whereas one every week is of tremendous value.

### Herbal Baths

Pleasant and relaxing, these are warm baths to which herbs have been added. They are rarely found in regular beauty salons, but are nearly always part of the treatments at a health farm. They are prescribed when heat treatments such as sauna or steam cabinet cannot be taken because of high blood pressure or related medical problems. One of the most beneficial is a peat bath, which provides long-lasting warmth in the tissues and is valuable in improving rheumatic conditions.

### Infra Red Heat

This is a concentration of warming rays that penetrates the tissues helps aches and pains, relaxes and encourages quick healing of any scars. It mustn't be confused with ultra violet rays that are used for tanning.

### Manicure

It is only by having a professional manicure that you can really assess if you are doing it all right on your own. A good manicurist will hold your hands and nails firmly, and you will feel, not only see what she is doing. She will ask if you want your cuticles cut – not just ignore them, as some therapists do. She should also thoroughly massage your fingers and hands beyond the wrists, pull your fingers so the joints are stretched and mobilized, rotate your wrist. Any manicurist who holds your hands limply and puts hardly any pressure on your nails whilst doing the various procedures, is no good. Also a reliable manicurist will give advice on what you could do for yourself; and anyone who looks at your nails in a condemning way (and many do) should never have your patronage again. (Self-care guide on page 43.)

### Massage

It is soothing and relaxing as well as being well known for its effect in increasing circulation and improving muscle tone. It is not going to make you thinner, but if you are on a diet, it certainly helps to keep the skin and muscle in condition. Because of the improvement in circulation, it helps to eliminate toxic matter from the body, so therefore is an important part of the counter attack on cellulite. I'm a great believer in the benefits of a weekly massage (see page 187 for therapeutic details). A massage lasts about half an hour, and again you can only assess a good masseur through experience. A firm, confident touch is essential; superficial skimming of the body is no good at all.

### Nailbuilding

A method of building with a cement-like substance an extension to your short nails. There are many women with problem nails that simply do not respond to treatment and break off before they have a chance to become longer and stronger. This is a worthwhile solution, because it is only the tip that is covered – the false nail extends beyond so the base is left free to grow. This system is far superior to sticking on false nails, which are really kiss of death to your own nails suffocating below. The idea is that as your own nails grow, you gradually file down the tip and finally reach a point when the entire longer nail is all your own. However, it doesn't always work that way, as weak nails often remain weak nails, but nailbuilding is a definite beauty asset when you are desperate about the state of your nails.

### Panthermal

This is a four-stage body treatment to help the skin. You lie in an oval-shaped capsule that looks like a space machine – your body is on a wood slatted bed, the machine closes over you, but your head is outside and the neck protected with a towel. This peculiar apparatus is just a way of being able to jettison steam, water and oils on all parts of your body at once. At first it is an odd sensation and you might feel a bit claustrophobic, but once relaxed you can lie back and enjoy it. Initially ionized vapour surrounds the body, this produces profuse perspiration even at a low temperature, it opens pores, helps remove impurities and cleanses. Next is exposure to ozone vapour, which provides additional oxygen to the skin. Then comes the conditioning product, depending on your type of skin, and is jettisoned in as vapour or liquid. Finally high-pressure jets of water massage the body. All this is programmed on a control panel with the therapist there to check procedures. It is relaxing and all body skin is exposed to the treatment.

## Pedicure

All therapists are trained to give a proper pedicure, but many of them will avoid checking on the rough skin on the soles of the feet and around the heel, also on tidying up any hardened spots that are almost corns and bunions. They should, although by law they are not allowed to touch and treat serious problems that come under the realm of the chiropodist. But when you go for a pedicure, you really should have your entire foot taken care of as well – smoothed with a pumice stone, massaged and creamed. As with a manicure, it is a firm touch that is an indication of someone who is good. Toenails should be cut straight, the rims thoroughly cleared of odd bits of skin. (Self-care guide on page 45.)

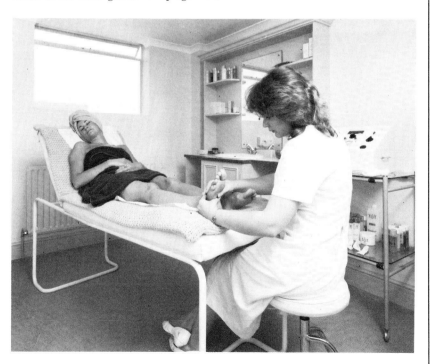

'reatment at Grayshott Hall

### Sauna

Many beauty and slimming salons have a sauna, but not enough take precautions to check you should have one, nor check how long you should stay in. Anyone with high blood pressure should never take a sauna. As for time, it is advisable to be in for ten minutes only at first (less if you feel too hot or breathless), then outside to cool in the air or preferably under a cold shower, for a few minutes, then back in for ten. A sauna is not really for slimming; though some pounds can be lost they are immediately gained. Because of the sweating, it helps eliminate toxic matter from the skin and improve its condition and circulation. A sauna is also said to be good for the nervous system.

### Slendertone

A very popular slimming treatment which works on the principle of artificial muscle stimulation by means of an electrical current. Protective pads are placed strategically on the body; these are bases for wires through which the electric current runs. Through electric impulses the muscles under the pads are forced to alternately relax and contract. The idea is that you lie there and do nothing, and your muscles happily work. That they do, but the degree of weight loss and reshaping is not nearly what it's made out to be. Your muscles may get toned, but you are not using up any energy. If this treatment is undertaken together with a diet and some physical exercise on your part, then it can be of some help. However, on its own, it is not a valid way to slimness for any health conscious woman.

### Steam Cabinet

A heat treatment that may be cited by some therapists as being weight reducing, but it is really for conditioning the skin, increasing circulation and eliminating toxic matter through the pores. Any weight loss will be quickly gained. A steam cabinet is a cone-shaped capsule; you step into it, sit on a wooden-slatted seat, closed in and the head is left outside. It has the advantage of bringing steam to the body and allowing normal breathing of air. Many women prefer this to a sauna. Some skins respond by more profuse perspiration in this damp heat, than in the dry heat of a sauna.

### Suction Cupping

A rubber cup, connected to an air pump, is applied to the skin and a vacuum is created underneath. This is said to suck up the subcutaneous fat. What it does is improve circulation, get the skin into renewed action and through that help the elimination of toxic matter which is often responsible for holding on to fat. Cellulite is a combination of toxic waste and fat, and improves greatly once the skin is free of impurities. Suction cupping will help this process, but it doesn't suck out fat per se, as the name implies.

### Sunbeds

These have gained greatly in popularity over the past few years with their promotion geared to safe suntanning – the harmful ultra violet

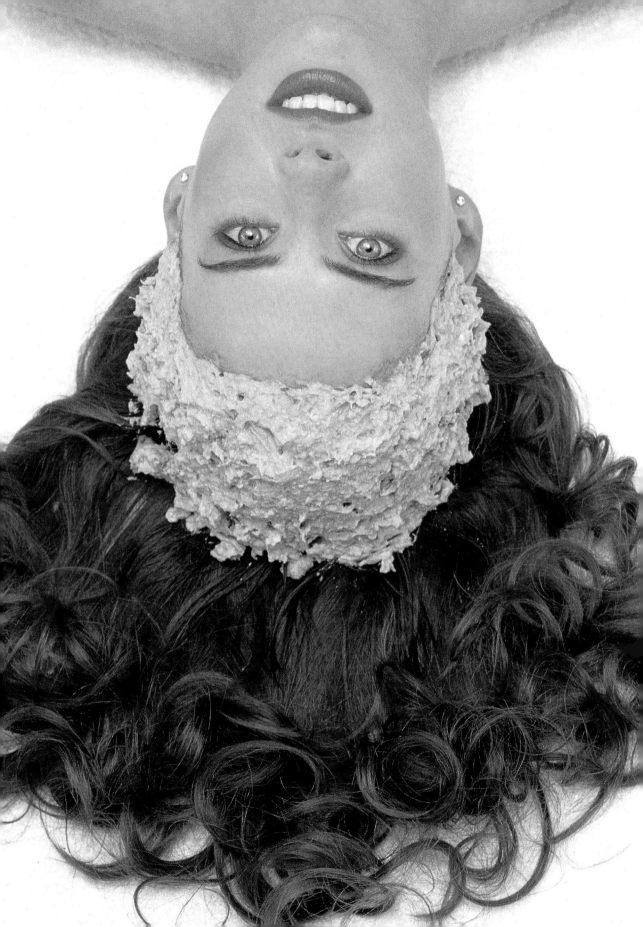

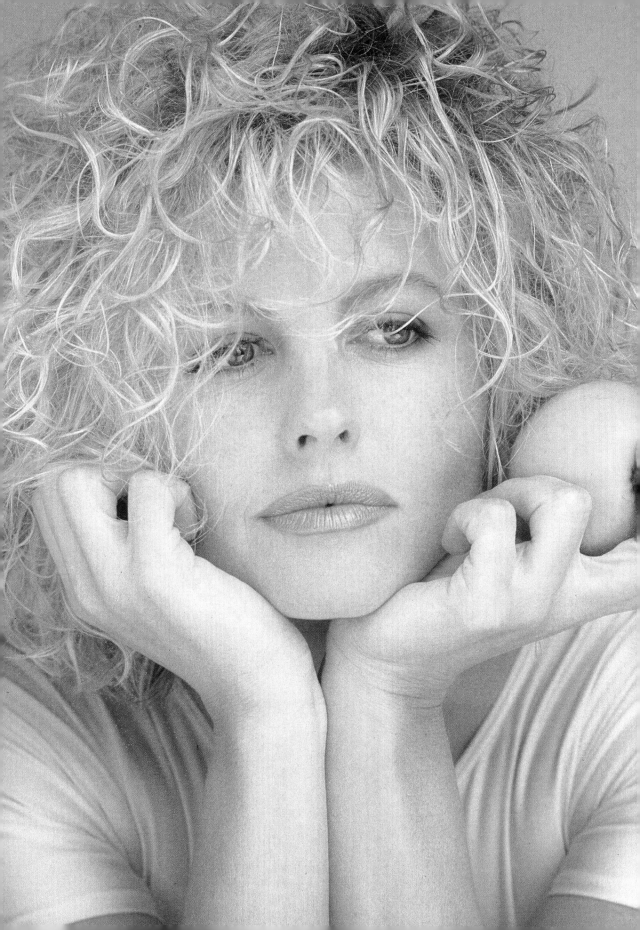

rays are eliminated, the good ones provide a tan. Frankly, I am nervous of any artificial means of tanning, and if timing goes even slightly astray there could be harmful effects. Remember that the safeness depends on the efficiency of the machines and the careful attention of the therapist. All too often, there is no-one around to check timing. I would use sunbeds with caution, if at all.

## Underwater Massage

Rarely available in salons, but can be found at most health resorts. It has been used on the Continent for years, but only over the past few years has been employed in Britain. It is similar in effect to hand massage, but a much higher pressure can be tolerated under water. You sit in an oversized warm bath, and the therapist literally hoses your body underwater, the water coming out under great pressure. It is particularly good for any circulation problem, and it does help break down and disperse obstinate fatty tissue. If you combine underwater massage with diet and exercise, it is amazing how quickly the body will shape up.

Treatment at Inglewood Health Hydro

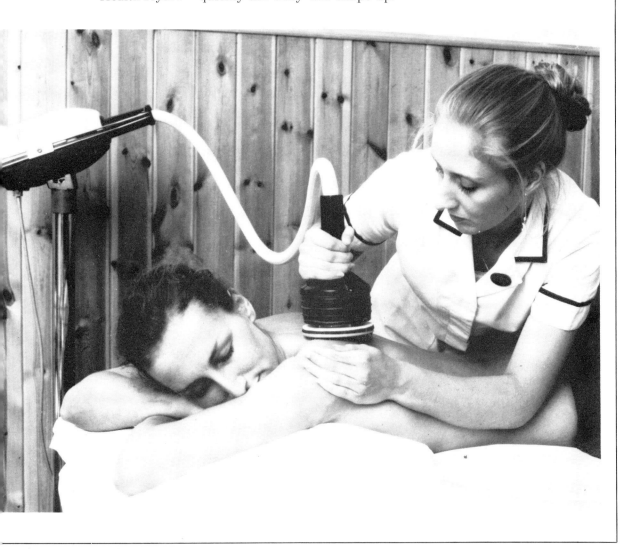

## Vibrator Treatments

These are for stimulation of the circulatory system, and at the same time they relax. The most well-known is G-5, where a head of rubber nodules is vibrated all over the body to help break down fatty deposits. Doctors say it does nothing of the sort, but there are an awful lot of women around who say one of the best ways to lose weight around waist, hips and thighs is to have a series of G-5 treatments. I'm inclined to agree.

## Waxing

Superfluous hair is more or less every woman's problem, and still one of the most satisfactory methods is to remove it with wax. At home this is a messy and not always a satisfactory operation, but in a salon it can be done quickly and efficiently. It is one beauty treatment I really consider being worthwhile. Granted the hair does grow back, but the more it is removed by wax, the slower the growth. It also leaves the skin really smooth. There are two methods – hot and cold. Hot wax is heated in a pan, applied in patches, allowed to cool for a few seconds and then quickly ripped off the skin. If it is ripped off quickly, there is not much pain though always a little. The skin can be smoothed with an immediate application of

Treatment at Champneys at
Tring Health Resort

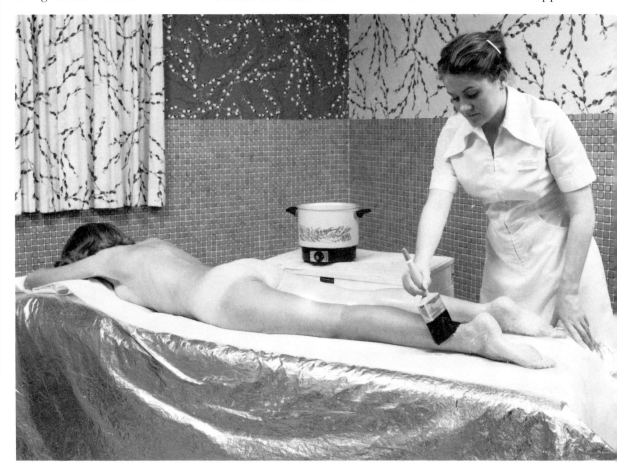

talcum powder. If the wax really burns at first, or if the ripping process is really painful, then the therapist is not doing a proper job. Almost any part of the body can be waxed except the nipples – arms, legs, underarms, face. A bikini wax is when part of the crotch area is treated, so no hair will show even with the briefest of swimming costumes; this can be painful, but it only lasts a few seconds. Hot wax dilates the hair follicle at its deepest point, just above the root. When it is ripped off, it takes the uppermost layer of dead skin cells with it, so can be an irritant for sensitive skin. Cold wax treatment involves the use of a honey-based liquid wax, which is smoothed over the area to be treated, covered with a layer of gauze, then the gauze is pulled away taking the wax and hairs with it. Cold wax is not so harsh on the skin, but it is not as good at removing thick and coarse hair. After either hot or cold wax treatment, the skin should be massaged with a rich lotion.

## Wax Treatment

Paraffin wax is used to cover the body, inducing sweating and thereby bringing out impurities and thoroughly cleansing the skin. You lie on a raised table, or in a sort of bath-tub container, covered with grease-proof paper. The wax – light, white wax similar to that of a candle – is heated and then poured or brushed over the entire body. The heart area should be left free, and pubic hairs are protected with a tissue. The wax quickly solidifies and you are wrapped like an Egyptian mummy in the greaseproof paper, then further wrapped with blankets. You can feel your skin sweating under the heat and restriction of the solid wax. After about twenty minutes to half an hour, the therapist unwraps you, and the wax simply peels away from the body, because between it and your skin is a layer of moisture. This is a marvellous way to cleanse all the body, eliminate toxins and give the skin a smooth, silky touch at the same time. It is not for the claustrophobic.

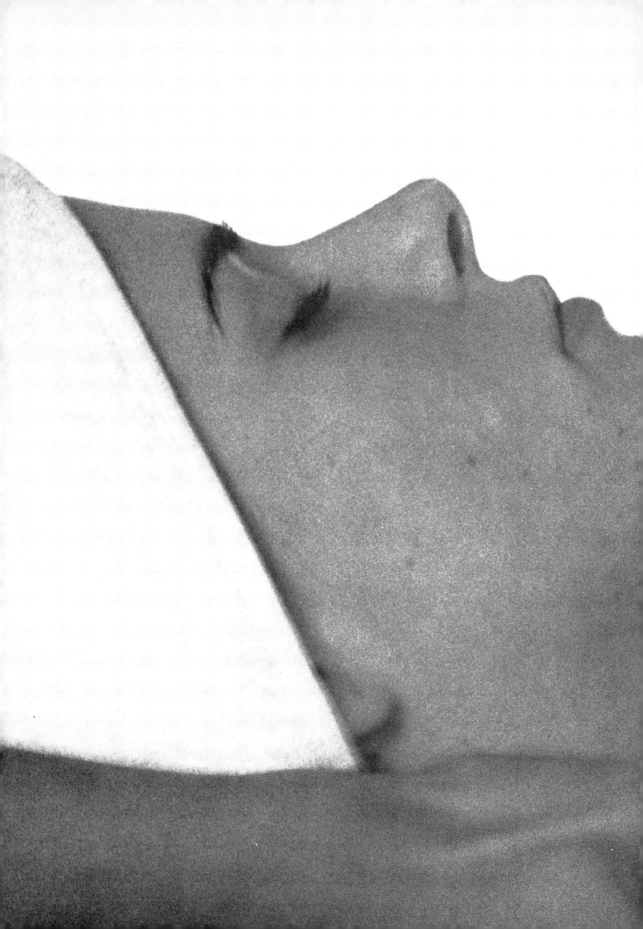

# HEALTH SPAS
## Guiding lights to staying young

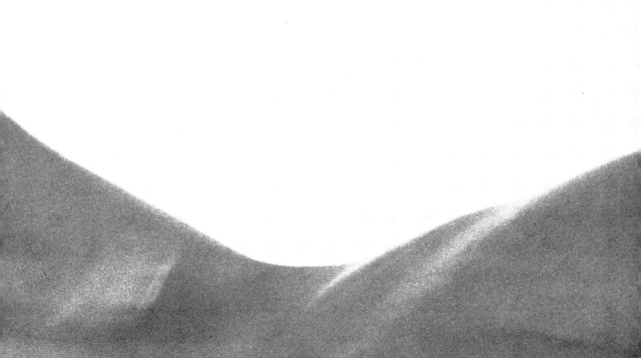

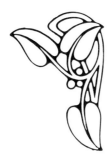

A stay at a health resort is one of the best investments you can make for your health. If you've never been to one, you may be inclined to think of it as an over-expensive slimming centre – all that money for raw carrot etc. – but that is not what health spas are all about. True, many women do go with weight loss as their prime goal, but the real benefits are far more reaching. The best spas are teaching as well as treatment centres. You learn through your daily regimen and from additional lectures how to become more conscious of your health, your diet, your body. You immediately put this new knowledge into daily action and thus re-educate your system to a more health orientated pattern. You will be amazed at how much better you can look and feel in just one week of discipline and concentrated effort on yourself. It could be the most beneficial holiday you've ever had.

So what exactly is a health spa and what goes on? There are various types of health resorts, ranging from medical clinics to establishments that are more like luxury country hotels with all the treatment and sporting facilities, plus a strict diet regimen. Diet, exercise sessions and hydrotherapy treatments are standard in all because the basis of care is founded on the belief in one or more forms of naturopathy (see page 189). The difference lies in the degree of seriousness and strictness of the approach. If weight loss and general body toning is the goal, then there is a wide choice because every health farm offers a slimming diet and body therapeutics. If you are recuperating from an illness or need special remedial treatments, then you have to be more selective – details of the various health centres are given later. One of the most significant aspects of health spa life is the peace and quiet, which is of equal importance to any treatment. You are forced to relax, to let go, to get away from pressures and worries. It does take several days to unwind, to benefit from the effects of a proper diet and treatments – this is why many clinics stipulate a minimum stay of a week. Then there's the additional bonus of fresh, uncontaminated air. Nearly all health farms are deep in the countryside, sometimes by a lake or near the sea where nature's resources are at their best. Air, sun, water and tranquillity all contribute to a health cure.

The naturopathic approach is an old tradition and today's institutions are based on the principle established in the famous watering spots. Water in particular has always been regarded as a regenerating element and because of this whole towns have turned themselves into medical centres based on the therapeutic value of hydrotherapy when specific minerals are present. This still remains the case on the continent, whereas in Great Britain the spas have been sadly neglected and health resorts are now more likely to be isolated country mansions. The word 'cure' is actually misleading; it comes from the German 'kur' which means treatment. Hence in English we are lead to believe that specific food and waters can cure which is what orthodox medical practitioners prefer to deny. What happens, in fact, is that they 'treat'; they can improve health, can ease certain conditions, can temporarily stall them and at times can eliminate many problems completely.

# Health Hydros in Great Britain

Detailed below is information about the leading health resorts in this country. Whether they are called clinics, farms, hydros, spas or whatever, they offer the same kind of regimen. As I mentioned before, a week's stay is considered the beneficial minimum, but many establishments do offer short breaks.

Sunday is the usual day of arrival, in the early afternoon. It is customary to be checked in either by a doctor or a registered nurse, who will take your case history, measure weight and blood pressure; there's also a discussion as to what you expect to gain from your stay; diet, exercise options and particular treatments are explained. Special medical consultations can be arranged. Most patients begin by spending two or three days fasting on hot water and lemon, fruit or a vegetable diet. This is individually prescribed, each patient collecting a tray at mealtimes. There are two dining rooms – one for those eating hardly anything, and the other where a buffet of mostly vegetarian raw food is the choice. After the first few meagre days, you generally graduate to the main dining room. Breakfast, however, is served in your room and early each morning you are given a slip denoting times and types of treatment during the day. Otherwise you are on your own to do what you want – rest, participate in exercises, walk, swim, arrange other sports.

The most common treatments are: sauna, steam cabinet, massage, underwater massage, electrical vibration, infra red heat and the sunbed. They are limited to two or three a day, and are usually included in the overall daily rate.

Beauty treatments – facials, aromatherapy, manicure, pedicure, hair, make-up – are generally extras. Clothing is very casual, to the extent of dressing gowns and slippers day and evening, though many women now wear track suits, and leotards are necessary for exercise classes.

### Champneys, Tring, Hertfordshire

Way back in the 1920s, Champneys was the pioneer of health farms and the same applies today. Since 1978 and under the management of Tanya and Allan Wheway it has led the way in providing a new image for health spas. The old idea used to be an annual fast to try to undo the cumulative damage of a year. Now the emphasis is on showing and teaching you how to adjust your day to day living with an aim to positive health through preventive medical methods. It is probably the best equipped and organized health resort in Europe offering a vast choice of leisure activities as well as treatments and diet control. The particular joy here is the recently added indoor heated pool with floor to ceiling glass windows. It is purified with odourless ozone instead of chlorine and because it is not too deep anywhere is perfect for the beneficial water exercises.

The original house is a Victorian mansion – once owned by the Rothschild family – set in 170 acres of parkland. The main house provides gracious public rooms and some bedrooms, while modern

*Barbra Streisand*
I have a problem with my weight, so I go to a health farm in Escondido to spend a few days doing exercises and following a strict diet. I continually have to do battle with my hips.'

extensions over recent years are efficiently designed for the treatments and leisure activities. A holiday environment has been created at Champneys which is light relief for those who get bored with a spartan health regime. Indoors there are facilities for swimming, table tennis, bar billiards, darts, a large variety of table games including chess, backgammon, scrabble and cards; then there's the leisure craft centre where you can do pottery, painting, jewellery making, fabric dyeing and many other crafts. Outdoors there's tennis, badminton, volleyball, cycling, jogging and walking trails, guided walks, golf driving net, putting and croquet. Indeed, few resort hotels offer as much. It is very much a place to get fit, not just lose weight.

Special programmes are available for stress and for smokers who are desperate to stop. There's also a 'well woman programme' which has been developed to extend preventive medicine in those areas specifically concerned with women.

In the stress workshop, there's a questionnaire which helps you to recognise what's causing you stress – check the list here:

- Do you feel that your confidence holds you back from doing what you would really like to do in your social life, your interests or your work?
- Are there people in your life whom you feel you cannot deal with and who leave you feeling frustrated or angry?
- Do you feel that people tell you that you are over-reacting to minor irritations?
- Do you become hesitant and unsure of yourself if you have to complain about bad service or work?
- Do you find it difficult to have a good night's sleep and wake feeling refreshed?
- Do you become nervous and hesitant if you have to talk to a group of people?
- Do you find it an effort to keep up with social demands?
- Do you feel that others will think you are burdening them if you talk to them about a difficulty you have?
- Have you become less interested in making love?
- Do you find you quite often feel physically tense and suffer pains in your back, head or stomach?
- When you sit back and try to relax do you feel guilty that you are doing nothing?
- Have you increased the amount you smoke or drink over the last year?
- Do you shy away from talking to people you do not know at parties or other social events?
- Do you sometimes get up feeling that you cannot face the day ahead of you?

If you answer 'yes' to five or more questions, then the pressure is on and your capacity for coping is being strained.

Apart from the scheduled treatments, the optional programme is planned to keep you doing something all the time – should you so wish. Your first day choice would be like this: 8.00–8.30 country walk, 8.00–9.30 breakfast, 9.30–10.15 morning exercises and 'start jogging safely' guide, 10.30–11.00 water exercises, 12.30–1.45 lunch, 2.00–2.30 country walk, 3.00–3.30 total relaxation session, 3.00–4.00 tennis group, 3.00–5.00 leisure crafts, 3.45–4.15 back mobilizing exercises, 3.45—4.15 water exercises, 4.00–5.00 tea, 4.30 to 5.15 abdominal exercises, 5.30–6.30 lecture on 'healthy eating', 7.00–8.30 dinner. 8.30 to 10.00 reception party. And finally to bed.

Whirlpool with ozone purified main pool in the background, Champneys at Tring

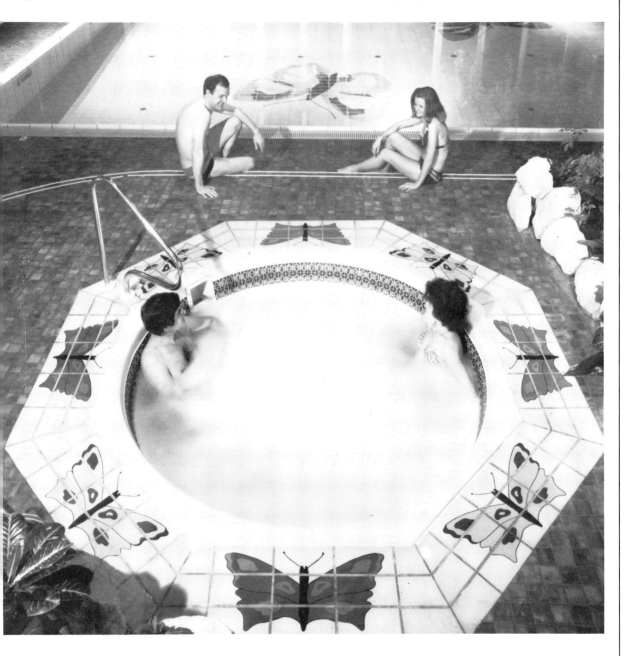

**Enton Hall, Enton, Nr. Godalming, Surrey**

This clinic was founded in 1949 by one of the deputy principals of Champneys and right from the start was very medically orientated with emphasis on healing through natural therapeutics, health education and organic husbandry. For thirty years the clinic's market garden of three acres has been run on purely organic lines and provides most of the salads and vegetables for the diet. Enton Hall has recently been purchased by an American association connected with the Seventh-Day Adventist church and its original health programmes now continue under the guidance of Dr Robert Dunn, who is a member of the American College of Preventive Medicine.

This is a place for patients needing help for chronic conditions rather than for those looking for a weight-loss and overall fitness programme. There's a fully qualified nursing staff throughout the day and night; a doctor is always on call and first thing in the morning you are always visited in your room by either a medical consultant or a sister. Osteopathy plays an important role in treatment and is indicated for low back pain, migraine, hypertension, gastric problems and traumatic injuries. The physiotherapy department provides treatment for early mobilization and short term rehabilitation after illness or injury; patients can also learn how to correct postural imbalances, ease breathing difficulties, strengthen weak muscles and loosen stiff joints. (Many medical insurance schemes will cover physiotherapy treatments.) The most recent addition is a biofeedback training course (see page 170). There are also programmes for stress control and stop-smoking.

Plans are underway to modernize both accommodation and treatment areas, which look as though they have been somewhat neglected in recent years. Chalets in the garden have already been redecorated. The current swimming pool is outdoors and very small.

The programme of natural therapies embraces the holistic view of medical treatment, the aim being to get body, mind, feeling and spirit in harmonious balance. Here it is called 'newstart' which stands for: nutrition, exercise, water, sunshine, temperance, air, rest and trust in God.

A change in dietary habits is the first principle, says Dr Dunn, but he has turned away from fasting. The diet is primarily vegetarian at the clinic and there are lectures and classes on vegetarian cooking. The importance of a nourishing – though not fattening – breakfast is stressed, particularly when patients are undergoing the stress or stop-smoking courses. The clinic's nutritionist, Mrs Audrey Ellison, has worked out the following menus for a week.

Beverages: you can choose from tea with skimmed milk or lemon, decaffeinated coffee, barley water, herbal teas of peppermint, rosehip, fennel, camomile or nettle.

Day 1:  fresh fruit with muesli
        slice wholemeal toast with peanut butter
        beverage choice

Day 2:   stewed prunes without sugar
skimmed milk yogurt
granola
slice wholemeal toast
beverage choice

Day 3:   oatmeal porridge with skimmed milk and prune juice
1 piece fresh fruit
slice wholemeal toast with peanut butter
beverage choice

Day 4:   granola
skimmed milk yogurt
1 sliced banana
slice wholemeal toast with butter and honey
beverage choice

Day 5:   muesli
glass skimmed milk
stewed apricots or 1 orange
slice wholemeal toast with butter
beverage choice

Day 6:   $\frac{1}{2}$ grapefruit
skimmed milk yogurt with wheatgerm, flaked wheatbran
milled nuts and grated apple
slice wholemeal toast with butter
beverage choice

Day 7:   dried fruit compote, wheatgerm, skimmed milk
slice wholemeal toast with peanut butter
$\frac{1}{2}$ sliced banana, or 1 orange or 4 dates
beverage choice


**Forest Mere, Liphook, Hampshire**

The setting of Forest Mere is one of the most beautiful and tranquil of the health spas. Even before you approach the main sweep of drive, you have to negotiate a winding lane that makes you realize immediately that this is one place that is really off the beaten track where no pressures could possibly invade. Water is always soothing, and here there is a large expanse of a lake with lawns dipping right down to it. The house itself is not so imposing as some of the other health mansions, but is graceful and formal, very English country-house. There's also a new wing providing rooms with private baths, treatment areas, a light dining-room with large terrace and a good-sized indoor swimming pool. There's also a lovely large pool outdoors – this is heated. Tennis, badminton and sailing on the lake are available, and arrangements can be made to play golf on the Liphook golf course. Inside there's also plenty of choice – table tennis, smooker, billiards and cards.

On your first visit, Forest Mere prefer you to stay for about ten days and this is always from a Sunday to a Wednesday week. The dietetic regimen is of the utmost importance, though constructive fasting may not be necessary for everyone. You are likely to start on the light diet – a combination of fresh fruit and home-made yogurt with wheatgerm and honey. After a few days you are usually eating full meals. Lunch is a particularly impressive selection of salads (some of the best I've seen), wholemeal bread, cheese and fruit. Dinner is an appetizing (though calorie-controlled) three-course meal.

Hydrotherapy and other treatments are usually in the morning – a nursing sister visits you in your room to check on your condition. Organized exercise includes water movements, a class in the well-equipped recreation gymnasium that emphasizes posture, mobility and stamina. Then later in the afternoon there's a Yoga and relaxation class.

Forest Mere from across the lake

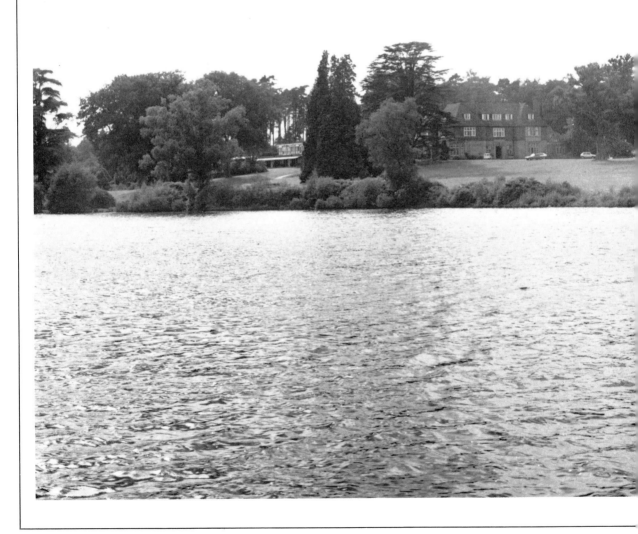

Forest Mere sum up their attitude to overall wellbeing in these few simple rules for health maintenance:

- eliminate all refined food and ensure an adequate intake of lean meat, grilled fish, vegetables and raw fresh fruit. Include some wholemeal bread or cereal daily. Justify the quantity of food consumed.
- reduce the quantity of animal fats eaten.
- eat slowly and chew thoroughly.
- avoid eating snacks in between meals, excepting fresh fruit.
- moderate tea and coffee consumption. Substitute fresh unsweetened fruit juices, decaffeinated coffee or water.
- simplify composition of meals.
- keep alcohol at a minimum and avoid smoking.
- apply physical activity daily within one's capacity but endeavour to stretch that capacity slowly. Brisk walking, controlled jogging, Yoga and regular swimming are the forms of exercise most recommended.
- practise relaxation once each day.

What would be an effective reducing diet to follow at home? Forest Mere have worked out this one that contains approximately 800 calories a day.

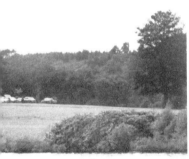

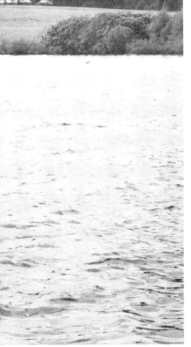

| During the day: | 5oz milk, preferably skimmed |
| Breakfast: | Tomato juice or 1 grapefruit |
| | 1 egg boiled or poached or 1oz All-Bran or |
| | 1 slice wholemeal toast and a little butter |
| | 1 cup tea or coffee |
| Mid-morning: | 1 cup tea or coffee |
| Mid-day: | $\frac{1}{2}$ grapefruit |
| | 2oz lean meat or 6oz baked or grilled fish; mushrooms, runner beans, broccoli, sprouts or cabbage, or salad ad lib |
| | 1 plain yogurt or 1 apple, orange or pear |
| Tea: | lemon tea |
| Evening: | clear soup or $\frac{1}{2}$ grapefruit |
| | 6oz cottage cheese or 4oz cold chicken or |
| | 2 hard-boiled eggs |
| | salad of lettuce, cucumber, grated carrot, celery, radishes and tomatoes |
| | orange, apple or pear |
| | decaffeinated coffee if required. |

### Grayshott Hall, Grayshott, Nr Hindhead, Surrey

Recent extensions and redecoration have turned this imposing Victorian mansion into a very efficient and luxurious resort. The grounds stretch for forty-seven acres, and then adjoining is a further 700 acres of National Trust woodland. This provides great scope for walking, jogging, cycling and riding. There's also a small golf course in the grounds, as well as facilities for tennis, badminton and croquet. All these outdoor possibilities, plus the high standard of treatments make Grayshott one of my favourite health spas.

There is a large indoor heated swimming pool surrounded by glass on three sides and providing good space and depth for continued lengths of swimming – something not always possible in smaller or shallower pools. There is a well-equipped gym, with a good daily choice of exercise regimes, though it is advisable to attend just one class a day at the beginning unless you are particularly fit. The selection is: general exercise class, body workout with music, suppleness, strength and aerobic exercise, abdominal exercises, exercises using the gym equipment, Yoga and relaxation.

The usual body treatments are available and in addition there's the panthermal apparatus (see page 222). The beauty department deserves special mention, because here you really can get good facial treatments of every type, which are individually selected and well applied.

Of course, food is very much to the fore – control of it, that is, though after the initial light diet days everyone is encouraged to eat three-course meals in the main dining-room. These appear substantial, but are rarely more than 1,000 calories in all for a day. Here is the Grayshott Guide for a slimming diet:

Grayshott Hall

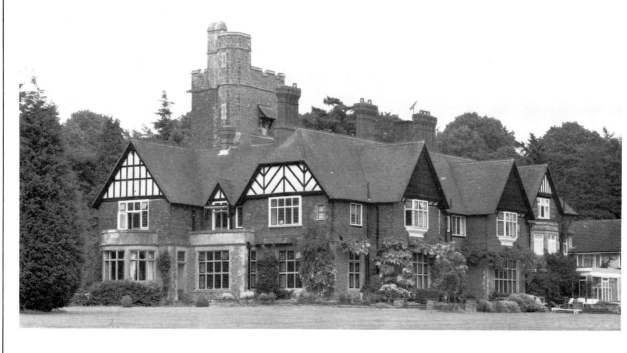

| | |
|---|---|
| Your daily allowance: | 4 crispbreads<br>$\frac{1}{2}$oz butter or margarine<br>$\frac{1}{2}$ pint skimmed milk |
| Your daily fruit allowance: | one portion only to be taken with each meal<br>2oz grapes, stewed prunes or apricots<br>3oz apple, pear, fresh pineapple or cherries<br>4oz raw plums, damsons, orange, peach, or stewed apples, pears or damsons, fresh strawberries, raspberries, apricots or grapefruit |
| Breakfast: | $\frac{1}{2}$ grapefruit, 1 orange or 1 glass of diluted orange juice<br>with . . . 2 crispbreads with butter from daily allowance<br>with . . . 1 boiled egg, poached or scrambled with tomatoes<br>or . . . 3oz fish, grilled, baked or steamed with tomatoes<br>or . . . 1oz lean grilled bacon with tomatoes<br>with . . . tea, coffee or herbal tea with milk from your daily allowance |
| Mid-morning: | glass of hot water and lemon, marmite, herbal tea or rosehip tea, tea or coffee with milk from your daily allowance |
| Lunch: | 3oz lean meat, chicken, tripe, liver or kidney with a large portion of green vegetables and a small amount of root vegetables or a mixed salad<br>or . . . 4oz fish, steamed, grilled or baked with a large portion of green vegetables and a small amount of root vegetables or a mixed raw salad<br>or . . . 2$\frac{1}{2}$oz cheese with a mixed raw salad or cooked green vegetables with a small amount of root vegetables<br>with . . . one fruit from daily allowance<br>with . . . tea or coffee with milk from your main allowance |
| Tea: | One crispbread with tomatoes and watercress with butter or margarine from your daily allowance |
| Dinner: | Clear soup or $\frac{1}{2}$ grapefruit or unsweetened tomato juice<br>with . . . 4oz fish or 3oz lean meat or 2$\frac{1}{2}$oz cheese<br>with . . . mixed raw salad or cooked green vegetables with a small amount of root vegetables<br>or . . . 2 boiled eggs, poached or scrambled, or an omelet with a raw mixed salad or cooked green vegetables with a small amount of root vegetables<br>with . . . one fruit meal from the main list<br>with . . . tea or coffee with milk from daily allowance |

## Henlow Grange, Henlow, Bedfordshire

This is a relaxed, unpretentious health farm – although the building itself is an impressive Georgian mansion with nine acres of surrounding parkland. The cosy atmosphere is due no doubt to the fact that it is a family owned and run enterprise – Bob, Dorothy and Stephen Purden. The underlying principle of treatment here is that you ease yourself gently into new health regimens. A fast of just lemon and water is discouraged, and the diet is not so strict as in some establishments, but it still follows the wholesome, fresh path wine is available on request at any meal.

The particular point about Henlow is that some beauty treatments are included in the daily rate – they are usually extras. For example, you get a facial every day; then there's a special instruction class on skincare and make-up, and if you stay a week, a manicure is also thrown in. It is one of the few places where you can get a complete body wax bath.

There's a good-sized indoor swimming pool flanked by the gymnasium where there's a daily choice of exercise classes aerobics, dance routines and yoga. It is up to you to decide which classes you wish to take, and for the enthusiastic there's supervised jogging every morning at 8.30 where the rule is to alternate twenty paces of jogging with twenty paces of walking to break you in gently.

To give you an idea of the more generous attitude towards diet here are some typical menus, which if you follow at home will probably give a weight loss of about three lbs a week:

Henlow Grange

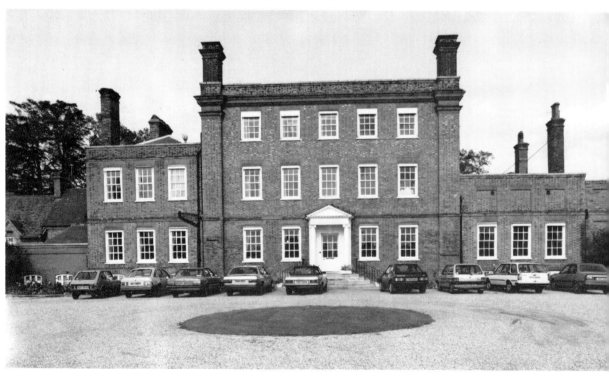

### Breakfast Plans:

$\frac{1}{2}$ grapefruit  
smoked haddock  
slice wholegrain toast

All Bran or Muesli  
small yogurt  
grated apple

sliced orange  
boiled egg  
slice wholegrain toast

slice melon  
poached fillet of fish  
slice wholegrain toast

### Lunch Plans:

vegetable soup  
cheese souffle  
green salad  
fruit jelly

leek soup  
bean and tomato casserole  
mixed salad  
jelly with yogurt

lettuce soup  
baked potato  
mixed salad  
fruit jelly

tomato soup  
cold turkey slice  
mixed salad  
fresh fruit

### Dinner Plans:

tomato and anchovy salad  
braised steak  
cabbage  
carrots

egg salad  
lamb chop  
courgettes and sprouts  
fresh fruit

sardine salad  
smoked haddock  
broccoli and carrots  
slice melon

leek soup  
chicken  
green beans  
compote of fruit

### Inglewood Health Hydro, Kintbury, Berkshire

Set in fifty acres, Inglewood has long been recognised as one of the great houses of England, going as far back as the Crusades. In 1975 it was converted into a health hydro and apart from gracious public rooms it offers a particularly wide range of accommodation – budget, large suites and even extends to a splendid separate five-bedroomed house which is secluded in the grounds and can be reserved by special arrangement.

After consultations with the clinical staff and dietician, you are prescribed four treatments a day. There are several optional exercise classes each day, and individual programmes can be worked out. Therapeutic activity centres around the heated indoor swimming pool, which is designed rather like the courtyard of a Mediterranean villa – all the treatment rooms conveniently surround it, and it serves as both a waiting and lounging area.

If you require special medical attention, there's a qualified nursing staff, and in addition to the initial consultation, full medical check ups can be arranged on request. There are facilities to take care of post-operative patients and general medical convalescence. Another plus: mothers with babies or children can have each child taken care of by a Norland Nanny, as this famous school is just a couple of miles away.

As at other health spas, you are either put on a light diet or allowed to select from mainly vegetarian food in the dining room – the selection is wide and imaginative. Losing weight under supervision is one thing, doing it alone is another, and so here is some advice from Inglewood's dietician, Carole Potter. She has devised the 'Little and Often Diet' which she particularly recommends for women who lead a sedentary life. You have six small meals within a 24 hour period; the order of the meals is not important, but it is best to space them evenly because it will reduce the chance of overeating and will keep the metabolic rate as high as possible on this number of calories. Here is a week's plan:

**Daily Allowance:**
1 pint skimmed milk
$\frac{1}{2}$ oz. butter or margarine
as much tea or coffee as desired, but no more than the milk allowance permits if taken white; no sugar, of course

**Allowed Extra Dressings:**

| | |
|---|---|
| tomato dressing: | $\frac{1}{4}$ pint tomato juice, 1 oz. dried skimmed milk, dry mustard, 2 tablespoons lemon juice, pepper, a little salt; mix in blender and chill. |
| slimming gravy: | puree carrots and cauliflower, add to a thin gravy stock to make a thick, low calorie gravy. |

**Monday**

| | |
|---|---|
| Breakfast | 1 slice wholegrain bread, poached egg |
| Mid Morning | 1 fresh fruit |
| Lunch | 2 oz. cold lean beef, crisp green salad dressed with lemon juice. |
| Mid Afternoon | 2 cream crackers, 1 oz. Brie cheese |
| Dinner | 2 egg omelet, broccoli, grilled tomato |
| Supper | 2 Rich Tea biscuits, herbal tea |

**Tuesday**

| | |
|---|---|
| Breakfast | 2 oz. muesli, $\frac{1}{2}$ grapefruit |
| Mid Morning | 1 crispbread, 2 oz. cottage cheese, tomato |
| Lunch | 2 oz. skinned chicken, beansprout salad with yogurt dressing |
| Mid Afternoon | 1 slice toast with marmite |
| Dinner | 3 oz. lean lamb chop, carrots and peas, thin gravy |
| Supper | fresh fruit salad |

**Wednesday**

| | |
|---|---|
| Breakfast | 1 slice wholegrain bread, grilled mushrooms and tomatoes |

| | |
|---|---|
| Mid Morning | ½ carton fruit yogurt or 1 carton natural yogurt |
| Lunch | 1 boiled egg, sweetcorn and green salad with tomato dressing |
| Mid Afternoon | 2 chopped fruits mixed with 1 oz. muesli and milk from allowance |
| Dinner | ratatouille, 2 oz. grated cheese |
| Supper | 2 crispbread and 1 oz. lean meat |

**Thursday**

| | |
|---|---|
| Breakfast | stewed fruit, 1 oz. All Bran, 3 oz. natural yogurt |
| Mid Morning | 2 Rich Tea biscuits |
| Lunch | 3 oz. tuna, tomatoes, French beans and peppers |
| Mid Afternoon | 1 slice wholegrain bread, 1 oz. lean meat |
| Dinner | 3 oz. skinned chicken, green vegetable, sweetcorn, thin gravy |
| Supper | fresh fruit |

**Friday**

| | |
|---|---|
| Breakfast | 1 slice wholegrain toast, 1 grilled rasher of bacon |
| Mid Morning | 1 crispbread and 1 oz. lean meat |
| Lunch | 2 oz. Camembert cheese, 1 apple, celery and tomato |
| Mid Afternoon | 1 piece fresh fruit |
| Dinner | 3 oz. lean beef, carrots and broccoli, thin gravy |
| Supper | 2 Rich Tea or Arrowroot biscuits |

**Saturday**

| | |
|---|---|
| Breakfast | 2 oz. muesli |
| Mid Morning | piece of fresh fruit |
| Lunch | 2 oz. ham sausage, green salad dressed with lemon juice |
| Mid Afternoon | 2 crispbread, sliced tomato and cucumber |
| Dinner | 4 oz. grilled fish, lemon, grilled tomato, mixed green salad |
| Supper | 2 plain biscuits |

**Sunday**

| | |
|---|---|
| Breakfast | 1 slice wholegrain toast |
| | 1 scrambled egg and grilled tomato |
| Mid Morning | tea or coffee only |
| Lunch | 3 oz. grilled pork cutlet, unsweetened apple sauce, green vegetable, carrots, small potato (baked) |
| Mid Afternoon | piece of fresh fruit |
| Dinner | 3 oz. cottage cheese, large green salad with celery, shredded cabbage, apple, chopped mint, dressed with lemon |
| Supper | 1 Rich Tea biscuit |

## A beginner's exercise routine from Inglewood

John Templeman is in charge of the fitness studio – a separate unit at the rear of the building – and finds that many women have not exercised for years, yet now are inspired by the new vogue for fitness. He has devised this simple routine which will gradually strengthen those unused muscles.

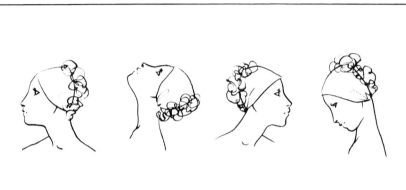

**Neck Rotation:** many of us forget how essential it is to keep the neck area supple; it is the main area of tenseness and unless this is relieved through movement or massages, headaches and increased tenseness result. Circle the head clock and anti-clockwise ten times in each direction; do it slowly, keeping the shoulders down and really stretching the neck in all directions.

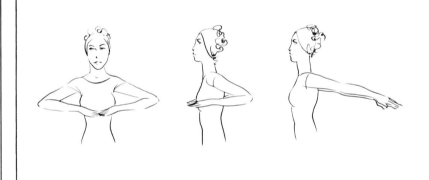

**Arm Fling:** this is a way to strengthen upper arms and chest area. Bend arms at shoulder level, fingers just touching. First push elbows back as if trying to make them meet pulling shoulder blades together, push twice, then straighten arms in a backward fling. Repeat ten times.

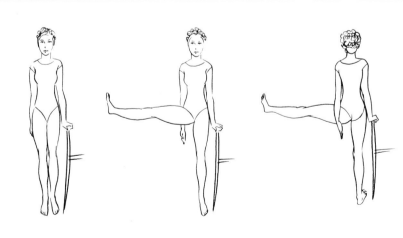

**Side Leg Raise:** start to get legs back into shape by doing high side kicks. Lean against any support, stand with feet a little apart and kick the outside leg sideways attempting a right angle. Do fifteen times with each leg. Concentrate on putting more control and speed in the leg raises before increasing the number of kicks.

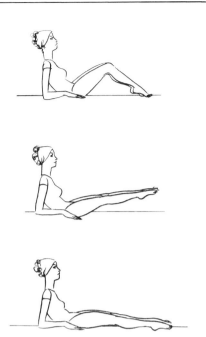

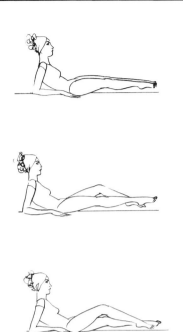

**Toe Tap:** for strengthening the stomach muscles. Sit on floor, rest body on elbows, legs straight in front, toes pointed. Bend legs to about 45 degrees, straighten legs then slowly toe tap the floor, one, two, three times. Bend and hold to the count of three. Repeat ten times.

**Pedal Push:** this is basically a stomach exercise but it also strengthens the legs. Sit on floor, support yourself with the elbows, stretch legs out in front, toes pointed. Lift both legs about six inches off the ground and start pedalling in the air. Ideally you build up to thirty pedals.

**Calf Push:** excellent for ankles, calves and Achilles' tendons. Stand on tip toes, support yourself with a chair, rock back slowly on to the heels, raising toes, then return to the ball of the foot. Do fifteen times – and you'll soon be ready to cycle, walk distances or jog without doing damage to those underworked feet and calf muscles.

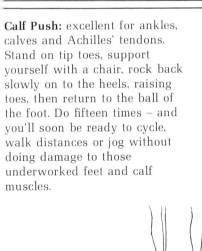

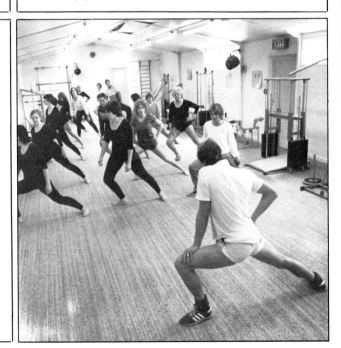

Exercises in the gym at Inglewood Health Hydro

### Shrubland Hall Health Clinic, Coddenham, Ipswich, Suffolk

Shrubland Hall was built in 1740 on one of the highest points in Suffolk. It was one of the earliest established health spas and although it has been fully modernized and equipped with a very comprehensive range of treatment rooms, it still retains the atmosphere of an elegant country house. Many of the original paintings and furniture remain. A particular pleasure is the large conservatory where semi-tropical plants flourish, and just outside is a heated swimming pool – unfortunately too small for energetic swimming – which is covered with a plastic bubble in cold weather. The extensive grounds and gardens are a delight – in fact they have been described as among the most spectacular classical gardens in England, laid out by Sir Charles Barry in the style of the Villa d'Este outside Rome.

Against this background of established grandeur, the regimen at Shrublands follows the established continental 'cure' philosophy under the practised eye of Lady de Saumarez, whose family home it is. She has a very strict attitude towards diet, believing it is fundamental to health revitalization. Fasting on liquids – at times just lemon and water – is done under careful supervision and is considered a major curative therapy assisting the cleansing of the entire system as well as a method of losing weight quickly. For all, a raw food diet is prescribed – fruit, vegetables, plus occasional additions of cheese, homemade yogurt, vegetable broths and wholegrain breads. Indeed Shrublands go out of their way to stress

Shrubland Hall Health Clinic

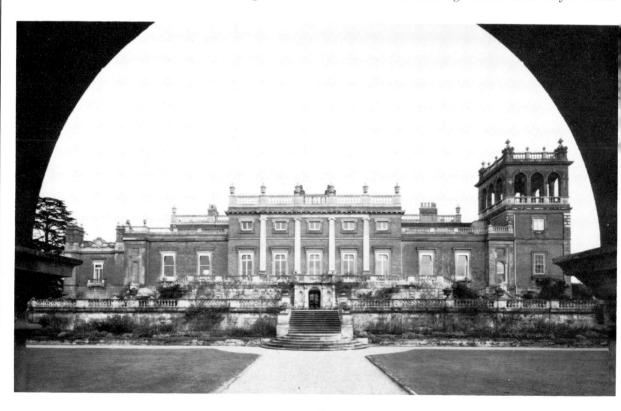

that a hotel-type menu is not available and cooked meals are not provided except on your last reward day. Food, however, is beautifully presented and looks as enticing as anything cooked – more so in fact. One special piece of advice: no matter what your diet, it is always recommended to have afternoon tea, preferably with a little honey.

When I stayed at Shrublands, I went on the following mainly fruit diet for six days, lost nine pounds, and came out with glowing skin and bright eyes:

**First Day:** Breakfast: grapefruit pieces
Herb tea with honey
Lunch: half a melon, 2 kiwi fruits
Tea: China tea with lemon and honey
Supper: Small bunch of grapes, 2 prunes, 1 pear

**Second Day:** Breakfast: grapefruit segments, herb tea and honey
Lunch: 1 slice pineapple, bunch grapes, 1 apricot (dried and soaked)
Tea: China tea with lemon and honey
Supper: 1 orange, 2 plums, 2 lychees

**Third Day:** Breakfast: grapefruit segments, herb tea and honey
Lunch: 1 pear, 1 plum, 4 lychees
Tea: China tea with lemon and honey
Supper: $\frac{1}{4}$ melon, 4 lychees

**Fourth Day:** Breakfast: grapefruit segments, 2 Ryvita biscuits, small pat of butter, little honey, herbal tea
Lunch: 1 orange, 1 kiwi fruit
Tea: China tea with honey
Supper: 1 cup vegetable broth, 4 dates with cucumber slices, 1 apple

**Fifth Day:** Breakfast: grapefruit segments, 2 Ryvita biscuits, small pat of butter, little honey, herbal tea
Lunch: cottage cheese, 1 orange, 2 dates
Tea: China tea with honey
Supper: 1 cup vegetable broth, pear, 1 kiwi fruit, 1 Ryvita biscuit

**Sixth Day:** Breakfast: grapefruit segments, 2 Ryvita biscuits, small pat of butter, little honey, herbal tea
Lunch: selection of raw vegetable salads
Tea: China tea with honey
Supper: reward meal of baked fish, 2 fresh vegetables, dessert mousse, glass white wine

On the treatment side, Shrublands was the first to bring in many of the continental ideas. It initiated the use of sauna as a regular treatment – and it still has the best plunge pool of all. Another first was the introduction of under-water massage, while Sitz baths are used for after the steam cabinet treatment, and pressure hosing of the body is a stimulating finale to underwater massage.

Although the clinic has a well equipped gym, exercise classes are limited and clearly the emphasis here is on raw food, hydrotherapy massage and rest – all backed by physiotherapy prescribed by an osteopathic practitioner.

### Tyringham Clinic, Newport Pagnell, Buckinghamshire

This clinic is rather special as it is the nearest equivalent Britain has to a naturopathic hospital, and as such goes way beyond the usual scope of a health farm yet incorporates the standard fare of fresh vegetarian food, exercise and sports opportunities, health and beauty treatments. It is housed in a striking Georgian mansion with a large ornamental pond in the rear and surrounded by thirty acres of landscaped gardens.

However, one of the most significant aspects about Tyringham is that it is a non-profit organization: patients pay for their accommodation, but treatments are free – whatever is needed. Accommodation ranges from luxury single and double rooms with private facilities to cubicled dormitories, the former helping to subsidize the latter. This system expresses the fundamental philosophy at Tyringham, which is to provide naturopathic treatment for as many people as possible irrespective of financial circumstances – the Tyringham Foundation was established in 1966 and apart from the

Tyringham Clinic

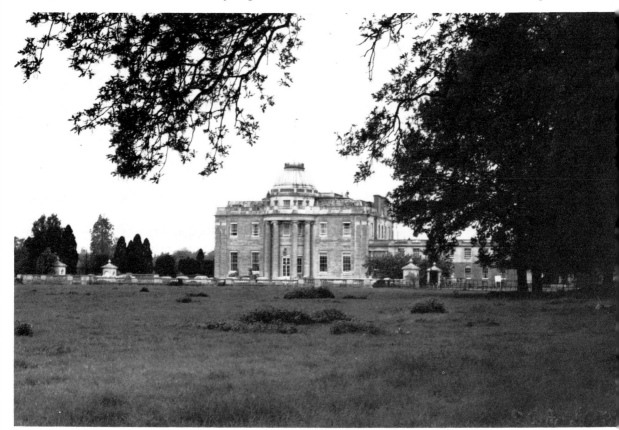

clinic there are complete research and teaching facilities.

Initial consultation is very thorough – the clinic has its own X-ray and laboratory department. There are specialists in acupuncture, osteopathy, chiropractic and physiotherapy. Medications include herbal, homeopathic and vitamin prescriptions. Wide use is made of hydrotherapy – mineral waters, brine, sulphur, alkaline, peat, seaweed and pine applications, also localized wax treatments.

The clinic is under the direction of Dr Ian Urquart who has an international background in rehabilitation and alternative medical practices. He stresses the need for an intelligent co-operation between orthodox and unorthodox medicine. He points out to patients that natural medicine is the maintenance of health in the least noxious way – he is particularly keen on mineral therapy, the use of zinc, gold, copper and magnesium. A stay at Tyringham is a way to health improvement through all the naturopathic channels – a regimen that has success with the chronically ill.

The basis of naturopathic treatment is, of course, a diet of fresh vegetarian food. There's always a wide selection on the buffet table and here are some recipes you can try at home:

### Humus (for four)
Drain the cooked chick peas, keeping the liquid. Put aside a few whole peas for garnish, liquidize the remainder into a puree, thinning if necessary with a little of the liquid. Add crushed garlic, lemon juice and salt. The mixture should be creamy and thick. Garnish with whole peas and parsley.

### Bean Salad (for six)
Any kind of bean can be used – kidney, red, brown, black eye, haricot, broad, butter, chick peas.
Chop the onions, add to the beans, mix in the tomatoes and crushed garlic; finally add the oil and vinegar dressing – if dry, use additional oil. It is best if this is made an hour or two before serving.

### Mixed Rice Salad (for eight)
Cook the rice until tender and cool. Chop into small pieces the apple and celery, also tomatoes and onions. Chop the herbs very finely. Mix all the ingredients together, finally adding the mayonnaise and enough of the oil-and-vinegar to moisten.

---

6 oz. chick peas (dry weight) soaked and cooked
uice of 2 lemons
pinch sea salt
3 cloves of garlic
fresh chopped parsley

½ lb beans (dry weight) soaked well and cooked
1 medium size onion or small bunch spring onions
1 clove garlic
1 chopped tomatoes
pinch sea salt
2 tablespoons olive oil blended with a little cider vinegar

3 oz. brown rice
1 apple
2 oz. chopped walnuts
1 stick celery
2 oz. raisins
3 tablespoons mayonnaise
3 tomatoes
1 small onion
1 clove garlic
small bunch of mint
small bunch lemon balm
small bunch parsley
olive oil and vinegar dressing
pinch sea salt

## Health Centres on the Continent

Continental hydros are centred in towns that sprang up due to the presence of beneficial spa water; then there are special clinics located in areas where the air is particularly pure and refined – in the Alps, for instance. Altogether it is a much more medical approach; diet, exercise and hydrotherapies are invariably used to help specific conditions, not just to lose weight and provide overall fitness, though both these are natural bi-products of the regimens. Many spas have a central treatment building, and patients can stay in various hotels where a doctor is recommended and special provision is made for dietary plans. Of course, all spas have in-patient sanitoriums for serious cases. The tourist bureaux of each country can provide detailed information as to the waters, type of treatment and accommodation available.

The important minerals in spa water are sodium, calcium, magnesium, bicarbonates and sulphates. A number of springs are also radioactive, but this does not afford any danger. External application can stimulate skin metabolism, thus improving circulation and muscle tone – two aspects that show early visible changes in condition and turgor of the skin. Internally, mineral waters can aid all disorders of digestion including liver and kidney complaints. Many gynaecological disorders can also be helped. Spas have come to specialize in specific problems according to the type of water available. Here's a check list of the most important:

**France:** There are over 1,000 mineral springs and all spa centres are under public supervision. In France the medical speciality of 'balneology' is considered very important and it is taught at university. One of the most famous spas is Vichy; the water here is particularly high in sodium bicarbonate which is considered very good for liver complaints and has often provided long-lasting results for digestive disturbances, diabetes, gallstones and gout. At Aix-les-Bains, the water is used to treat all kinds of rheumatic problems, neuralgia and the after effects of fractures and difficult wounds. There are many thalassotherapy centres in France, where the sea water and marine climate are used for therapeutic purposes. Mud baths and baths containing seaweed are often part of the treatment. Thalassotherapy particularly helps rheumatism, back problems, tension and stress.

**Germany:** The Germans have always been keen on the value of spa treatment for diseases, and still today it is often medically prescribed as an essential part of recuperation from practically any illness. The best known are: Bad Nauheim where the rich carbonic acidic waters help heart and circulatory problems, also alleviate rheumatic pain and improve mobility of joints. Bad Homburg is held in esteem for the treatment of heart problems; Bad Pyrmont aids metabolic diseases. Baden-Baden is possibly the best known, and its brine water, sulphur springs, mud and peat are said to be helpful for general rejuvenation and arthritic complaints in particular.

**Switzerland:** Because climate and altitude is considered to be of equal importance to the mineral waters, many health centres have been established in the Alps. They are ideal convalescent centres and are also recommended for aging symptoms, tension, stress and disorders of the pulmonary and respiratory tracks. St Moritz has the highest medicinal springs in Switzerland and the highest content of carbonic acid and iron of any waters in Europe. Bad Ragaz has a hot spring which helps rheumatism, paralysis and back problems.

**Italy:** In addition to many mineral waters, there's a great deal of therapeutic volcanic mud in Italy and it is widely used to help anything to do with movement – mobility of joints, problems with muscle and bone function after injury, arthritis and rheumatism. Abano, together with the Montegrotto spa, is the most important mud therapy centre in Europe. (See below for details on the best hydro-hotel.) At Salsomaggiore (near Milan) the iodine waters are used for gynaecological conditions and treatment also includes mud baths. Montecatini is another well known Italian spa; treatment is given for liver and bile duct disorders, problems of the digestive system and urinary tract. At Ischia, an island off the coast near Naples, the waters are highly alkaline, containing sodium chloride and bicarbonates; they are also highly radioactive and so is the volcanic mud in this area. Again there are good results for injuries, for gynaecological problems resulting from hormone disturbances that often arise in the pre-menopausal years.

As I mentioned before, it is possible to get very detailed information from the various tourist centres as to what is available in the way of treatment and accommodation in the many resorts. However, below are details of three particularly important establishments that offer different regimens towards the same goal: improved allround health and a boost to help you to keep looking younger for as long as possible. All three are treatments that many women undertake on a yearly basis as a preventive measure, as a way to tone up the entire body.

### Klinik Buchinger am Bodensee, Uberlingen, West Germany

At this clinic you can undergo the most respected and valued fasting therapy in Europe. It is not simply a method of losing weight, although it is a most effective way to do so, but it is essentially a cleansing and detoxifying process under constant medical supervision which enables the physician to treat specific ailments. The original clinic was established in the 1920s by Dr Otto Buchinger, whose own illness, chronic arthritic rheumatism, led him to study all the available literature on fasting methods and he applied his findings to his own case. After a strict, self-imposed 28-day fast, he recovered completely and was still active well into his late eighties.

The approach at this modern clinic set in southern Germany is thoroughly medical combining the multifaceted naturopathic cure of fasting and diet, physical training and relaxation with the scientific precision of modern diagnostic facilities. Every stage of treatment is under the supervision of a physician. On the premises there is a well-equipped laboratory that can also handle specialized tests. After an initial medical examination and laboratory analyses the emphasis is on natural medicine: Kneipp and Priessnitz hydrotherapy and medical baths, sauna, lymphatic drainage massage concentrating on connective tissues, reflexology and acupressure. Homeopathic medication, ozonification and neural therapy are also complementary.

It is strongly suggested that a patient spends at least a fortnight at the clinic. A three to four week stay will provide even better results. Fasting is undertaken from the start (see details below) together with a specialized physical training programme graded according to your fitness level and capabilities. In addition, specific exercise sessions demonstrate spine and foot exercises, also breathing techniques. Twice a week patients are asked to take part in rhythmic gymnastics, dances or ball games. Only with the doctor's permission can other active sports be practised. Guided walks are organized each day – and Lake Constance is extremely beautiful.

The clinic is now run by Dr Otto Buchinger's daughter Maria Wilhelmi-Buchinger and her husband Helmut Wilhelmi. And for those of you who prefer sunnier climes, you'll be pleased to hear that recently they built a clinic near Marbella on the Spanish Costa del Sol, where exactly the same treatments are given.

An extended fast has proved to be a great health benefit and general rejuvenator, but it should only be taken when medically controlled. A fast doesn't necessarily mean nothing at all – a limited intake of fruit and vegetable juices is considered more beneficial. This is the basis of the Buchinger regimen, which you can safely follow on your own for a few days. At the clinic an enema is given every morning or every other morning. Daily plan:

9 am:  Cup of herb tea, warm not hot – choose from peppermint, rosehip, camomile

11 am: glass of fresh fruit juice, diluted 1:1 with water

1 pm:  glass of fresh vegetable juice or a cup of vegetable broth (see recipe below)

4 pm:  cup of herb tea

7 pm   glass of fresh fruit or vegetable juice, diluted 1:1 with water

9 pm:  cup of vegetable broth

Plain water or mineral water can be drunk when thirsty.

Vegetable Broth: should be made freshly each day; it is an alkalizing drink, supplying vitamins and minerals and is a great cleansing tonic.

2 large potatoes, unpeeled and chopped
1 cup carrots, unpeeled and sliced
1 cup celery including leaves, chopped

1 cup red beets, finely sliced
1 cup any other available vegetable – cabbage, spinach, courgettes

Put $1\frac{1}{2}$ quarts water in a pan (not aluminium or copper). Slice the vegetables right into the water so as not to expose them to the air. Slow cook for 45 minutes; stand for 15 minutes then strain.

### Grand Hotel Royal Orologio, Abano, Italy

Abano is one of Europe's leading spa treatment resorts; its thermal waters are rich in healing biological and mineral matter, but it is for its mud that Abano is chiefly known. The town itself is picturesque and ideally situated for a cultural holiday as well as for health, as the cure takes place in the mornings and the rest of the day is free. Afternoons can be spent in Padua, Venice (only forty-five minutes by car) or in the historic Euganean Hills that surround the town and where you can find some of the most splendid Palladian villas.

The Grand Hotel Royal Orologio is like a small palace in the very centre of town, surrounded by a park. It is a health centre as well as a luxury hotel (beautifully furnished) and they pay special attention to ensure that their mud is the most beneficial in the area. Not that it is basically different than anybody else's, but it is specially matured in extensive tanks for three years. Treatment is medically pre-scribed, but apart from that you are on your own even to the extent of diet. The dining room offers the most sumptuous food, so it is up to you to have reasonable discipline and not eat and drink too much. The food, though not limited as to type or quantity, is absolutely fresh and when cooked is done so with finesse but not richly.

The medical specialist prescribes and supervises the treatment of each patient on arrival. Suggested programmes last for twelve days, two weeks or three weeks. Whatever the cure, morning treatments are systematically scheduled: mud, ozone therapy, rest, massage, hydrotherapy.

But the main treatment, of course, is mud, combined with thermal applications and inhalations. The body is entirely covered with mud except for the heart area. The length of application depends upon the condition being treated. The mud looks like a greyish homoge-neous slime. Its value derives from the volcanic origins of the subsoil and the mineral elements of the thermal water. Being radioactive, it retains heat over long periods. One of its basic characteristics is a luxuriant growth of special algae, which act on the minerals and transform the mud into valuable therapeutic material.

How does it work? The combination of mud and water does give positive results, but reasons for them remain obscure. The stimuli produced by the mud and water travel into the skin through the nerve receptors and are passed on to the inner organs via the blood and nervous systems. Inhalation of the steam is very effective as a complementary treatment.

A programme of lymphatic drainage is recommended before the start of the mud-water treatment; water exercises are also an

important part of the treatment. The outdoor pool is one of th
loveliest I've seen anywhere. Set in woods, the water comes from
natural source and is very warm at 30 degrees centigrade. There
also a large indoor pool for therapy that is kept at a constant 3
degrees. The Abano cure particularly helps problems of movemer
after injury or due to rheumatism, arthritis or gout; it is also good fc
nervous disorders, defects of the peripheric blood circulation, afte
effects of surgery and skin complaints. However, it is becomin
more and more recognized as a way of maintaining health an
preventing body failures: a way of preparation for a better middle
life and after.

### Thalamer Institut de Thalassothérapie: Front de Mer, Le Touque France

This is one of the leading spas for an invigorating sea-water cur
The treatment centre is literally perched on the rim of the sea and
an impressive modern structure designed with decks and terrace
to afford maximum access to sea, air and sand.

The treatment centre has all the water therapy treatment
including a huge covered swimming pool. Thalassotherapy
hydrotherapy plus the additional advantages of sea air and wate
The climate at Le Touquet plays an essential role – it is modera
and extremely rich in iodine. Baths and sprays are rich in the varie
sea salts of sodium, chloride, calcium, magnesium, sulphur, iron an
potassium; they are also loaded with negative ions. This particula
therapeutic cure is recommended for arthritis (for both pain an
immobility), bone decalcification and any stiffness of movement.
relieves locomotive problems due to accidents, fractures or strain
helps fatigue and overweight, and aids intoxication from tobacco

A medical examination is obligatory prior to treatment. You
daily programme could include any or all of the following:

- bubble bath – micro and macro bubbles agitate the wate
  relaxing muscles and activating circulation.
- underwater massage – sea-water hosed with high pressure o
  your body whilst immersed in a bath.
- seaweed baths and sea-mud applications – this mud is rich i
  silicates and their effect on the system is sedative. Either whe
  mixed with water or applied directly, it is anti-inflammatory an
  eases pain, particularly bringing relief to those with rheumatisr
  or arthritis.
- sea breathing – fresh sea water is vaporized and negativel
  ionized in a special room, where you breathe in this saturate
  atmosphere of fine beneficial particles. Asthmatic, bronchitic an
  sinus troubles can be helped.

As far as food is concerned, there is the choice between the dieteti
restaurant at the centre and the more usual French fare at th
adjacent hotel. The hotel offers all the facilities of a good resort
tennis, golf, riding, and there's the additional enticement of a casino
For health seekers, the pine forests and miles of bracing sand
beach encourage long revitalizing walks.